Thinking nursing

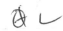

Thinking nursing

Tom Mason and Elizabeth Whitehead

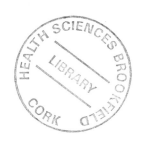

Open University Press

Open University Press
McGraw-Hill Education
McGraw-Hill House
Shoppenhangers Road
Maidenhead
Berkshire
England
SL6 2QL

email: enquiries@openup.co.uk
world wide web: www.openup.co.uk

First published 2003

A catalogue record of this book is available from the British Library

ISBN 0 335 21040 6 (pb)   0 335 21041 4 (hb)

Library of Congress Cataloging-in-Publication Data
CIP data has been applied for

Typeset by RefineCatch Limited, Bungay, Suffolk
Printed in the UK by Bell & Bain Ltd, Glasgow

This book is dedicated to Kelly, Sarah, Lois, Lucy and India

Contents

Preface

As knowledge expands there is an ever-increasing amount of concepts, perspectives and literature to be covered in any course of study, and nursing is no exception. As nursing does not appear to have a unique theoretical body of knowledge specific to itself, it has traditionally drawn upon many other fields of study to provide the basis of nursing education. These traditional areas would include anatomy, physiology, pharmacology and so on, and many of these topics are replete with appropriate textbooks for student nurses to draw upon. However, there are other theoretical spheres of study that are highly pertinent to the contemporary education of nursing students, and these include, for example, sociology, anthropology and philosophy. These subjects broaden the curriculum base significantly and students may not have either the time or the inclination to grapple with the numerous sources outlining the relative perspectives. We felt that what is required, in these conceptually difficult areas, is an accessible source of basic knowledge, brought together into one book, which the student can access relatively quickly.

It is well appreciated that nursing is first and foremost a practical endeavour, but one that is understood in many cases to incorporate a dynamic social interaction rather than merely pragmatic action. However, what is often overlooked is the ever-expanding, and diverse, theory that informs the application of this complex nursing activity. The authors of this book have been nursing across a wide range of areas for over 55 years in total, in clinical practice, education and research, in both universities and higher educational settings. Having taught many hundreds of students over this period, we realized that the majority of student nurses found studying for the traditional components of nursing courses relatively straightforward. As we mention above, these areas include anatomy, physiology, pharmacology, genetics etc. Access to these textbooks is reasonably easy and most students did not generally find these topic areas overly difficult to relate to nursing practice. However, in the modern nursing curriculum other perspectives are brought into focus to broaden the students' field. These disciplines include the contents of this current book. They are considered to be more abstruse and conceptually difficult to grasp if the student has not dealt with them before, and often students cannot see the relevance of them to their clinical practice. It has been noticed that students generally find them more difficult to come to terms with and spend long troublesome periods of time trying to access works from a wide variety of sources or, as mentioned above, neglect them to their cost. As educators we have long known that an amalgamated source for this material, at a conceptually basic, straightforward but comprehensive level, would be a valuable addition to the student literature.

Drawing this material together will provide the student with a general source of knowledge in what are considered to be conceptually difficult areas of nursing study. This book is specifically targeted at nurses studying at degree and diploma levels, including nurses who are studying for a combined honours degree and registered nurse qualification. It will also be beneficial to those students who are working towards a diploma in higher education, as well as qualified nurses undertaking additional specialist training; for example, a mental health or health visiting qualification. This book will also be relevant for those nurses studying at a masters level who require an outline of disciplines that may be new to them. Furthermore, this book will be beneficial for those involved in planning, designing and implementing educational courses for nurses. In nurse education today tutors and lecturers are expected to teach across a wide curriculum and this book will provide a good source of reference.

Although this book is primarily aimed at the UK market, its contents reflect an appreciation of nurses working abroad and collaboratively with colleagues from other countries within the European Union and beyond. Finally, it is envisaged that as more nurses from overseas work in the UK, they too will find this book a valuable tool. Although clearly there are many books on all the topics covered in this text, its uniqueness is that it draws these perspectives together within one source. It has been our intention to be as comprehensive as possible, within a restricted space, which meant that the topic areas needed to be succinctly stated, and having avoided 'dumbing down' this inevitably resulted in a text that is highly challenging for all students of nursing.

Tom Mason and Elizabeth Whitehead
Blundellsands

Acknowledgements

We would like to express our thanks to a number of people and organizations for their much appreciated assistance in the writing of this book. First, to Elsevier Science for allowing us to reproduce Box 3.4. Second, to the staff of University College Chester School of Nursing and Midwifery, the Caswell Clinic Bridgend, the University of Glamorgan and the Robert Baxter Fellowship, who have all supported this project, in one form or another, from its beginnings to its completion. Third, we are grateful to the Library staff of University College Chester for their time and assistance. Finally, we would like to thank the staff of Open University Press for their encouragement and expertise.

1

Introduction

1.1 Introduction

Like the many other professions and disciplines both within and outside health care, nursing is developmental. That is, from its early beginnings nursing has evolved in relation to both theory and practice. The practice of nursing does not develop in isolation but as a result of theoretical developments in many areas of work that are then related to patient care. Thus, modern day nursing activity is a combination of many aspects of theory and practice that are brought together to form an intimate, intricate and frequently intense social interaction, often accompanying a practical objective, usually with someone who is feeling vulnerable. While there are some who believe that nursing is merely a practical endeavour, comprising basic human actions, operated by someone, for someone who cannot do them for themselves, there are others who believe that there is more to it than that. In fact, the modern day nurse is acutely aware of the complex nature of contemporary nursing as it embraces growing technology, theoretical advancements and increasing accountability (United Kingdom Central Council 1999).

Traditional nursing practice largely developed through trial and error, with personal views about how nursing should be undertaken dominating the practice. The 'scientific' basis of such nursing practices may well have been dubious, but what is important is that presumably some thought accompanied this. It may well be viewed that these thinking processes surrounding early nursing, as well as many other practices, were more mythical than scientific, but none the less at least they were attached to some theoretical explanation. In modern times the professions allied to medicine, as well as medicine itself, are more geared towards practices that can be grounded in evidence (1:2, 9:4). Thus, the focus of nurse education is to base nursing practice alongside a critical enquiry as to its relevance and efficacy, particularly in terms of striving for higher standards of patient care and a quality health care service delivery. We, as nurses, are engaged in a quest to balance limited resources with our personal and professional desire to achieve a high standard of nursing practice in relation to growing expectations from increasingly demanding public and political arenas (Asbridge 2002).

In developing this book on 'thinking nursing' we are using the term 'thinking' not as a cognitive process involving electrical and chemical neuronal activity, but as a type of mental set or attitude towards nursing. Thinking nursing is an emphasis on the constant need to scrutinize the practice of nursing in relation to the wide and varied theories that might pertain to it. We feel that it is necessary constantly to ask the question 'why?' in nursing and that this requires a specific mental focus. This is in no way to suggest that the practice of nursing is inferior to theory, but to argue that practice without theory is limited. We consider that, in terms of the production of literature, there are ample numbers of excellent books and journals related to the practice of nursing. Furthermore, there are more than sufficient books on all the topics covered in this text. However, we do believe that they have not previously been brought together into a book on nursing to provide the overall focus on thinking about nursing in relation to both theory and practice.

1.2 Growth of knowledge

The exploration of our world, and our role in it, has always been considered to be a natural human quest, from the early ventures out into new lands or the precarious voyages on open seas, to the frontiers of space and the depths of the oceans. This desire to explore and understand our world also includes an exploration of the human body and our functioning as human beings living together in various communities, albeit often hostile to each other. A great deal of energy, time and money are expended on exploring the internal workings of the body, as well as the more external visible human behaviours that we engage in. This human exploratory drive has brought us to where we are today in terms of the extent of knowledge that we have about ourselves, and one certainty is that we know more today than we did yesterday, and that we will know more tomorrow than we do today. The growth of knowledge appears to be inexorable, with advancements being made in many walks of life, and nursing is no exception (Simpson and Kenrick 1997).

Of course, the growth of knowledge does not occur at a standard pace, as there appear to be long periods of time during which little advancement is apparent. However, it is fair to say that the speed of advancement appears to be the greatest over the previous century, particularly so since the Second World War, and especially over the past two decades. The reason for this latter surge in knowledge is largely attributable to the developments in information technology and the use of computers (10:7). In Western societies there are few areas of life that have not been touched by the creation of the microchip. This development in information technology has had an impact not only in relation to the technology of *how* information is processed but also in relation to *what* information is managed. For example, computers are used in many areas of health care delivery, from managing patients' clinical notes and medical/nursing care to storing information in libraries regarding books, journals, dissertations and so on (Thede 1999). Some journals and books are now available, electronically, via the computer. The modern emphasis in health care, for all disciplines, is concerned with evidence-based practices, and this shifts the focus from what someone may believe is best for the patient to what the scientific world considers to be the best practice. Information technology is now used to manage vast amounts of 'evidence', from the scientific literature regarding patient care to the wealth of experience from patient groups via the Internet (Nicoll 2001). Clearly, with this massive expansion in knowledge of clinical conditions, and the growing access to this information, there is some concern as to how reliable it is and how it should be used. Therefore, the teaching of skills in accessing, managing, reading and synthesizing data is considered to be essential in contemporary training and education, and the ability to draw upon a vast array of data sources, as well as theoretical perspectives, is now central to professional practice.

The growth in knowledge and the developments in information technology have also had an impact on health care from a global perspective, and we are here concerned with nursing. Through more effective communication systems we are now increasingly aware of the many cultures around the world, their health belief systems and the ways in which their health needs are met, or not as the case may be. The health problems associated with disease, poverty, prejudice, war and political systems are now more widely known and their impact across the world is more readily felt. Nuclear fallout, biological and chemical warfare are global concerns as they affect everyone, once released. Furthermore, it is the suffering associated with disease and poverty, created through unjust systems and the greed of a few, that usually generates the conditions of war. As our knowledge grows, and continues to grow, it must take account of the differences in cross-cultural health care issues, including the impact that their political as well as religious systems may have on their health. We must be both aware of and concerned about the domination of one health belief system (say Western) over another equally respected health belief system (say traditional) in another culture, as this creates a tension for all concerned. As Richman (1987: 19) pointed out, 'with immigration from former colonial territories, cosmopolitan medicine is being jostled, intellectually and practically, by it [traditional medicine]. Closer inspection of traditional medicine has revealed "scientific" ingenuity'.

The growth in knowledge has also had an impact on the professions that are involved in delivering health care, particularly in Western medical systems. It is not expected that one person can hold all the knowledge relating to medicine, nursing, psychology etc., which has led to the creation of a growing number of specialities. While most professional training maintains a knowledge baseline, it is becoming increasingly expected that people will eventually specialize in a particular area of practice. The knowledge is so vast that it is only through this specialization that a person may be able to manage the amount of information that is available in that speciality. However, a corollary of this is the need to rely on many professionals in an overall team approach to patient care. Multidisciplinary team working is now a necessary feature in the delivery of care in order to ensure that patients receive the necessary treatment in an overall, or holistic, manner, which is to the highest standard available. Although we still experience problems with this, in relation to professional statuses and personal egos, public expectations and the increased possibility of litigation ensure that multidisciplinary team working is necessary.

1.3 Curriculum

The term curriculum is employed to describe the overall plan or design of an educational programme, and it encompasses all the activities usually associated with the umbrella terms of education and training (Quinn 1994). The importance of curriculum cannot be over-emphasized, as it is the link between the knowledge base of a particular profession and the professional practice itself. As we saw above (1:2), we cannot know everything, and therefore we must be selective as to what we put into a curriculum, and decisions surrounding this are important ones. In terms of nursing these decisions involve at least two serious considerations. First, the nursing curriculum must fulfil the requirements of our professional body, which is now the Nursing and Midwifery Council (NMC). Most professions have evolved over a long period of time and usually adapt in response to events occurring in the society in which they are rooted. They also change as knowledge grows and technology is developed, and curriculum design should respond to this. Second, decisions regarding curriculum design should also reflect the need to address issues of patient safety. The highest standards of care require highly skilled practitioners and the curriculum needs to take this into account. The content of a particular curriculum ought to be grounded on the most up-to-date knowledge, which should be evidence-based and accepted as the best practice by the professional body.

Traditionally, nurse training took place in schools of nursing, which were usually attached to a hospital. However, nurse training is now located in universities and colleges of higher education, which has brought both advantages and disadvantages. The advantages include an increase in professionalization whereby nursing sits alongside other educational courses in health care. There are also the advantages of a raised academic profile, with nurses completing their programme of study with a diploma or degree. This makes nursing a more attractive choice for applicants, as there are increased opportunities for career developments; for example, into research. However, there are some who consider that the transition of nurse training into higher educational settings has brought considerable disadvantages. These include the belief that the subject matter of nursing is more practical than theoretical and the 50:50 split between theory and practice of most nursing courses does not allow students to enjoy the full benefits of student life. Furthermore, some student nurses may not be academically capable of fulfilling the requirements of a rigorous degree programme but none the less would make very capable nurses. Furthermore, there are some who believe that modern nurse training in universities and colleges of higher education has 'invented' academic nursing knowledge in order to fit it alongside the other professions. Although we readily accept that there are both advantages and disadvantages, we believe that the advantages do outweigh the disadvantages and that a reading of this book should provide the evidence for this.

Curriculum also develops through changes in both how nursing is perceived and how it is organized structurally. For example, the generalist versus specialist debate is concerned with whether nurses should have a basic level of knowledge and skills to enable them to work across a wide range of patient conditions or whether they should have a higher level of knowledge and skills to allow them to work in specialist areas of patient need. Again, there appears to us to be a need for a balance between the two as the political pressures to increase generalist nurses in the UK sit alongside the development of the nurse consultants. Thus, curriculum design needs to be flexible and respond to these events, which brings us to the design and purpose of this book.

1.4 The contents of the book

As we pointed out in the preface to this book, nurses tend not to have too much difficulty with learning the traditional theoretical nursing topics such as anatomy, physiology or pharmacology, or with learning practical nursing skills such as the sterile procedure or bandaging. Furthermore, there are numerous books to cover all these topics in great detail. However, nursing students do appear to have some difficulty with the more abstruse theoretical perspectives, particularly in relation to how their principles impinge on nursing practice. The nine main chapters of this book, Chapters 2 to 10, are the perspectives that we consider nursing students to have the most difficulty with in understanding their application to nursing practice. Each of the nine chapters stands independently but it will be noted that there are certain elements of overlap between all of them, and it is this overlap and linkage that makes them so important to an understanding of contemporary nursing practice as it impacts on patient care. Furthermore, it is the fact that they interlink that makes it important to understand each of the perspectives in relation to thinking about nursing.

Chapter 2 deals with sociology. Much of health care work is at a face-to-face level, and it is well accepted that there is a huge infrastructure servicing such health care delivery, with much of this being social by nature. From the notion of a 'bedside manner' to the forming of therapeutic relationships, the social nature of nursing work is clearly apparent. Therefore, sociology is extremely valuable to us, not only in helping us to understand how illnesses and disease processes are dealt with in various communities but also in its contribution to the therapeutic process. Psychology, in Chapter 3, has long played a part in health care courses, including nursing and medicine, and its importance has remained undiminished. It is focused on the study of human behaviour (although psychologists often study animals as well) in relation to individual and group processes. However, it is primarily concerned with the processes that function within the mind, whether in response to external factors or derived from internal forces. Chapter 3 outlines the central role that psychology plays in understanding human behaviour in relation to disease, disorder and illness.

Chapter 4 is concerned with thinking about anthropology in relation to health care. When groups of people come together to undertake a common goal over a period of time, and when that objective is passed down over generations, those involved will usually form strategies of human behaviour that are open to anthropological understanding. It is common to study tribes and groups within anthropology who have developed their social structures, beliefs and traditions, and in this sense nursing is no exception. Anthropology now features on many nursing courses as a method of under-standing contemporary health care practice. Chapter 5 focuses on public health and in this chapter we set out the principles of how the health needs of a given population are defined, identified and met. We discuss the prin-ciples of public health and inform the reader of the challenges met by those in the public health field. We also inform our audience of the new focus on public health and discuss its significance in health care practice both in the UK and abroad. We articulate the significance of having a breadth of public health knowledge and emphasize its impact upon nursing practice. Within the public health agenda there are a number of major issues that deserve particular attention; for example, epidemiology and health promotion and their specific theories and applications to health provision are discussed.

In Chapter 6 we deal with the role of philosophy in nursing practice. Despite the common understanding of the term philosophy, its relationship to modern health care delivery often goes unappreciated. Given its central role in medical ethics it is, perhaps, surprising that it has not featured as prominently in professions allied to medicine as it ought to. We outline this importance throughout the chapter and relate the philosophical perspectives to issues such as the right to life and the right to death. Economics plays a large part of modern health care delivery and we examine this in Chapter 7. We are called upon to question the cost of care and all nurses are prompted to address this at some point during their professional careers. The econom-ics of health care covers a very wide field from the price of a bandage to the annual expenditure of the National Health Service. Whichever aspect of care is under scrutiny, the expenditure of health is of interest to all users and providers. In this chapter we aim to provide an overview of the importance of economics to the professional nurse and highlight how such knowledge will provide greater understanding of the economics of caring in the UK, Europe and beyond.

Chapter 8 deals with the thorny issue of politics in health care. Past generations of health care workers were fond of attempting to separate politics from care. Over the past 20 years we have come to realize that the two are inextricably linked, in fact health care *is* politics. We outline the importance of dealing with politics at both a theoretical and a practical level. In Chapter 9 we are concerned with the expansion of science in nursing. In the modern world the role of science in health care practice is central to effective, rational and pragmatic service delivery. In this chapter we outline the role of science and its importance to both basic and complex nursing care. We indicate the relevance of scientific principles to treatment application and innovation in the progress and development of nursing. Chapter 10, a short chapter in relation to the others, deals with writing, which has become increasingly important in nursing. The commonly heard phrase 'I just want to nurse, I don't want to write' is, in contemporary health care delivery, an anachronism. This is due to a number of factors, including the bureaucratization of the NHS, the professionalization of nursing and the increase in litigation. All of these factors contribute to the necessity of nurses and other allied professions being able to write and construct reports. Increasingly nursing reports are becoming public documents and poorly presented material diminishes the professional status and is not acceptable.

1.5 The structure of the chapters

As we have mentioned above, there are numerous books written on each of the nine areas that we have outlined in this text, and therefore attempting to reduce each of these perspectives to a single chapter is a very difficult, if not impossible, task to undertake. This is one reason why the main chapters are unusually large ones (Chapter 10 being the exception), in that we have attempted to be as comprehensive as we can, given the limited space that is available. This comprehensiveness entails highlighting the major aspects within each perspective that relate to nursing, in our opinion. By this, we mean that each particular aspect that we cover is not covered in depth, but by covering them across a number of theoretical perspectives we can provide the breadth of knowledge that is required. A second reason why the chapters are so large is that we have divided them into two main parts. The first deals with the main theories of the perspective being dealt with, while the second is concerned with their application to practice, from a nursing point of view.

The second major structural component to each of the chapters concerns the subdivisions within both the theoretical part and the application to practice parts. Clearly these subdivisions constitute what we believe form the major relevant aspects of these nine perspectives, as they relate to nursing practice, but we could well have included more. A cut-off was required. The subsections are all given a number (example 7:12), with the first number preceding the colon referring to the chapter number and the second number following the colon relating to the numerically ordered subsection within the chapter. Each of these small subsections could well constitute a chapter in a book, if not a book in themselves, and therefore, we have had to be succinct. This has meant relaying the main points without too much elaboration and we have provided references as supporting evidence and to offer additional reading.

The third main structure to the chapters is the use of the numbered subsections within the text. You will note as you read through the chapters that we insert these numbers to represent where in the book a particular issue can be cross-referenced in the same chapter or in another one. In doing this we have attempted not to break up the flow of reading with copious numbers in brackets but to give as short an indication as possible where the main cross-referencing takes place. This should provide a further breadth of appreciation of the relevance of these issues to each other as well as to their importance on nursing practice. Thus, it is hoped that knowledge will expand and perspectives will broaden through a reading of the book. However, it should be undertaken correctly if the maximum is to be gained from it (1:6). Finally, in structural terms, there are two other elements. First, at the beginning of each chapter we have provided a box with the glossary terms that are used in the chapter, and this is supported by a full glossary at the end of the book. Second, at the end of each subsection we have provided a further reading reference, which will provide a much more in-depth look at the topic under study.

1.6 How to use the book

The book covers a huge breadth of knowledge and if used correctly will provide a good reference source. These chapters brought together, here in a nursing text, offer a wide array of perspectives that if studied carefully should offer the opportunity to develop an appreciation and understanding of nursing in a different light. As we say above, it was not intended to cover any of the topics in depth, as these are adequately dealt with in numerous books, but to provide a wide solid theoretical base that pinpoints the major aspects underpinning the perspective. From this we attempted to indicate where and how these aspects impinge on nursing practice. Therefore, the first way in which this book should be used is as a quick reference source to provide the basics of, say, psychology and anthropology as related to nursing. This will be useful for planning projects, assignments and so on, and will provide sufficient material to aid structuring, indicating other references and providing further reading. The breadth of perspectives within the book should provide enlightening ways of looking at nursing practices, which will offer the student the potential for creativity and lateral thinking. Thus, the book can be used to provide both structural thinking and perspective thinking.

The second way to glean the most out of this book is to use the cross-referencing subsection numbers appropriately; that is, as needed. It is not necessary to cross-reference constantly while you are reading the chapter, but better to cross-reference when needed for specific reasons. If time permits it may well be better to read the book in its entirety first and then to re-read for cross-referencing purposes as required. Use the cross-referencing carefully by reading and then drawing your own conclusions as to the relationships between perspectives. Note how they overlap and interlink with each other, and also note how they form an intricate web of ideas and concepts. In short, they should eventually weave a pattern to reveal at least one part of an overall process, and that is *thinking nursing*.

2

Thinking sociology

Glossary terms used in this chapter

Aetiology · Alienation · Anomie · Ascites · Asthma · Base · Bourgeoisie · Capitalism · Class consciousness · Conflict · Conscience collective · Dialectical materialism · Disseminated strongyloidiasis · Exchange value · Iatrogenesis · Latent function · Manifest function · Moiety · Multiple sclerosis · Nosology · Palliative · Proletariat · Reification · Teleology · Superstructure · Surplus value · Use value

---

2.1 Introduction

No man, or woman, is an island. The forming of relationships between individuals is central to our lives and these relationships may be of many different kinds. They may range from the intense love of lifelong partnerships, to the briefest friendship established by chance. The fact that *Homo sapiens* has developed as a herding animal, living in groups, gatherings and communities, is testimony to the contemporary view that we are fundamentally social beings. Within any social gathering relationships are formed, developed, altered and broken, as the spate of TV documentaries following groups of people forced to live together has shown (for example, *Castaway*, *Big Brother*, *Survivor*). Numerous theories abound regarding how social groups structure themselves and operate according to sets of values and normative prescriptions. Some of these theories are highly complex and deal with relationships between divine beliefs and secular needs. In the first part of this chapter we outline a number of the central social theories that are relevant to an understanding of how societies function, but we emphasize to the reader that many more theories exist.

In the second part of the chapter we highlight the role of the social in helping or hindering people's mental and physical health. Much of our work in health care is social by nature, from the well established notion of the 'bedside manner' to the forming of specific therapeutic relationships. It is not only important how a procedure is undertaken but also relevant who is doing it. This says something about the social nature of the interaction between the patient and the health care professional. Health and illness are viewed differently, not only between individuals, but also between cultures and communities. Therefore, sociological theory and practice are extremely valuable to us in helping us to understand how health, illnesses and disease processes are defined and dealt with in various communities, and also in their contribution to the therapeutic process.

It can be said that most animals merely act on instinct, and even those who learn to respond in certain ways from human conditioning are unlikely to appreciate fully the extent of their learning. People, on the other hand, or at least most of them, have a curiosity regarding how they themselves act and how others behave in society. Sociologists would probably go a step further and suggest that this level of understanding ought to lead towards some advancement of the human condition and analysing how societies are structured and operate should improve conditions for future generations. The following major theories are examples of this sociological progress.

PART ONE: THEORY

2.2 Marxism

Introduction

Although we have located Marxism primarily within the chapter on sociology, this is not to suggest that this restricts his work to this science alone. On the contrary, Karl Marx (1818–83) is a major figure in economics, political science, philosophy and history, to name but a few perspectives, and it is this diversity that makes a synopsis of his work extremely challenging. However, we focus here on Marxism as related to sociology, and we visit his work later in the book in other relevant chapters where we can be more specific.

Marxism has two distinct parts that fall neatly into theoretical and practical perspectives. The theoretical aspects combine to form the central ideas that Marx developed throughout his life and involve his political commitment to proletarian revolutionary drives. The proletariat refers to the class of labourers formed under capitalist industry who, technically, have little to sell other than their labour. The revolution, in Marxist terms, refers to two, possibly compatible, types of revolutionary movement. In the first, the forces of production, having continuously repressed the workers, begin to crack under the strain, and the system ceases to function. In the second, class struggle grows until there is open conflict where one class replaces another. The practical perspective concerns the bourgeois state and its preparedness for revolution, rather than the revolution itself, in terms of social and institutional structures of society. For Marx, the bourgeoisie denoted the class created by the relations of production and represented by property owners. Thus, the nature of Marxism is set in a conflict between the classes, modes of production and the theoretical and practical perspectives.

Marxist origins and definitional terms

Karl Marx was born and educated in Germany and following the completion of his education he married and gained temporary employment as a journalist. He emigrated to Paris in 1843 where he met Friedrich Engels (1820–95), a German born industrialist with family connections in a textile business in Manchester, England. This was the start of a life-long friendship, and a writing partnership that was to make them both significant key players in the field of sociology. Marx mixed with the Parisian socialist radicals and was a keen student of the German philosopher G. W. F. Hegel (1770–1831). However, he was exiled in 1849, having supported the French revolutionary activities that had occurred in the middle of that decade. He was refused entry into Germany and Belgium and settled in London, where he remained for the rest of his life engaged in writing and political activity. He lived in relative poverty supported mainly by Engels and some temporary journalism. Only 11 mourners attended the funeral of Karl Marx, which took place on 17 March 1883 (Wheen 2000). Death in poverty, only finding wealth posthumously, has been the fate of other famous people from other walks of life, including Mozart, who was buried in a pauper's grave in Austria.

The works of Marx have had such a profound impact, as was said above, in many walks of life that some of the terms now applied to his work have tended to become almost meaningless. Furthermore, the numerous thinkers who have developed, reinterpreted and expanded his thoughts have been so prolific that many of his original ideas are unrecognizable. However, what we would like to do here is briefly to define some of the major terms that are associated with his name. When reference is made to 'Marxist' it is usually a statement pertaining to the theory or practice of Marxism, while 'Marxian' usually means adhering to some element of the complex revolutionary movement rooted in the writings of Marx. Therefore, one could well be a Marxist but not considered a Marxian if one were opposed to the revolutionary spirit. Marxism/Leninism is a term that was adopted in the USSR to denote the combination of Marx's analysis of capitalism and Lenin's revolutionary ideology. Some believe that the two theories are incompatible, while others suggest that when combined they form a distinct doctrine. Finally, Marxizing is a popularized term to indicate the use of Marx's terminology in one's own speech or writing in order to portray the image of being a member of the intellectual left (Scruton 1982).

Key themes

As was stated above it is difficult to compartmentalize the extensive work of Marx, particularly as it has been expanded upon in such diverse areas. However, for the purposes of this chapter we have located his central concepts under five subheadings.

Alienation

It is fair to say that the fundamental position in Marxist theory is concerned with the relationship between man and labour. Marx believed that there was a tension between man's essence towards self-fulfilment as subjective beings and when men are compelled to see themselves as objects of labour. In capitalist societies workers are powerless and exploited, they work for wages in order to survive and they are unlikely to own the machines, tools or factories with which they work. They are told when to work, for how long, and when they may stop. They do not own the materials that they use, or have any say in what is produced, and they have no control over what becomes of the end product. They must produce more than what they themselves would need and manufacture sufficient to maintain their own wages, the maintenance of the factory and the profits of the owner. On the other hand, the owner possesses all these items and controls the means of production. Furthermore, he has the power over time and the control of hiring and firing. The conflict of interests is obvious, as the worker attempts to acquire high wages and more control over his labour, and the owner attempts to acquire high profits and more control over the means of production.

Alienation refers to the estrangement of workers from both themselves and others through the means of production and the relationship between man and labour. The schism is caused through a split between the subjective essence of fulfilment and the objectification of production. Marx identified four types of alienation:

- where the worker is alienated from the product of his labour (no say in what he produces);
- where the worker is alienated from the act of his work (work for money rather than satisfaction);
- where the worker is alienated from his human nature (creativity versus commodity);
- where the worker is alienated from his fellow men as capitalism transforms social relations into market relations (judged by status of employment in the market rather than on human qualities).

Alienation is a complex concept that is rooted in the notion that workers become commodities in the operation of capital and are controlled and dominated through the requirements of profitability. Since Marx outlined his theory of alienation it has now been developed, in labyrinthine fashion, to incorporate many aspects of social isolation from many social institutions. Thus, for some it has become too non-specific to be of much analytical use (Scott 1979).

Base and superstructure

These Marxian concepts are grounded in his understanding of the relationship between economic life and other social structures. Marx noted that in many societies the economic base was of paramount importance and composed of three central elements: first, the worker in relation to production; second, the means of production, incorporating the control of materials, means of manufacture and outcome of the product; third, the non-worker who appropriates the product and contributes to the market forces. Although he argued that all economies had these basic elements, what differentiated one economy from another was the relationship between these elements and the way in which they combined to create social forces. This base is, then, pivoted on the relations between men and the extent to which they can influence, determine or control the means of production and the distribution and exchange of products. These relations are of two types, the first concerning possession and the second concerning property. In the former relations, it is a question as to the extent to which the worker, or class of workers, has the power (possession) to control and direct the means of production, distribution and exchange through which productive forces operate. The second relation involves the extent to which the non-worker owns the means of production and the labour force (property), which will ultimately determine his ownership of the product.

The superstructure comprises legal, political and social institutions that often express the relations of economic power in relation to the base, and can enforce and consolidate such relations. Superstructures within these institutions can incorporate such social systems as the state, family and political ideologies. Within Marxist thought it is the relationship between base and superstructure, and the extent to which one influences the other, that differentiates between fundamentalist and dialectical versions of the bas/superstructure model. Traditional Marxists believe that changes in the base relations can explain corresponding changes in the superstructure, but do not believe the reverse to be the case. This is the fundamentalist position. In the dialectical version of the later Marxists it is suggested that developments in the superstructure can influence changes in the base. However, this latter position is highly complex and beyond the scope of this current overview.

Social class and relations of production

Marx saw society as a dynamic system rather than a static one, and the movement he envisaged was a unidirectional one, from capitalist to socialist. The basis of this struggle from a capitalist system in which the owners, the bourgeoisie, who controlled the means of production, towards a society organized by the proletariat, the workers, would be conflict. Marx saw capitalist societies as systems based on these two classes, i.e. the bourgeoisie and the proletariat, in which the conflict of interests would lead to a revolutionary movement based on class struggle. Thus, most Marxist revolutionaries align themselves with the lower class, the oppressed. However, within this two-class system Marx made another division. He made a distinction between the capitalists and the petit-bourgeoisie, and between the proletariat as a class *in* itself and as a class *for* itself. Within the bourgeois subdivision he argued that the capitalists were the ones who had all the wealth and controlled the means of production, and thus acquired the power and influence. The petit-bourgeoisie, on the other hand, were the managers of production and its support systems such as finance, law and technology, and they managed on behalf of the capitalists. With regard to the proletariat the class *in* itself group comprised those workers who continued to share in the idea of selling their labour to the bourgeoisie. The class *for* itself were those workers who had become aware of their common interests and saw their responsibilities as a collectivity, and believed that members had to operate not for their individual benefits but for the good of the group as a whole. Those in the latter group were said to have class consciousness, i.e. awareness of their common shared responsibilities in relation to the bourgeoisie. Those in the former proletariat group were said to be under a false consciousness, i.e. they saw their work situation in terms of personal problems as they had succumbed to the propaganda and ideological conditioning that had persuaded them to think and behave in ways that would maintain their position in the lower class, thus maintaining the bourgeoisie–proletariat system (Nichols and Beynon 1977).

Conflict and contradiction in the class struggle

Having set society apart, in terms of bourgeoisie and proletariat, the owners and the workers, Marx put forward a theory of social change that was rooted in the class struggle. He called this the 'motor of history'. In capitalist societies, Marx suggested that the rich get richer and the poor become poorer. Furthermore, he argued that the basis of the relationship between the bourgeoisie and the proletariat was one of exploitation. In this scenario conflict, for Marx, was inevitable. Change would not follow without the active intervention by human beings, and thus the notion of revolution lies centrally within Marxist theory. Marx saw the natural move from capitalism to a more egalitarian system as inexorable and the basis for this change would emerge out of the contradictions of the two-class system. The change was based on what is termed dialectical materialism. This process is comprised of three elements, or stages – thesis, antithesis and synthesis – and Marx employed these ideas to explain historical and social change.

The term dialectical materialism was not used by Marx himself but was later applied to his theory of history and consciousness. Dialectics is concerned with the emergence of resolution, or change, from competing or contradictory forces, with the emphasis on progress, or dynamic movement. Marx's early view was that the contradiction within the means of production led to class struggle, and that the tension within this was rooted in possession, products and materials. This materialist view is propounded on the notion that it is a human activity which involves the material, or physical, transformation of nature. In short, it does not have a divine, or spiritual, element, but is based on the physicality of existence.

Capitalism

Marx rarely used the term capitalism but none the less the theory is in essence his. Building on the earlier concepts of owners and workers another distinction can be drawn between two categories of labour: (a) *necessary labour* and (b) *surplus labour*. The former is concerned with the necessary, but minimum, amount of labour required to secure the basic means of their subsistence, while the latter is the labour that produces a surplus above basic subsistence. For Marx the bourgeoisie accumulates all the surplus and the proletariat accumulates nothing. Capitalism is, thus, a system based on commodity production that is used for exchange rather than direct use or need. The *exchange value* is the quantity of some other commodity for which it can be exchanged in conditions of equilibrium. *Surplus value* is the term used to represent the exchange of commodities that the bourgeoisie appropriate from workers through the means of production. *Use value*, on the other hand, refers to the value that is determined by the needs it will satisfy. When viewed in relation to need, use value simply equates with the satisfaction of that need. However, use value becomes a highly complex and scholastic concept when it is applied to notions of desire. For example, a loaf of bread has a use value when it satisfies hunger, but so does a work of art when it satisfies a desire. Notwithstanding this complexity we can summarize the Marxist structure of capitalism as the production of exchange value, with the surplus value being retained by the capitalists, and the rate of extraction of this surplus value determines the rate of exploitation. Thus, Marx saw in capitalism its fundamental flaw and its inherent means of its own downfall, the ever-increasing conflict of interests. However, the fact that Marx's prediction regarding the downfall of capitalism has not come to fruition has led to criticism and revision of some of his premises (Lee and Newby 1987). These are briefly dealt with below.

Critical analysis

The main criticisms of Mark's ideas can be summarized within the five broad areas identified above. However, the reader is cautioned that a full critique of Marxism is both complex and diverse. In relation to Marx's concept of alienation this has received considerable sociological as well as psychological attention, and is itself viewed as an elaborate representation. To some extent it has now been abandoned in favour of understanding the relationship between man and labour, the basis of alienation, in terms of such socio-psychological human elements as powerlessness, meaninglessness, isolation, self-estrangement and exploitation. Thus, alienation is now viewed as too all-encompassing to be of much analytical use. The debate on base and superstructure pivots on two criticisms. The first concerns the way in which the relations of production are defined in legalistic terms that, for Marx, are fixed in the superstructure. This leads to the criticism that it is then difficult to separate base and superstructure analytically. The second criticism refers to the question of economic determinism, which views all social phenomena as explainable in terms of economic factors or relations of production. The argument is that other factors contribute to social change, not just economic ones.

The major criticism of Marx's class structure is seen in relation to its two-tier formation. This leaves it difficult to fit the middle-class element into the model and also difficult to explain that class of persons who own and control the means of production when the capital passes into institutions. This lessens the impact of Marx's conflict theory, which in his view is required to create change. This Marxist theory has, in turn, proved controversial, as it has been argued that class struggle is unrelated to change from one society to another. Furthermore, Marx's prediction that in capitalist societies the working class become increasingly disintegrated, polarized and impoverished has not occurred. However, despite these criticisms Marx's theories have remained useful and have been adjusted to overcome some of these theoretical difficulties.

Evolution and impact

If it is correct that the three founding fathers of modern sociology are Marx, Weber and Durkheim, it is perhaps Marx who has had the biggest impact. However, because of the voluminous nature of his work and the fact that he wrote extensively with his colleague and friend Engels, even a modest outline is difficult. Furthermore, as we have pointed out, an enormous amount of literature has grown around his work from many perspectives and in the light of the critical analysis of his central tenets his theories have evolved over the years. These too are extensive and we can only briefly state the main developments here.

New theories of social class have evolved to take account of different patterns of property ownership and to explain the rise and dominance of the middle classes. Furthermore, later Marxist analyses have developed the notion of class consciousness as a prerequisite for class struggle and suggested that in contemporary society superstructures, such as the church, the family and even trade unions, are apparatuses of capitalism holding down the working classes (Gramsci 1971). Revisions have also been made in the analysis of Marx's economics by distinguishing between different modes of capital fractions, and also in politics with a different emphasis on the subtle relationship between democratic governments and the sophisticated manner in which they 'satisfy' the working classes in relation to favouring the interests of capital (Lukács 1971). A further development that resonates with contemporary views of the world is in relation to the imperialistic expansion of capitalism into Third World countries. This now suggests that capitalism needs such expansion in order to maintain it, and once it has expanded around the globe it will ultimately exhaust itself and die (Lenin 1951). Finally, Marx's method has received serious critical attention and application in the analysis of social change, particularly, and recently, in the utility of the means of production (Anderson 1976).

Major works

The Poverty of Philosophy (1847), *Capital* (1867); with Engels, *The German Ideology* (1845), *Manifesto of the Communist Party* (1848); posthumously, *The Economic and Philosophic Manuscripts of 1844* (1964), *Grundrisse* (1973).

Further reading

Feuer, L. S. (1981) *Marx and Engels: Basic Writings on Politics and Philosophy*. London: Fontana.
Francome, C. (2000) *Karl Marx: Hero or Zero?* London: Carla Francome Publications.
Turner, B. S. (1999) *Classical Sociology*. London: Sage.

2.3 Functionalism

Functionalism has a long history in the development of social theory and has received close attention over the past century or so. Society has often been likened to a human body that is made up of independent parts or organs that work together to maintain the overall human system. Employing this organic analogy some functionalist sociologists analysed societies by establishing interdependent aspects of their systems and interpreting how they were related to each other in maintaining the overall society. Just as the liver of the body has an independent function, it is related to the overall maintenance of the person. In a similar vein a social activity, such as marriage, can be seen as independent of another social activity, say the law, but we can also see how they are related and what their function might be in maintaining the overall social system. Thus, as a very basic definition of functionalism we can say that it is concerned with the analysis of social activities in relation to their consequences for the functioning of both other social activities and the society in general. Contemporary functionalist sociologists no longer employ the organic analogy and refer to society as a system, while its parts are viewed as subsystems. These subsystems may include such social structures as politics, economics and cultural formations. However, a further distinction can be made in relation to what are termed social institutions, and these would include social processes such as marriage, the family, religion, law and education. What is important to remember is that functionalism, as a theoretical sociological discipline, is concerned with the relationship between these social subdivisions and how they maintain the overall functioning of society.

Historical developments

As was noted above, functionalism has a long history and in fact it can be argued that one of the founding fathers of sociology, Émile Durkheim (1858–1917), was also a functionalist in his analysis. An early English sociologist, Herbert Spencer (1820–1903), applied the organic analogy to social understanding and can also be viewed as a functionalist. Although these, and other, early sociologists can be labelled as adopting a functionalist perspective, modern day functionalism owes much of its more sophisticated analytical framework to the work of anthropologists (Chapter 4). Through the work of Alfred Radcliffe-Brown (1881–1955), a British anthropologist, and Bronislaw Malinowski (1884–1942), a Polish anthropologist, functionalism became a celebrated approach to understanding how societies maintain both their systems and their evolutionary existence. However, functionalism was perhaps at its most popular between the 1950s and the 1970s with the work of the American sociologists Talcott Parsons (1902–79) and Robert Merton (1910–2003). Parsons's work was, basically, to achieve an overall conceptual structure for all of sociology, which would incorporate the entire range of social sciences. Needless to say he did not achieve this, but his work has received some considerable attention and has been influential in developing a critique of functionalist sociology. His major works include *The Structure of Social Action* (Parsons 1937), *The Social System* (Parsons 1951a), *Social Structure and Personality* (Parsons 1964) and *The System of Modern Societies* (Parsons 1971). Merton too was a prolific academic sociologist who produced a wide ranging series of essays, of which his most influential have been on anomie, bureaucracy and functionalism (Merton 1957). Merton also developed the distinctions between manifest and latent functions within the functionalist perspective, which we outline below.

Social action and its functions

Understanding society from a functionalist perspective involves an appreciation of the differentiation of the subsystems of society and the ways in which they are integrated into the overall social system. A good starting point would be the work of Émile Durkheim in his classic book entitled *The Division of Labour* (1893). In this treatise Durkheim makes the case for viewing how societies bind together in a state of social cohesion in two ways. The first he referred to as mechanical solidarity, in which primitive societies operated on common beliefs, common interests and a collective conscience, which formed the consensus of that society. The second state of social cohesion Durkheim termed organic solidarity, based on the interdependent social parts working together to maintain the viability of the overall complex society. Durkheim believed that industrialization and urbanization led to the breakdown of mechanical solidarity through the division of labour, thus forming organic solidarity via the establishment of new economic ties, occupational associations and a collective restraint against self-interest (Moore 1979). However useful Durkheim's distinctions of social cohesion might have been they have received some criticism in relation to the lack of credibility of his concept of mechanical solidarity, as it is unlikely that any society, primitive or otherwise, would not have some degree of internal differentiation; for example, based on sex and age.

Later functionalists developed this perspective further. Merton (1957), in developing the concepts of manifest and latent functions of social action, gives us the example of the Hopi Indians of New Mexico and their rain dance. In this social activity (ceremonial dance) the manifest function is the production of rain to water the crops and despite the fact that other societies may believe that the relationship between the dance and rain is a spurious one the belief system is strong enough to maintain the social activity (dancing for rain). However, Merton also identified latent functions of a social activity, which refers to the unrecognized and unintended consequences of the activity. Taking the rain dance further Merton argued that the latent functions of this social activity included enhancing the social cohesion of the Hopi Indians and reinforcing the traditional identity of the tribe itself (4:2, 4:3, 4:4, 4:5, 4:6). Merton also established a distinction between functions and dysfunctions. The former are adequately covered by the manifest and latent functions outlined above and pivot on the social activity that contributes to the production, maintenance and reinforcement of social cohesion. On the other hand, dysfunctions refer to social activities that threaten social cohesion and produce the conditions for creating change to the social order. For example, while the social activity of religion can be understood in relation to its manifest content of gaining access to eternal spiritual life in a state of heavenly ecstasy, and its latent function can be understood in terms of its mechanistic force in maintaining good behaviour and social cohesion, it can also be seen to have a dysfunctional element; that is, its capacity to create conflict and social disharmony, leading, as we sadly note, to war and suffering.

Another mid-twentieth-century functionalist writer is Talcott Parsons. Although we will revisit his work in relation to personality and culture outlined below in this section and in relation to 'sick-role' in 2:14, we would like to mention briefly one aspect of his work that has relevance here. This concerns his notion that social interactions have a systematic character; that is, he believed that a connection existed between a social action and the social system. Parsons termed these connections *pattern variables* and argued that they were dilemmatic frameworks that faced social actors in social situations. He claimed there were four such frameworks of dilemmas:

- *Particularism versus universalism*, in which social actors must make decisions regarding how to judge others in a social action, either by general criteria (universalism) or by criteria specific to the individual being judged.

- *Performance versus quality*, in which social actors must make decisions whether to judge another by what they do (performance) or by their personal characteristics (qualities).

- *Affectivity versus absence of affectivity*, in which social relationships are formed with personal feelings attached to them or social relationships are operated for instrumental reasons without personal feelings being connected.

- *Specificity versus diffuseness*, in which social actors must decide whether to engage with others across a range of social activities or whether to engage only for specified purposes.

Parsons believed that these dilemmatic frameworks structured all social interactions, and their relevance for health care professionals can be seen in relation to how they inform interactions with patients as well as other colleagues within the many hierarchical structures of medicine.

Social activity and functional prerequisites

Parsons claimed that systems of interactions had a number of needs of their own that needed to be satisfied. This was required by both the social system and its external environment, as well as by the internal mechanisms of the system itself. To make clear this linkage between what may appear as concrete entities, such as social action and social systems, we need to recognize Parsons's focus on personality (3:3) and culture (4:5). This begins to unravel the complex relationship between psychological cognitive mechanisms (3:8) and socialized values and norms (4:6) from wider societal traditions. In simple terms social interactive systems, according to Parsons, require four functional needs.

- Adaptation: a basic requirement to respond to the environment by employing and interacting with its resources.

- Goal attainment: the establishment of aims and objectives for the social system.

- Integration: the regulation of an internal order through rules of engagement.

- Latency: the requirement for motivation to perform social tasks.

Social subsystems such as cultural formations and economics will fulfil the systems prerequisites; for example, economics will satisfy the need for adaptation in using environmental resources in the productive process (2:2, Chapter 7). However, it can be seen that each subsystem will also require the fulfilment of each of the prerequisites (AGIL) in turn. Thus, we are faced with an infinite regression of prerequisites and the production of further subdivisions. Although, to be fair, this is a theoretical possibility only, it has received both some degree of criticism (Giddens 1989a) and some defence (Alexander 1985).

Criticisms of functionalism

Functionalism has lost some of its earlier support as its limitations have emerged. However, these criticisms of it have lessened somewhat in recent times. The major criticisms of the functionalist perspective can be grouped under three headings. The first refers to social conflict. Within functionalism there is an implicit assumption that societies have common values or interests that are satisfied by the maintenance of that culture. It is as if they have achieved a state of social cohesion or social order that is ideal, and the perpetuation of that society is achieved through the self-reinforcing systems that have produced the ideal state. Thus, functionalism is often criticized for not incorporating, as fully as it ought to, the division, conflict and social tension that abound in many societies. The second area of criticism is one of reification. Many functionalists are said to speak of abstract social systems and institutions as if they have a material, or concrete, existence in their own right. This process of making things 'real' is called reification and in functionalist terms does not take into account the dynamic forces in which humans often create, redefine and recreate the processes of social interaction. They often speak of societies and institutions as having 'needs' or 'purposes' as if they existed in themselves, when in fact it is the individual human beings that have needs and purposes. However, functionalists counter this by pointing to concepts such as differentiation, which they argue account for these changes. The third area of criticism concerns the focus on consequences of social activity. It is suggested that functionalism ignores, or underplays, the meaning that individual actors attribute to their social activity and by emphasizing the consequences of action, critics suggest, functionalism is a form of teleology. That is, it is concerned with the purpose and design of society as if it were destined towards an ideal end state.

Despite the strengths of these criticisms some functionalists have attempted to counter many of the arguments or have adapted their theories to absorb the contradictions. For example, Levy (1952) developed a sophisticated analysis of society from a functionalist perspective and made the case for a persistent and self-subsistent social system composed of a plurality of interacting individuals who were, generally, focused on reinforcing the system. This persisted throughout the life span of the individuals and in part was centred on sexual recruitment. Thus, societies were perpetuated. This incorporates a form of neo-evolutionary perspective that accounts for change in social systems. Although functionalists, even neo-functionalists, may accept some need for theoretical refining of their perspective it is none the less a useful paradigm for opening up various levels of interpretation regarding extant social activity, social institutions and social systems in both general society and specific health care settings.

Further reading

Turner, B. S. (1999) *Classical Sociology*. London: Sage.

2.4 Structuralism

Structuralism is a term that is found in various fields of study, including literature, art, linguistics, anthropology, psychology, philosophy and sociology. Therefore, it could well have been located in several chapters of this book and is certainly interrelated, as are many conceptual perspectives in nursing, to numerous scientific disciplines. In sociology structuralism has several levels, or layers, of meaning and in its most basic form is concerned with the identification of the social structures of any given society, which can be studied through an examination of the ordered and patterned relationships formed in human behaviour. For example, we may study the social structure of marriage in different cultures by examining the elementary parts of courtship, arranged marriages, bonding, ceremonies, wedding vows and divorce proceedings. Although huge differences occur throughout the world the social structure of some form of 'marriage' partnership remains constant. However, in structuralist approaches there is another level of analysis, which refers to a hidden, or implicit, 'area' of meaning that is encapsulated in the phrase the 'relation is more important than the parts'. Although a lot more can be said about this, the central message is contained in that statement. At this holistic level something is created above and beyond the constitutive elements of the individual parts. Thus, we may analyse all the elements of marriage outlined above, including the roles of all the players in the ceremony, and claim that beyond all the parts the creation of the social structure of 'marriage' itself has a higher level of meaning. Furthermore, we can then make a claim that this hidden meaning can actually influence our behaviour and attitudes to marriage, and may well govern, in a self-reinforcing way, how we engage in courtship ourselves, and how we respond to our actual marriage itself. Although for our example we have used the very obvious social structure of marriage, sociologists and anthropologists have studied a large array of social structures, from myths (Lévi-Strauss 1966) to the exchange of gifts (Mauss 1954), and these have highlighted a complex interplay of meanings.

Key theorists

The quest to search for, and identify, the structures of society has fuelled an impetus to formulate models based on organism analogies. As we saw in the functionalist perspective (2:3), viewing elements or parts of a society in terms of the overall operation of the whole has been popular from the early Greeks onwards. However, other models have also assisted many generations of philosophers, sociologists and anthropologists; for example, mathematical and mechanical models. Certainly the pre-Socratic Pythagorean school formulated a mathematical model of reality based on irreducible geometrical patterns (Bottomore and Nisbet 1978) and mechanical models enjoyed a renaissance in the sixteenth and seventeenth centuries with the rise of the physical philosophers such as Galileo and Newton (Lange 1967).

However, structuralism in our sociological framework begins with the founding fathers of sociology, or at least some of them: Auguste Comte (1798–1857) and Émile Durkheim (1858–1917). Comte is often referred to as the first sociologist, but it should be remembered that he was influenced by many others. We can make a single statement regarding Comte's sociology that it is centred on the priority of relationships to individuals (Bottomore and Nisbet 1978). Comte believed that sociology was a science, like all the other sciences of that time, and involved observation, experimentation and comparison. He believed that societies evolved through three stages – primitive, intermediary and scientific – and used an organic analogy to explain how societies, through the *division of labour*, become more complex, differentiated and highly specialized. Comte argued that sciences, like societies, flow historically in structure and possess both a social dynamics and a social statics. The former is concerned with the general laws of social development, while the latter focuses on the connection of social relationships in which human beings engage. Durkheim, some 70 years later, was having difficulty in making a distinction between Comte's social dynamics and statics and began to see social structures not in terms of entities in themselves but in terms of their constant formation and dissolution. This gave them a focus of evolutionary *becoming*. Durkheim saw societies as moving through stages of solidarity, which he called mechanical solidarity and organic solidarity. Mechanical solidarity was the dominant form of social relations in primitive societies that were based on common values, beliefs and norms in a form of *conscience collective*. Through the division of labour Durkheim believed that industrialized societies destroyed this mechanical solidarity and a different form of social relations developed. These were built on economic ties, occupational associations and moral restraints to the rise of egoism, and this Durkheim termed organic solidarity. The discerning reader may well be reminded of Marxist thought here (2:2), particularly in relation to the concept of alienation.

Extending the longstanding tradition of French structuralist thought, two others will be mentioned here: Claude Lévi-Strauss (1908–) and Jean Piaget (1896–1980). The latter, a Swiss psychologist, produced texts on the development of thought processes and concepts of space and movement, but the seminal works for which he is famous involve logic and reasoning in children, and are dealt with further under 3:2. Lévi-Strauss is known as a structural anthropologist and his work essentially involves an analysis of the relationship between nature and different cultural groups in relation to language. Although fundamentally cognitive, Lévi-Strauss's approach involves establishing the underlying regularities and patterning of social phenomena that indicate the functioning of the physiological constitution of the brain. Lévi-Strauss sought, as did Freud, universal structures, or principles, by which all human minds operate, and he attempted this analysis through study of what he viewed as primitive thought processes involved in myths (Lévi-Strauss 1964, 1966). To what extent he has achieved his aim is for others to judge.

Structuralism and language

As we have noted, the search for 'structures' is not confined to society alone, as many subjects have received attention by structuralists. However, two areas are worth noting here, as they relate closely to the field of health care. The first area is linguistics. Ferdinand de Saussure (1857–1913) was a Swiss linguist who argued that language was a collectively produced and shared system of meaning very much like, say, a culture is. Having worked on the structures of language for most of his adult life he radically claimed that the meaning of language is determined by those who have mutually defined the relationship between what is spoken and what is spoken about. For example, we might believe that the meaning of the word 'rock' is the item itself, i.e. the hard stony object to which the word refers. However, for Saussure this is not so. We can understand this, as there are many words in many languages that do not refer to anything, such as, in English, 'and' or 'but'. Furthermore, as Giddens (1989a) points out, there are plenty of mythical objects that have no existence in reality at all, such as a 'unicorn'. So, we ask ourselves: if the meaning of the words do not come from an object to which they refer then where do they come from? Saussure's answer is that the structure of the meaning of words is derived from the *difference* between related concepts. For example, the meaning of the word 'rock' is derived from the difference between 'rock' and stone, pebble, boulder, brick and so on. Meaning is established in a self-referential way based on the relationship between a signifier (the word) and a signified (mental concept). This brings us to the second area, structuralism and semiotics.

Structuralism and semiotics

Semiotics, or semiology, is the study of signs. Saussure claimed that it was not only words that create meaning but also writing and drawings, and in fact any object that can be systematically distinguished. Take, for example, the colours of a traffic light that create the meaning to stop, get ready and go. In semiotics the fundamental starting point is making the distinction between signifier, signified and sign. The red traffic light is the signifier, the mental concept of stopping the car is the signified and the relationship between them is the sign. This latter point may be better explained by saying that you would not stop your car at a red telephone box or a red post box but only at a red traffic light. The meaning is created by the context, and by the convention that we apply to stopping at red traffic lights. Any red object other than a traffic light would not carry that meaning. Furthermore, signifiers may also indicate different signifieds at different levels of meaning. For example, a photograph of a baby may signify a human child, but at another level it may signify innocence, and at another level it may signify the future generation, family values and so on. Roland Barthes (1915–80), who is often regarded as a French structuralist, suggested that there are two approaches to understanding the function of signs at this second level of signification. First, there is a mythical function in which signs have meanings that represent traditional cultural values that change little over time. Second, signs can not only indicate a relationship between an object and a mental concept but also evoke feelings in the perceiver.

In conclusion, structuralism, or structural analysis, has been employed in many areas of life and is now considered more suitable for some fields, such as communication, media and cultural studies, than for others, such as economics and politics (Giddens 1989a). However, in terms of the health care arena we would consider it a useful approach to understanding the hidden, and not so hidden, elements of human behaviour. These may include the inter- and intra-professional power dynamics, the ranking of hierarchical statuses and the abundance of signifiers, signified and signs that have structured layers of meaning in the institution of Western medicine. We deal with some of these in Chapter 4.

Further reading

Caws, P. (1988) *Structuralism: The Art of the Intelligible*. Atlantic Highlands, NJ: Humanities Press.
Robey, D. (1973) *Structuralism: An Introduction*. Oxford: Clarendon Press.

2.5 Feminism and gender

In this section we link feminism and gender together, but clearly, as we will see, they are not necessarily theoretically connected. Equally, we could have incorporated sexuality in the title, as there is a common understanding that the three terms are somehow interlinked. However, we deal briefly with sexuality within the notion of gender in this section, and deal with it more comprehensively in the next chapter, on thinking psychology. Briefly stated, feminism is a doctrine that views women as systematically disadvantaged, subjugated and oppressed by male-dominated social systems. However, although this is starkly expressed, and indeed some structures and systems of society bluntly operate in this manner, most strategies are now viewed as more subtle and sophisticated, and function at an implicit level to dominate women. We cannot do justice to the complex reticulate of social relations that manoeuvre this interactive mechanism in this short section. But what we can do is sketch the main principles and hope that the reader will be motivated to pursue this important line of enquiry in the many social relations in which they operate. We do not wish to labour the point but feel that it is important to link the theoretical position of feminism with the status of nursing (as a predominantly female occupation) within the medical (predominantly male occupation) profession. Many of the issues within feminism pertain to the status of nursing, both in popular culture and in professional health care settings. A starting point for our sketch is to attempt to define and delineate some of the terms that are often associated with feminism, and often used incorrectly, leading to some degree of confusion.

- *Feminism*. A term that is grounded in the belief that women are dis-advantaged in comparison to men. Feminism has changed and adapted throughout its history in response to changing societal mores. It is not a single philosophical position but has many variants; however, they all share the common theme of an inequity between females and males in modern society.

- *Femininity*. This term, as employed by sociologists, is used to attribute certain generalized characteristics to females, such as kind, caring, warm and therefore sexually attractive. We need to question whether these characteristics are biologically or socially determined, and to what extent they may be employed to maintain male power.

- *Feminization*. In sociological terms this usually refers to an occupation that is predominantly populated by females, and can be associated with proletarianization (2:2), in which certain elements of work within the division of labour become less skilled, leading to cheaper employment of women. Feminization in non-sociological terms usually indicates someone taking on the attributes of a female.

- *Feminist*. This usually denotes someone who upholds the principles of feminism and, depending on perspective, who is actively engaged in behaviour aimed at addressing the female–male power imbalance.

Feminism has a long history. Giddens (1989a: 513) tells us that 'Marie Gouze was executed in 1793, charged with "having forgotten the virtues which belong to her sex".' The suffragette movement (women's suffrage bills placed before and defeated by Parliament between 1886 and 1911), particularly the militant campaigner Emmeline Pankhurst, can be located under the rubric of the early feminist movement (first wave). However, contemporary feminism has its roots in the resurgence of the feminist movement in the 1960s (second wave) but, as we noted above, the broad doctrine of feminism now embraces diverse philosophies. For example, specific disciplines include feminism and social science, feminism and psychoanalysis, feminism and aesthetics, feminist epistemology, feminist ethics, feminist jurisprudence, feminist literary criticism, feminist philosophy of science, feminist politics and feminist theology. Although all are important, many of these perspectives are not relevant to us in this current text, and we restrict ourselves to a brief outline of feminism and social science, feminism and psychoanalysis and feminism and postmodernism in this section, while dealing with feminist ethics (6:14) and feminism and politics (8:7) later in the book.

Gender

While we can be reasonably comfortable that sex can mean the biologically determined category of either male or female (hermaphrodites are an exception) or refer to the physical act of 'having sex', it is often confused with gender. Gender is predominantly concerned with the psychological, social and cultural differences between the biologically determined sexes. The major debate in gender studies concerns this very point. That is, to what extent are the behaviours of men and women determined by sex or gender? Or, put another way, are the ways in which males and females behave due to nature or nurture? One line of argument suggests that there are differences in the ways that males and females behave that are the result of innate tendencies, and socio-cultural studies would point to such male behaviours as hunting and aggressive tendencies as examples. In most cultures it is the males who hunt and in most cultures it is the males that are the most aggressive. However, antagonists to this line of argument would counter this by pointing to cultural differences in which expectations as to the aggressiveness of women vary (Elshtain 1987). Furthermore, it is universal that women have the children, and almost universal that they care for and rear them; therefore they do not have the time to do the hunting. As an aside we could add that mothers forced to protect their children can be extremely aggressive indeed!

It seems reasonably clear, then, that what makes male and female behaviour more or less masculine or feminine is determined by a wealth of social, psychological, cultural and biological factors consisting of ideas, beliefs, attitudes and desires that have been laid down in childhood (Lewontin 1982). Thus, we see wide differences between some males who are more masculine than others and some who are more feminine. Similarly, there are differences with females, with some having more feminine traits and others more masculine ones. It cannot merely be a question of biological size or chemical differences, as some small males are extremely aggressive while some larger men are often called 'gentle giants' and considered kind and caring. Furthermore, some larger women are extremely feminine while some more petite females are considered 'butch'. We can now turn our attention to examining the factors that might contribute to the process of learning the characteristic traits of gender roles, this process often being referred to as gender socialization.

Parental and adult influences

We are all familiar with the social fact that baby girls are predominantly dressed in pink and baby boys in blue, and there is no reason, other than a social one, why the reverse could not be the case. Furthermore, specific toys are given to girls, such as dolls, and others to boys, such as cars. Will *et al.* (1976) carried out an experiment with a 6-month-old baby and a group of young mothers, and depending on whether the mothers thought that the child was a boy or a girl they reacted differently towards the child. When they were told that her name was Beth they said that she was 'sweet' and had a 'soft cry', they smiled often and gave her toys such as dolls to play with. When a second group of mothers were told that the child's name was Adam their reactions were different and they gave the child 'male' toys to play with, such as a train. The child was, in fact, the same child.

Learning gender

If parents and adults have an influence on children's gender then we need to understand the process by which children become socialized into their gender roles. Giddens (1989a) assures us that this process is unconscious. It almost certainly occurs through a range of pre-verbal cues: through boys and girls being handled differently, parental scents being dissimilar, differences in dress and hairstyles and so on (Oakley 1985). By the age of 2 they have some understanding of gender differences and as they grow, toys, books, peer groups and television all contribute to their processing of gender differences (Zammuner 1987).

Effects of neutral gender rearing

Neutral gender rearing is, of course, nigh on impossible due to the huge social influences on growing children. However, some studies do exist in which this has been attempted, or at least they have gone some way in approximating to this situation. Statham (1986) studied a group of parents who were committed to bringing their children up in as gender neutral a state as is possible. The parents were mainly middle-class lecturers and teachers and the children's ages ranged from 2 to 12 years. They reported that overcoming traditional gender roles was extremely difficult. Reactions from the children were often severe, with one 5-year-old boy complaining to his mother that 'she did not like boys, she only liked girls'. The peripheral power of socialized gender influences from friends, relatives, peers and the media have such force that they impact on the children despite parental desires to fuse feminine and masculine stereotypes (Lorber 1994).

Gender roles are grounded in everyday practice, as Lorber (1994) has shown, and nowhere is this more clearly indicated than in evidence from those who have changed their sexual identity. Transsexual Jan Morris reported how different it was to go to a restaurant as a man and then later as a woman. The difference emanated from how he/she was expected to behave by others around him/her, and these differing roles were gendered expectations (Morris 1974). Throughout life our genders are reinforced through the social relations established in schools, workplaces and leisure activities (Sharpe 1994).

Feminist peregrinations

As we have noted above, the ground to be covered in feminist thought is wide and diverse, and in an attempt to introduce the topic in such a restricted space we have limited ourselves to three perspectives.

Feminism and theoretical social science

We cannot understand feminist social theory as a distinct entity from the feminist social movement over the past century, as they are inextricably linked. In short, feminist social theory seeks to understand the subordin-ation of women in society, particularly from a patriarchal perspective. Philo-sophically, this is located in Wollstonecraft's (1792) *A Vindication of the Rights of Women*. More recently, the wave of feminist social theory since the 1960s has attempted a radical change of society through a reinterpretation of Marxism (2:2) and psychoanalytical theory, and through an association with such movements as black, civil and gay rights campaigns. The Green-ham Common opposition to the location of US missiles in the UK was rooted in the feminist movement against male militarism (Young 1990). A wide range of critiques emerged concerning gender bias and patriarchal power. These reflected two strands, one of which concerned the male-dominated conceptual frameworks in which scientific questions were posed and the methods by which they were researched. The second concerned the male-dominated social institutional objectives and practices that were con-sidered to perpetuate sexism and gender bias. Key publications focused on sex and its relationship to these male-orientated institutions, including de Beauvoir's (1949) analysis of women as the second sex, Millett's (1970) analysis of sexual politics, Firestone's (1970) understanding of the tensions and conflicts rooted in the sexual relationship and Greer's (1970) exhort-ation for women to reclaim their right to assert their own sexual freedom.

Feminism and psychoanalysis

In short, Freudian psychoanalytical theory of gender centres on the pres-ence or absence of the penis. The learning of the gendered roles, according to Freud, begins with the equation 'I am a boy, I have a penis' or 'I am a girl, I lack a penis'. However, Freud develops his theory from this anatomical beginning to a symbolic representation of masculinity and femininity. Understandably, feminists have ferociously attacked Freud's theory on a number of counts. First, there is too strong a focus on the genitals, and they argue that in childhood other body parts are equally fascinating. Second, the presence or absence of the penis debate suggests that presence equals superior and absence inferior, and why should the reverse not be the case? Third, in Freudian theory the father is seen as the central figure of authority and discipline, but in many cultures it is the mother who has these defining qualities. Finally, Freud suggests that gender learning takes place around the age of 4 or 5, whereas later theorists have argued that it actually begins much earlier, in infancy (Wright 1984).

Rather than simply consigning psychoanalysis to the waste bin, some feminists have developed this perspective, but from a feminist point of view. Notably, Nancy Chodorow (1978, 1988) argued that gender learning arose from parental attachment at an early age and that the role of the mother was central in this process. The attachment to the mother, as the dominant force, allows for emotional involvement and expression, but this attachment has to be broken at a later age as the child grows. Breaking this attachment differs for boys and girls. Girls stay closer to the mother, Chodorow argues, learning her feminine skills by imitating her. Girls develop their own sense of self, which is more continuous with others: first the mother, then peers and, in most cases, finally a male partner. Boys, on the other hand, gain a sense of self by a more radical rupture of the mother attachment. Boys quickly learn not to be 'sissies' or 'girly' and forge their own masculinity. This, it is argued, means that they do not develop their skills in relating to others as much as girls do, and that they become more self-directed and repress their ability to understand their own feelings in relation to others. Chodorow's feminist psychoanalytical theory has been criticized by other feminists (Sayers 1986; Brennan 1988) but, notwithstanding this, her ideas remain important for feminist thought.

Feminism and postmodernism

Postmodernism (2:8) would suggest that we have reached the end of the era of Grand Narratives (Lyotard 1979). Feminism can be viewed as such a narrative, in a similar vein to Marxism or psychoanalysis. If this is so then postmodern feminists are understandably anxious that their cause will be diluted and their criticism of patriarchy undermined. Furthermore, this would then weaken their entire political movement (Weedon 1987). The postmodern argument of extreme relativism would challenge the main thrust of feminist opposition to male domination and lay claim to the idea that equality has, by and large, been achieved. However, other postmodern feminists argue that forms of male domination have merely become more subtle and sophisticated in the face of males feeling that they have lost some ground to females over the past three decades (Evans 1995). The contemporary postmodern position on feminism pivots on two approaches. The first concerns feminists who focus on equity between the sexes and attempt to progress society towards fairness and justice for all. In this, they argue, males and females can live and work together and a state of relative happiness is, at least potentially, achievable. The second refers to feminists who focus on gender and aim to overturn the structures of male domination and acquire ever-increasing areas of liberation for women. However, by attempting to free women, it is argued, they must subjugate males, and this causes a constant conflictual state in which anger on all sides pervades.

Further reading

Evans, J. (1995) *Feminist Theory Today: An Introduction to Second-wave Feminism.* London: Sage.

Davies, C. (1995) *Gender and the Professional Predicament in Nursing.* Buckingham: Open University Press.

Minsky, R. (1996) *Psychoanalysis and Gender: An Introductory Reader.* London: Routledge.

2.6 Symbolic interactionism

It can be said that sociology grew out of a concern with society, and certainly the early pioneers tended to focus on the macro-structures and processes of the various societies that they studied. A central issue throughout the history of sociology is a question that relates to the extent to which human nature is shaped by society or the extent to which society is influenced by human action. Put another way, the concern is the extent to which rational human beings can be considered free to act, and to which social structures and processes constrain human action (6:5). Functionalist and structuralist approaches moderated the creative side of the individual in their sociologies, but in symbolic interactionism this receives a much greater emphasis. Like structuralism, symbolic interactionism was born out of a concern with language but has developed in a strikingly different way. The person most commonly regarded as the leading proponent of symbolic interactionism is George Herbert Mead (1863–1931). Mead, an American intellectual in the Chicago School, published little in his lifetime and would probably have called himself a philosopher, or a social behaviourist, rather than a sociologist. However, his work has been hugely influential in the field of sociology that is now called symbolic interactionism with his posthumously published work and that of his students.

Key themes

The starting position for symbolic interactionists is the *location of the self*. Numerous sociological perspectives relegated the role of the self to social forces and suggested that individual behaviour is determined by social pressures. However, symbolic interactionism offers a new solution to the age-old philosophical conundrum of freewill and determinism (6:5) by raising the role of the self to new heights. Often contrasted with psychoanalysis, in which Freud had located the self in the unconscious mind with its drives, repressions and resolutions, symbolic interactionism located the self in the conscious, and thus made it a more social affair (Fisher and Strauss 1978). By doing so it is said that the self has a conversation with itself, which is termed the 'dialectic of the self'. However, it is not strictly a one-way conversation, as the mind contrasts the self, the individual 'I', with how we perceive others might see us. This is the 'me'. Thus, this conversation, the dialectic of the self, comprises of both 'I' and 'me', which means that although we are not totally free agents acting as we would wish, as we take into consideration others' view of us, we are relatively autonomous in symbolic interactionist terms (2:6). Symbolic interactionism employs a number of metaphors to highlight how individuals manage this dialectic, such as 'looking-glass self', 'social mirrors' and 'social masks'. The suggestion is that they are symbols of identity in a close relationship, or partnership, between the self and society (Mead 1934). We view not only ourselves but also how others perceive us, and we don social masks to portray to society a different view from what we really are and feel.

The second theme is *reflexivity*. Mead's approach to social behaviourism was to focus on actual behaviour rather than social structures or processes. He believed that it was the human being's capacity for self-reflection that set it apart from the rest of the animal kingdom. This capacity 'enables us to reason and learn on the basis of past experience, to stand outside that experience as it were and look at the present situation in the light of it' (Lee and Newby 1987: 317). This reflexivity is a complicated affair but is best understood as the ability of the human mind to 'bend back' on itself, or put another way the mind can apprehend itself. In a strange way the mind can not only think, but can also hold itself up for thinking about what it is thinking. It can bring into focus its present state and relate it to both past experiences and future possibilities. It learns to learn. This brings us to the third theme, which is concerned with *selectivity*. The mind chooses its focus and selects, intelligently, what it wishes to focus on. Out of the infinite number of possible items it selectively brings into view is choice. This choice has its history in relation to past experiences and present situation through the interaction with others. Mead saw the identity of the individual as developing from this interaction with others in the present and, through culture, with individuals of the past. He believed neither that individuals were totally programmed by social interaction nor that they were totally at the behest of biological impulses. He did believe that individuals possessed *intentions* and that these needed to be communicated back to society via gestures. These gestures, or symbols, have meaning, which may be interpreted by others; for example, a wave of the hand or the clenching of a fist. Although these are simple forms of symbols, Mead believed that more complex gestures were represented in language form.

The fourth theme is probably the single most important aspect of symbolic interactionism, and that is *taking the role of the Other*. All symbols have a double trajectory; on one level they are common property for all and on another level they are part of each person's individual personality. This is often referred to as the internalization of symbolic meaning and is what guides an individual's behaviour in relation to their intentions and what is culturally expected. This is learnt in childhood through play and helps the growing child to master the concepts of both the *Generalized Other* and the *Significant Other*. The former is all those people that the child will learn to distinguish from itself, and the latter is those closest to the child, such as parents, siblings and other family members, as well as peers. As the child plays, for example, a game of 'mummies and daddies', he or she will adopt the parental roles and play at being them, which allows the child to incorporate others' roles within their own private 'map' of the social world. This suggests that, in Mead's terms, the mind is a process by which the self interplays between the 'I' and the 'me'.

Most theoretical perspectives tend to change and develop with succeeding generations of academic interpreters, and symbolic interactionism is no exception. Herbert Blumer and his followers developed Mead's work and this can be set out in three main propositions identified by Blumer himself (Blumer 1969: 2).

- 'Human beings act towards things on the basis of the meanings that things have for them.' Blumer and his followers argued that meanings do not reside in the objects being referred to, or in the psychological process of the person, but in fact emanate from the social processes of interpretation by which definitions and meanings are formulated and employed.

- 'The meaning of things is derived from, or arises out of, the social interaction that one has with one's fellows.' This proposition stands in opposition to the functionalist view that social structures order social behaviour. Blumer and his co-workers argued that social order should be understood as a process, a dynamic entity, which is more adaptable, malleable and pliant than structural functionalism would suggest. Thus, at an interactive level the dynamics of human behaviour are much more susceptible to the vagaries of action and response.

- 'Group action takes the form of a fitting together of individual lines of action.' For interactionists, individuals share, and interpret, each other's symbols and meanings, and explain social order through the Generalized Other. Individuals adjust their behaviour in response to adopting the roles of others.

Symbolic interactionism has had a big influence on how society, and social behaviour, have been studied, and in relation to the health care context we can identify, at least, two central workers.

Relevance to the health care context

The first author to be mentioned is Erving Goffman (1922–82). Like his work, or loathe it, as many sociologists do, he has made a significant impact on how we understand social interaction. His major works that are relevant to our field are in relation to how we present ourselves in society (Goffman 1959) and how stigma is created, managed and reacted to (Goffman 1964). The stigma of illness and disability in health care contexts is a complex affair and can be as much created by health care professionals as it can be by members of society (Whitehead *et al.* 2001). Goffman also studied in-patients in mental institutions and identified how formal and informal rules were employed by both staff and patients (Goffman 1961). He showed how 'total institutions' absorbed the individual and encapsulated them within their social sphere, controlling and managing both staff and patients in a self-reinforcing cycle of 'government'.

The second author of significant relevance is Talcott Parsons (1902–79), an influential American sociologist in the post-Second World War period. Again, as often criticized as supported, his central, and probably most important, work was in relation to social action. However, it is the notion of 'sick role' that we wish to focus on here. The 'sick role' was first outlined by Henderson (1935) but received much closer and more elaborate attention from Parsons (1951b). The concept of the 'sick role' is said to have four components.

- The sick person is exempt from social responsibilities. They are not expected to fulfil social roles such as being a father, wage-earner, repairman etc. As long as they are ill they are excused from their usual obligations.
- The sick person is not held responsible for being sick. They are not blamed for their illness.
- The sick person is expected to seek out relevant and appropriate health professionals. They cannot ignore their sickness and accept their fate.
- The sick person is expected to comply with medical treatment. They must attempt to get better, they must desire non-sickness.

The 'sick role' is a legitimized social status that applies to those who comply with these four conditions. However, if they do not they may be labelled as malingering, manipulative or mad. The 'sick role' has been criticized on a number of counts and these can be listed as follows:

- It fails to make a clear distinction between the 'sick role' status and the patient.
- It does not take into account the conflict of interests that often exist between the doctor and the patient.
- It lacks universality, as some conditions do not result in an automatic suspension of social responsibilities, e.g. alcoholism, physical disabilities.
- It is more applicable to acute conditions than to chronic ones.
- Definitions of illness can vary between doctor and patient, e.g. Munchausen's syndrome.
- It does not describe the experience of being sick.

Despite these criticisms, Parsons's work on the 'sick role' did initiate a greater sociological critical enquiry into health-related matters, and particularly in relation to the medical model (2:13).

Further reading

Blumer, H. (1969) *Symbolic Interactionism: Perspective on Method*. Englewood Cliffs, NJ: Prentice Hall.
Mead, G. H. (1934) *Mind, Self and Society*. Chicago: University of Chicago Press.

2.7 Phenomenology

Phenomenology is well over a century old and is now considered an established philosophical doctrine that has its roots in the philosophers Georg Hegel (1770–1831) and Edmund Husserl (1859–1938). However, it was the

Austrian-American philosopher and social scientist Alfred Schutz (1899–1959) who popularized phenomenology by penetrating the dense work of these two earlier authors and made this perspective more accessible to the general student. The reader may well ask why we place this philosophical perspective here in a chapter on sociology. Our response would be that phenomenology is primarily concerned with the philosophy of the self in relation to society, and it has had a big impact on how we analyse social relations and social action. Furthermore, we could add that it has become a popular scientific research strategy for many nurses over the past two decades who have studied nursing procedures from this socio-philosophical perspective. Finally, because of its focus on the micro-components of the human mind and its relationship to social action it has been hugely influential on both sociology and psychiatry.

Major theoretical constructs

The voluminous work on phenomenology is difficult to précis, as it has been interpreted differently by a number of authors, such as Heidegger (1889–1976), Sartre (1905–80) and Merleau-Ponty (1908–61). Therefore, in this short section on phenomenology we restrict ourselves principally to the work of Alfred Schutz and his phenomenology and social relations. As we have noted above, sociology was predominantly concerned with the large, or macro, structures of societies and left the small, or micro, aspects of the mind to psychology. However, phenomenology, as a philosophical perspective, was taken up by Schutz, who was also considered a social scientist, and he began to analyse the micro aspects of the individual but in relation to the macro structures of social relationships. As we have seen in the previous section (2:6), George Herbert Mead had gone some way towards this with symbolic interactionism but his work was only published later and posthumously. Furthermore, later workers, such as Harold Garfinkel (1917–), were to employ a similar method, in a slightly tangential way, in his ethnomethodological approach. However, for the moment let us focus on Schutz and his phenomenological sociology.

The first major theme to be dealt with is the *stream of consciousness*. The starting point in phenomenological enquiry is to distinguish between temporal dimensions. Two types of time can be said to exist. The first refers to the cosmological clock; that is, the time that exists external to the individual experience of it, time that is 'out there' but that we are a part of. Second, there is our internal experience of time, our inner duration (Bergson's *durée*), which is our stream of consciousness. Without becoming too esoteric we can say that the external time is constant but that our internal time can at least appear to pass at different rates, e.g. faster when we are enjoying ourselves and slower when we are not. This stream of consciousness pivots on the notion of Now, the instant moment of Now that immediately passes and becomes the past, making way for the next Now that was in the immediate future but now becomes the new Now. In Schutz's terms, 'I cannot distinguish between the Now and the Earlier, between the later Now and the

Now that has just been, except that I know that what has just been is different from what now is' (Schutz 1970: 61). In short, this is the unidirectional, irreversible, stream of growing older!

The stream of consciousness is, of course, not just consciousness of everything but consciousness that attends to something specific. This specificity is the second key element of phenomenology and is called *intentionality*. It is said that our minds attend to what is relevant to us and there are *zones of relevance*. For our purposes there are said to be four regions of decreasing relevance. First, there is the primary zone of relevance, which is that part of the world within our reach and can be dominated by us; that is, it can be manipulated, changed and rearranged and we have some degree of control over it. The second zone of relevance comprises those parts of the world that are not directly open and available to us for control and manipulation but are connected to the primary zone of relevance. We are usually familiar with the fields within this secondary zone of relevance, even though we have less control over them. The third zone of relevance involves those fields of life that 'for the time being' have no connection to our present interests, and we can call them relatively irrelevant. Finally, we have the fourth zone of relevance, which consists of those aspects of the world that are absolutely irrelevant because whatever occurs in them will not affect us, or at least that is what we believe.

Taking the stream of consciousness and its attention to the zones of relevance, we can now appreciate that with every changing moment of Now we are adding to our experience of the world. In phenomenological terms this is the next key element and is called the *stock of knowledge*. This stock of knowledge is said to be structured according to our interests in relation to what our particular problem at hand might be and what tools we require to solve them. This stock of knowledge is also in a continual flux and grows with every experience. If a new moment (Now) brings forth a new object in the world, a new experience or a new event, it is said that we reflect on the novel moment and refer it to our stock of knowledge to see if it has typical features that we recognize from our past. Thus, if we perceive an animal for the first time (medium-sized, four-legged creature) we will typify it according to it being an animal and not an inanimate object, and dog-like rather than giraffe-like or rat-like. From this we will anticipate certain behaviours, i.e. ways of eating, biting, running, being friendly or unfriendly and so on. (An important point here for those readers who may go on to be phenomenological researchers is the fact that we may not actually see, for example, the animal's teeth but, as we have the previous experience of dog's teeth and what they can do, we view the animal as typically having them. This is known as apperception.)

The final theme that we wish to deal with is *meaning-endowed conduct*. From this phenomenological understanding of the micro operations of the individual Schutz built up a complex web of social interactions (influenced by the works of Husserl and Weber). Much of this is beyond the scope of this briefest of outlines but the linkage between this micro and macro perspective is what Schutz termed meaning-endowed conduct. This involves two different types of lived experiences. The first is distinguished by its passivity: it is 'undergone' or suffered. The second consists of an attitude or action towards it. For example, I may experience pain, or someone lifting my arm and letting it fall, but these cannot be regarded as behaviours or conduct. However, if I fight the pain, suppress it or even abandon myself to it, these are considered attitudes, behaviours or in short conduct towards pain. Similarly, if I resist or submit to someone lifting my arm that too can be viewed as conduct. Thus, in short, conduct carries meaning for the person who motivates the action.

Relevance to modern day practice

The relevance of phenomenology to us today can be briefly summed up under three areas. First, phenomenology has helped to open up the micro aspects of the life-world. Whereas the great social structures of given societies have been fruitfully attended to by sociologists, the mundane was largely neglected. Phenomenology (and later ethnomethodology) has opened up the micro aspects of daily living and revealed them to be just as highly complex as the macro social structures. For example, phenomenology has enabled us to analyse the complexity of shopping at the supermarket (Garfinkel 1986), as well as the experience of breastfeeding (Bottorf 1990). Second, phenomenology has, possibly more than any other perspective, managed the subjective. Whereas most scientific approaches attempt to relegate the subjective element of humanity to the objective component of natural sciences, phenomenology has not only convincingly incorporated it within its perspective but in fact has made it the central pivot. Finally, it is a mechanism that has been employed in a number of traditional disciplines other than sociology and enabled a reinterpretation revealing new insights; for example, in Marxism (2:2) (Tran-Duc-Thao 1951), in psychoanalysis (Lacan 1977), in economics (Chapter 7) (Bell and Kristol 1981), and in religion (Westphal 1984). Of course, like all perspectives phenomenology has received some criticism, and this criticism is largely esoteric. The main thrust of criticism against phenomenology revolves around the philosophical notions of essence and appearance. That is, the critical debate concerns whether the perceptions of the mind can be trusted enough to convince ourselves, and others, that things are real, or things are as we perceive them to be. Some say a qualified yes, while others offer a resounding no. However, notwithstanding the criticism of phenomenology, it appears to us to be a useful perspective to begin to analyse many of the mundane practices in health care settings and offers the discerning student a lively and energetic social scientific perspective.

Further reading

Embree, L. (1966) *The Encyclopedia of Phenomenology*. Dordrecht: Kluwer.

2.8 Modernism and postmodernism

The only single agreement concerning modernism and postmodernism is that there is no single agreement as to what the terms represent. However, their importance and influence on today's thinking are both large and growing. Ways of thinking about the world, including our arena of health care, are set in longstanding traditions, and those traditions are often held preciously and defended against intrusion by alternative interpretations. Take, for example, the time when it was a generally held truth that the world was flat and antagonism was felt towards those who suggested that it might be round. When traditional ways of thinking are challenged, ridicule, derision and disbelief are the norm. There is no clearer example than in the shift from modernist to postmodernist thinking.

Modernism

We can view the concepts of modernism and postmodernism along several trajectories. For example, we may distinguish societies along economic, political, social and cultural lines and define them in terms of pre-modern and modern. We may view modern societies as developing out of the move to capitalist economies (7:3), democratic rules of government (Chapter 8) and societies that are socially structured according to class and labour (2:2, 2:9). Or we may focus on the cultural fragmentation of experience, a commodification of events and a rationalistic approach to life as the turning points (Hall and Gieben 1992). However, if we wish to locate modernity as a period in time we can provide a loose chronology between the industrialization of Western societies and the Second World War. But it should be emphasized here that it all depends upon what field is being referred to when we speak of modernism. For example, modernism is a term that refers to the movement in Western arts between 1880 and 1950, in which traditional approaches were fragmented and overthrown by different ways of thinking and interpreting. These could include the paintings of Picasso, the poetry of Eliot, the music of Stravinsky and the architecture of Bauhaus. At one level it is represented by novelty, difference and rupture from tradition, but we can see that this soon becomes yet another norm. Thus, we are in a position to view (Western) societies as being pre-modern, modern and postmodern depending on whose point of view we are taking as the anchor point.

Postmodernism

We will briefly distinguish between postmodernism and postmodernity, although for the purposes of this short section we can use them interchangeably. Postmodernism is, again, a movement that is said to emanate from the arts in general, including literature, painting, poetry, film and television. Identifying its main features is difficult, as there is little agreement on what postmodernism is; in fact, as we will see, some do not even believe that it exists at all. However, we can establish some common elements that are useful in helping us to understand this perspective.

- *Mixture*: the drawing together of a blend of elements from different fields, contexts and epochs to form a radically different style.
- *Reflexivity*: the capacity to undertake self-reflection, and to evoke this in others, in order to challenge and overturn traditional ways of thinking.
- *Relativism*: the challenge to notions of objective standards of truth and an awareness of the role of the subjective.
- *Counteraction*: the challenge to traditional techniques attempting to portray one reality.
- *Disregard*: a lack of respect for traditions and a desire to cross established boundaries of style, cultures and authorities.
- *Scepticism*: a disbelief in the central position of the author, or the importance of the person as an authority, in any created work.

Postmodernity is a broader term that covers not only the arts but all of society, and is often contrasted with, or opposed to, modernity. Postmodernity is seen as a new condition of society, or a different stage in social development. However, many suggest that it is better understood as an extension to modernity rather than something inverted to it (Turner 1990a). Again, like modernity, postmodernity ranges across many contexts of social life, from works of art to forms of advertising, and from academic essays to architectural structures. However, it is usually characterized under the four main headings of:

- *Social*. In postmodernity social structures are less important, more fragmented and complex, and focus as much on gender, ethnicity and age as they do on class.
- *Cultural*. There is a focus on the aesthetic and the construction of personal identity based on choice rather than tradition.
- *Economic*. In postmodernity there is a challenge to mass production, with markets being more diverse and personal. Human relations are seen as central and the commodification of life is opposed.
- *Political*. There is a reversal of several elements, such as big government, well established welfare states, public ownership of utilities and intervention techniques into the economy. There is more attention to small-scale markets and competition.

Key postmodern themes and relevance to health care

To understand postmodernity in relation to its relevance for us in health care we need to set out some key themes. The first is *technology*. Since the Second World War (the period of postmodernity) we have witnessed supreme advancements in technology, which have redefined such things as labour forces, surveillance techniques and warfare management. Such high status technological weaponry as 'smart bombs' or 'star wars defence shields' have moved the 'front' from the trench to the computerized level of 'cockpit cognitions' (Harvey 1990). In medicine similar technological advances have made possible *in vitro* fertilization, the mapping of the human genome, and the cloning of sheep, moving bedside medicine through to the laboratory test tube. A second theme is that of *surveillance*. With the explosion of the 'plastic card', PINs and postcodes it is said that we are under scrutiny from 'big brother' organizations at all times (Davies 1996), and at any moment can be targeted for commercial reasons. Shockingly, it has been reported that of the many hundreds of satellites orbiting the Earth only a small fraction are looking outwards towards space, with the remainder spying downwards on us all (Davies 1996). In health care, surveillance of the body and mind is almost complete. From the earliest palpation of bodily structures and the early speculums and probes penetrating orifices we now have sophisticated fibre optics that can traverse living tissue and magnetic resonance techniques that can map the structures of the brain. Surveillance of the body can be undertaken via samples, specimens, signs and symptoms, and through the taking of measurements, biopsies and blood. We noted that this surveillance of the body and mind was *almost* complete, as it is not quite, as yet, total. The brain and the working of the human mind remain the last bastions of defence against this medical onslaught of surveillance. Despite voluminous psychologies and grand narratives, such as psychoanalysis, the brain continues to defy medical attempts to reveal its secret.

The third theme involves the *power/knowledge ratio*. The postmodern period has witnessed large-scale growth in Western capital and the expansion of institutional organizations that control more and more of everyday life. As knowledge increases, more of this everyday life becomes specialized and this fragmentation produces a situation in which trust increases. For example, due to *globalization* travelling around the world is a much more common practice and the expectation is that this can be undertaken safely. Trust is required on a large scale to achieve this. We trust that the machines that carry us are constructed safely, with the correct components, in the correct order. We trust that the operators of the machines we are travelling in are suitably qualified. We also trust that the system of travel is safe and secure. This trust now permeates ever-increasing areas of everyday life, and health care is no exception (Giddens 1989b). The belief in medical knowledge has increased manifold and expectations of the power of health professionals to effect cures and relieve symptoms are considerable. The fact that a tension exists between societal expectations and medical realism only serves to enhance the probability that the trust placed in health care professionals is often greater than their efficacy (Richman 1987).

Criticisms of postmodernism

Criticisms of both modernism and postmodernism abound. The first line of attack is usually that they are merely periods of time, histories and present, and that applying terms to them is arbitrary and fictitious (Eagleton 1996).

It is true, the argument goes, that things happen in any period of time but that circumscribing social past and present with defining terms merely gives the illusion of 'knowing' what modernity and postmodernity are. Eagleton (1996) suggests that, at best, postmodernity is merely a possibility and that we can get on quite well without it. Another critical line is that even if postmodernity exists it is irrelevant for those trapped in racial conflict, poverty, cycles of abuse; in short for the majority of the world. As esoteric concepts they may well be fashionable but, it is suggested, in 'real life' they are meaningless (Lash and Urry 1987). Another criticism is that even if they exist, and even if their elements are as we have identified above, there is nothing to suggest that the constituent parts are in any way related. Why, it is asked, should one affect the other in any meaningful way? Furthermore, in transitional terms there is no empirical evidence for the movement from one period to another, i.e. from modernity to postmodernity. Finally, the question is often posed: what comes after postmodernity? Post-postmodernity? However, despite these criticisms there continues to be an increasing number of postmodern thinkers who are analysing an increasing number of fields in relation to this perspective, including medicine and health.

Further reading

Eysteinsson, A. (1990) *The Concept of Modernism*. Ithaca, NY: Cornell University Press.

PART TWO: APPLICATION TO PRACTICE

2.9 Social stratification and social exclusion

As a discrete discipline sociology is a vitally important scientific perspective in helping us to understand not only the practice of nursing but also the professional position of its status in society. As we have noted above, nursing is predominantly a social event, with its human interaction lying centrally to its practice. An analysis of this is highly complex, as it incorporates the status within the wider social domain as well as its status within the professional health care arena. Therefore, sociological principles are excellent theoretical tools that aid us in highlighting the functional dynamic of nursing practice. Furthermore, the sociology of medicine now covers the areas that were previously termed applied sociology and clinical sociology and in which sociologists were employed in clinics working alongside psychiatrists, psychologists and social workers (Wirth 1931). The more modern sociology of medicine now covers a wide range of areas, which include the following:

- the sociology of health care professions;
- the sociology of illness, illness behaviour and 'help-seeking' behaviour;

- the sociology of health care settings (hospitals and clinics) and service organizations;
- sociological factors in the aetiology of illness and disease;
- sociological factors affecting the uptake of medical facilities;
- the sociological study of the doctor–patient (health care worker–patient) interaction;
- the sociology of health belief systems and their delivery of services;
- the sociology of global patterns of illness and health services;
- the sociological study of specific health care issues, such as fertility, mortality, pregnancy and disability.

The world of health care, like many other areas of life, such as the armed forces, police, religions and schools, consists of hierarchically structured organizations with divisions of labour (2:2), rank and status. In this section we will deal with social stratification as a sociological concept and show how its principles can reveal the features of division within the profession itself. We will also briefly introduce the issues relating to social exclusion.

Social stratification

Social stratification is a term that sociologists employ to denote the ways in which groups of people can be categorized vertically in terms of power, wealth, status, influence etc. It is a term that is borrowed from the field of geology, from the different types of rock strata. There is no known society that does not have some form of social stratification and there are said to be five main ways in which societies are divided.

- *Slavery*. This is the oldest and most extreme form of stratification and emanates from the early civilizations of Babylon, Egypt, Persia, Greece and Rome (Marsh *et al.* 1996). More recently, between the fifteenth and nineteenth centuries, European power was closely related to the slave trade, and in contemporary times there remains considerable concern regarding the continuance of slavery through war, trade, kidnapping, prostitution and debt repayment.
- *Caste*. This is closely related to Indian society and the Hindu religion. It is a complex division of labour with a rank ordering, which is not necessarily related to power or wealth but is related to traditional values going back some 3000 years. There is no movement between the castes, as one is born into one, divinely, based on a previous incarnation.
- *Estate*. This is a term that denotes social stratification based on the feudal system throughout Europe in medieval times (aristocracy, priesthood and commoners). It was more related to property and political power than to religious doctrines and therefore did allow for some social mobility through the divisions.
- *Class*. This social stratification system is based on property and authority (but is also closely related to prestige; see below). There are a number

of class systems and the reader is referred to any introductory text on sociology (for example, Marsh *et al.* 1996). We will briefly mention Max Weber's (1864–1920) theory of class, which is an elaboration on Marx's (2:2). Weber believed that class divisions were based not only on the means and control of production (2:2) but also on other resources, such as skills and qualifications. Weber related class divisions to professional and managerial occupations, more favourable conditions of work and qualifications such as degrees and diplomas. These skills that were learnt made them a more marketable commodity.

- *Prestige*. In Weber's theory the differences between social groups can also be based on the extent of social honour, prestige or status that is accorded to them by other members of society. This prestige may be positive or negative. High prestige groups are positively privileged: doctors and lawyers, for example. Low prestige groups are negatively privileged (called pariah groups) and are prevented from taking up opportunities available to others; for example, medieval Jews.

There are a number of ways in which modern British society is socially stratified; for example, upper class (capital ownership), middle class (educational credentials) and working class (labour power) (Giddens 1973). Or upper, upper-middle, middle-middle, lower-middle, skilled working, unskilled working, underclass (Runciman 1990). Or the Registrar-General's social divisions of professional, intermediate-skilled, partly skilled and unskilled occupations. There are, of course, many more, but we finish this section with an emphasis on the extent of prestige or status that is applied by society to any social stratificatory system in terms of the pyramid structure. That is, those at the top are fewer in number but carry the greater prestige, as well as the greater wealth and power.

Professional health care stratification

Differing professions have different statuses depending on the extent to which society values their skills. Well established professions, such as medicine and law, have great status and power due to a number of factors:

- they operate independently;
- they decide who will join their ranks;
- they control their single portal of entry;
- the body of knowledge is unique to that profession;
- they control the conduct and discipline of their members (Thompson 1982).

The power of medicine is rooted deep within the social structures of society, no matter what society it is (Turner 1987): Chinese medicine, Australian aboriginal medicine, the 'North American Indian medicine man', witchcraft or our own cosmopolitan medicine (Richman 1987). Whatever the health belief system, those with the perceived power over life and death, pain and relief, and disease and cure are awarded a high status in their society. The fact that this power is often attributed to women and men of medicine without them having any real power in reality to influence certain disease states is frequently overlooked, and society members are often shocked when they realize medical limitations. Notwithstanding this, the medical profession enjoys the highest prestige in Western health care settings.

Depending on setting, other health care professions also enjoy a high status, but not as great as the medical profession. These include psychologists, social workers, radiographers and occupational therapists, but these are viewed as a secondary stratum within health care delivery. Although it may be fair to say that from the patient's perspectives they may be held in high esteem, as the patient is in need of their services, members of the wider society differ in their view of their level of prestige.

Nursing as a 'profession' is in a sociologically complicated position. First, although we popularly refer to nursing as a 'profession' it does not adhere strictly to the professionalization principles outlined above. For example, it has several portals of entry and does not have a unique body of knowledge (as this book is testimony to the numerous disciplines that it draws upon). Second, nursing is held in high regard, generally, by both patients and members of the wider society (non-patients). Nursing carries a high social status. However, nursing is not considered a prestigious profession, as it does not have a high financial reward, nor is it considered a powerful professional group. Third, historically nursing has been linked to a 'vocation', a 'calling', which resonates with a dedication to a religious group. Religious groups are known for their lack of secular rewards in favour of a more divine (posthumous) reward (hence nurses as 'angels'). Finally, although some contemporary nursing is increasingly a technological practice, historically it is related to the care of the sick, particularly in relation to bodily excretions (low status work – hence a vocation). Thus, in terms of social stratification nurses enjoy a high social regard but nursing is considered low prestige in relation to other professional groups.

Social exclusion

We are introducing the notion of social exclusion here, as we can begin to see that as groups within society are stratified according to the principles outlined above, this raises questions concerning how individuals are incorporated into or excluded from certain groups. However, we merely introduce this issue of social exclusion here as it is covered more fully in other areas of the book (4:11).

Social distance is a term that is employed to denote the extent to which certain groups perceive a feeling of separation from other groups. The Bogardus Scale is a measurement tool that aims to establish the degree of tolerance or prejudice that is felt between social groups in society. This instrument is said to be cumulative. That is, a white subject who has positive views about mixed marriages is more likely to be tolerant towards black neighbours, and of course vice versa. What is important is that social distance can often lead to hostility between the groups concerned.

Gendered labour is of particular concern for us in relation to the male domination within medicine and the female domination within nursing, highlighted above (2:5). Although we can see the 'public' world of paid work as separate from the 'private' domain of the family, some feminist thinkers argue that gender labour relations in paid employment largely reflect the gender labour relation in the family environment (Morgan 1991). This, feminists argue, is why females have, historically, been excluded from, and disadvantaged in, many areas of employment. Nursing is an exception because of its linkage with the caring, nurturing role of the mother. However, it is interesting to note that despite the fact that nursing has far more females than males, the higher management positions in nursing are predominantly occupied by males.

Eugenics refers to the improvement of the human race through a policy of selective breeding. This involves identifying certain groups and individuals who would be considered to have some aspect that was considered to be 'inferior' and discouraging them from breeding. It also incorporates identifying others who are considered to have qualities that are deemed 'superior' and encouraging them to procreate. Despite the fact that there is little agreement about what the negative aspects of the human condition are, it is an extreme form of social exclusion. Furthermore, it is prone to abuse, as the eugenics policy of the Hitler regime showed in the 1930s, when doctors and nurses were closely involved in the killing of handicapped children and adults.

The relationship between the role of the health care professional and the creation and maintenance of stigma and social exclusion was clearly highlighted by Mason *et al.* (2001). In this text many areas of modern day health care working were shown to perpetuate the exclusion of stigmatized groups of patients, from surgical disfigurements to congenital abnormalities, and from teenage pregnancies to mentally disordered offenders. It is not surprising that the Labour government of 1997 immediately launched a new initiative, the Social Exclusion Unit (SEU), in response to its assessment of what the consequences are for those who are socially excluded from our society.

Further reading

Giddens, A. (1989) *Sociology*. Cambridge: Polity Press.
Hardey, M. (1998) *The Social Context of Health*. Buckingham: Open University Press.
Mason, T., Carlisle, C., Watkins, C. and Whitehead, E. (eds) (2001) *Stigma and Social Exclusion in Healthcare*. London: Routledge.

2.10 Deviance and difference

We have already begun to see how individuals and groups can be classified and categorized into groups (2:9), and while this process can be considered benign, and even helpful at times, it can also be viewed as negative and damaging. Putting individuals into groups can diminish their individuality by depersonalizing their traits and characteristics, which eliminates their personhood. Furthermore, placing a person in a particular group attributes to them certain social characteristics and semantic meanings pertaining to that group, which may, or may not, be accurate. For example, allocating an individual as 'left wing' or 'right wing' on the political spectrum would attribute to them certain ideological beliefs that are traditionally held in society about those categories. The fact that these 'positions' can be viewed as radically opposed, or closer to the centre, or even mixed (i.e. someone considered 'right wing' with certain 'left wing' views and vice versa), only goes to show that such categorizations are sometimes unhelpful. We could have employed a different allocation of categories as our example, which have more serious connotations to them; for example, 'racist' or 'sexist'. The important point is, and the political spectrum highlights this, that much allocation of groups is a question of placement along a continuum *between* certain categories rather than at the extremes of the polarized ends. This may be normal–abnormal, equilibrium–disequilibrium, right–wrong, good–bad and so on. Of course, these polarizations are often merely value judgements, but they are none the less judgements that are constantly made by all those in health care settings. Finally, we should note that there are many gradations on these continuums and it is often a question of degree as to which one is allocated to a particular group. In this section we now concentrate on a continuum that we often use in health care settings, that of deviance and difference.

Deviance

In a straightforward sense deviance simply refers to a deviation from the norm, the norm being understood as a set of scores that are characteristic of a particular, clearly defined, sample (Robinson and Reed 1998). Thus, we can take a series of measurements of people's heights, establish the average (mean distribution), or norm, and say how far one person deviates from this. However, the concept of deviance that we wish to deal with is predominantly a sociological one, and one that largely refers to aberrant behaviour related to gender/sex and/or crime. It is worth noting that deviance can also refer to other behaviours: drug and alcohol abuse, football hooliganism and certain religious cult formations, for example (Downes and Rock 1989). Deviance in health care matters has been associated with a wide range of behaviours from the habitual failure to keep appointments to manipulating a surgical operation without an actual disorder, and from abusing substances known to cause harm to engaging in strategies to maintain ill health (Mason *et al.* 2001). This complex mosaic of human behaviours requires grand theoretical explanations in order to understand and help those so afflicted, but this lies outside the remit of our book.

Here we focus on some discourses from the wider society in order to highlight the way in which deviance is used, and then focus more sharply on health care settings. If we take the basic sociological concepts of norms, conformity and sanctions as our starting points within the concept of deviance we may be able to define deviance as 'non-conformity to a given set of norms that are accepted by a significant number of people in a community or society' (Giddens 1989a: 173). However, we can see immediately that we may have semantic problems with the concepts of 'accepted' and 'significant' within this definition, and therein lies the main difficulty with the notion of deviance. We are dealing with deviance as a social term, which means that members of society socially construct it, and we are all well aware that establishing social agreement is extremely difficult. Thus, what one person may consider deviant in society another may not. However, to those who are considered by the majority to be deviant in some way certain sanctions may be applied. Sanctions can be both formal and informal. Formal sanctions are usually encapsulated in laws, rules, regulations and policies, while informal sanctions tend to be spontaneous and less organized, such as the mob outcry against a particularly heinous crime.

To highlight this complex area Giddens (1989a) sets out the 'careers' of two people who may be considered deviant. The first is Howard Hughes, the successful businessman who made a vast fortune and then became a recluse. He let his hair and beard grow long and became obsessed with avoiding being contaminated by germs. He looked more like a deviant than a successful businessman. The second is Ted Bundy, the serial killer who worked for the Samaritans. He was an extremely clever person who prepared his own defence at trial and was complimented by the judge for his excellent presentation (before being sentenced to death!). In short, he looked more normal than deviant. Of course, the dividing line between serial killing and growing one's hair long is clear, but the point is that deviant behaviour often lies deep within a set of other human behaviours and can be kept hidden from view. The question now raised is: where does deviance begin and difference end?

Difference

It is probably in the notion of difference that the roots of prejudice, stigma and social exclusion lie. The sociology of difference tends to focus on two main areas, the first referring to the difference between gender (2:5) and the second relating to differences in ethnicity (2:11). As we have covered these two topics elsewhere we will limit our discussion of difference to drawing a distinction between the terms deviance and difference. We would all probably agree that the distinction between the two is a question of degree. That is, it appears as if difference exists somewhere between what would be considered the norm, the same, the uniform and what would be considered clearly deviant, deviance being more extreme than mere difference. This then would suggest that difference is somehow more acceptable than deviance. However, the areas of overlap are not quite as easy to discern. For example, a female wearing trousers may be considered different, but a male wearing a skirt would be more likely to be considered deviant, unless the skirt was a kilt (Marsh *et al.* 1996). Here we can see that the apparent continuum from same, through difference to deviance is a question of what society would consider acceptable. The social context is central to our understanding of difference and whether the difference is accepted as mere difference and not perceived as unacceptably deviant depends upon what values of normality are being transgressed. For example, body piercing is an accepted form of human adornment and single pierced ears have a long history in Western, as well as other, societies. However, in contemporary times it is a common sight to see pierced tongues, noses, eyebrows and navels that may be seen as different from the traditional norm. The more common it becomes, the more normal it will be seen to be. Yet when we see someone with multiple piercing done to an extreme it goes beyond 'different' into another realm that may be considered deviant.

Difference can also have another level of analysis that focuses on the supposed human need to establish demarcation points in terms of belonging to either in-groups or out-groups (2:9, 4:11). It is said that this primitive need is reflected in one of the earliest biblical accounts, that of the murder of Abel by Cain (Foucault 1973). The motive for this murder was that Cain had fallen out of grace with God, who then favoured Abel, and Cain was envious of this. The establishment of this 'them and us' (in-group/out-group) situation is said to have remained a basic human characteristic down the centuries, with out-groups said to be manifesting the signs of their fallen grace. For example, we could cite leprosy, plague, epilepsy and mental illness, to name but a few historical out-groups (Foucault 1967). The fact that the difference established by the 'them and us' scenario has allowed, and continues to allow, for all manner of atrocities towards those deemed part of the out-group is often overlooked.

Overlap into practical areas

Nosology is a branch of medicine that is concerned with the systematic description and classification of diseases and disorders. This forms the basis of the diagnostic textbooks and manuals that are seen in medical circles, as well as nursing books. In general medicine it forms the structure of contents in the majority of textbooks through a series of categories, subcategories, sub-subcategories and so on. In psychiatry nosology forms the basis of the International Classification of Diseases, 10th version (ICD-10), and the Diagnostic Statistical Manual, 4th edition (DSM-IV). Nosology is based on establishing differences between conditions. An example might suffice. We may begin with the cardiovascular system as a major category construct of the body, with the heart as a subcategory, then subcategorize the heart into disorders referring to the four chambers. We may then subcategorize one chamber into subdivisions of different electrical dysrhythmias and then subdivide these according to the different cells that might be responsible and so on, *ad infinitum*. Nosological frameworks are useful if they deal with cause and effect relationships between events within a subcategory, relationships between subcategories and relationships between a subcategory and the overall functioning of the body. However, without the establishment of these relationships nosological frameworks merely give the illusion of knowledge. This is an important point given that they form the basis of diagnosis and ultimately treatment. Thus, the location of someone, or their signs and symptoms, as deviant or different can have profound effects. This brings us to labelling theory.

Labelling theory is a term that is used to describe a cluster of inter-related ideas rather than a single entity and some theorists argue that it is a *process* rather than a set of characteristics. This process is based on an interaction between those that are labelled deviant and those that are not, in short between 'them and us' (Downes and Rock 1989). Focusing on deviance in relation to crime, Lemert (1972) suggested that deviance consisted of two types, primary deviance and secondary deviance. Primary deviance is said to be the point when the initial transgression actually occurs. As people are labelled as deviant they are stigmatized accordingly, people react differently towards them and they then begin to act out the label attributed to them; this is known as secondary deviance. The important point for us in health care settings is that these concepts can hold true for people labelled as 'sick', 'diseased' or 'disordered', and they may begin to act out the label attached to them.

Labelling people in health care settings is, of course, necessary, particularly, as we have said, in relation to diagnosis and establishing interventions. However, referring to individuals according to these labels depersonalizes them and obscures the importance of their individuality. For example, referring to someone as the 'laparotomy in bed four' or 'a bad shoulder in cubicle two' ignores the importance of viewing the person and his/her need for health care in a holistic manner. At one level this is often viewed as a harmless aspect of human behaviour, but this belies the possibility of serious consequences that may follow this stigmatizing process. Health care workers are in a rich stigmatizing environment and may easily succumb to the pressures of such labelling, due to the fact that by the nature of the patient requiring health care services they differ from the norm. This difference is usually their ailment or injury. Mason *et al.* (2001) collated a series of essays written by health care professionals, some of whom had stigmatizing conditions themselves, and a chapter by a user of health care services, in which the focus was on how health care professionals both initiate and maintain the stigmatizing process, this process being grounded in the identification of deviance or difference. Examples are in areas of congenital and surgical disfigurements (Farrell and Corrin 2001), in areas of mental health (Shaughnessy 2001), terminal illnesses (Donovan 2001), speech defects (McArdle 2001) and breast feeding (Smale 2001). Some of these areas would not normally be seen as indicative of a condition that readily attracts stigma. However, often this process of labelling deviance and difference within the stigmatization of patients occurs at an unconscious level. If we are to prevent adding this burden to the patient then it is vital that nurses and other health care workers become aware of how this process develops, and are sensitive to the impact that it can have on patients. Raising this awareness is the first step towards prevention and reparation.

Further reading

Mason, T., Carlisle, C., Watkins, C. and Whitehead, E. (eds) (2001) *Stigma and Social Exclusion in Healthcare Settings*. London: Routledge.

Pattison, S. (2000) *Shame: Theory, Therapy, Theology*. Cambridge: Cambridge University Press.

Sumner, C. (1994) *The Sociology of Deviance: An Obituary*. Buckingham: Open University Press.

2.11 Ethnicity and race

In the previous sections we have been building up a picture in which we can see some of the sociological processes by which people in society can be viewed as different, and excluded because of this. We have noted how society can be stratified (2:9), causing divisions, how in-groups and out-groups can be created (4:11), causing conflict, and how people may be viewed as deviant or different (2:10) and treated accordingly. In this section we go one step further and deal with the issue of ethnicity as related to race, prejudice and discrimination, particularly in relation to health and health care. However, before we do this we spend a little time in defining the relevant terms, which often cause confusion, as they are sometimes used interchangeably, and incorrectly, in sociological, as well as lay, parlance.

The terms that do cause confusion include 'ethnic group', 'racial group', 'ethnic minority', 'caste' and 'social stratum'. The latter two have been dealt with above (2:9, 2:10) and we focus on the first three terms here. The first term, 'ethnic group' refers to the cultural practices and perspectives that are distinct from other groups. It is usually a two-way affair in which the ethnic group sees itself as set apart from other groups and in return the other groups generally agree that it is different. The characteristics that are most usually apparent in setting an ethnic group apart from others include: (a) a separate language; (b) a long history or ancestral roots that may be real or mythical; (c) a historical religion; and (d) a distinct style of dress or adornment (Giddens 1989a). Ethnic differences are said to be '*wholly learned*, a point that seems self-evident until we remember how often some groups have been regarded as "born to rule" or "shiftless", "unintelligent", and so forth' (Giddens 1989a: 210, emphasis in the original.

Whereas ethnic differences are learnt behaviours, racial differences are said to be 'physical variations singled out by the members of a community or society as socially significant' (Giddens 1989a: 212). Most sociologists do not believe that human beings can be separated into biologically different races or categories and prefer to focus on the social relations between culturally diverse groups. For example, they prefer to talk about ethnic relations and race relations rather than ethnicity and race *per se*. Clearly, there are different physical attributes between racial groups, but there are just as many different physical attributes *within* those groups (Banton 1988). It is worth noting that in contemporary times the concept of 'race' is used in three broad ways:

- *Race as classification.* Historically the term race has been used in an attempt to categorize people according to their common origin, as if it was fixed and permanent. Darwin despatched this theory, although his idea was slow to be accepted, and showed that no forms in nature were ever-lasting. Darwin preferred the term subspecies of *Homo sapiens*. Sadly, the term 'race' is still inappropriately used today as a form of classification in both legislative and governmental documents, as well as by members of society.

- *Race as synonym.* There are four ways of using 'race' as synonym. The first is a historical usage of dividing humans into subspecies such as Negroid, Mongoloid and Caucasoid. However, we now know that this is inaccurate due to the mixing of gene pools. Second, it has been used to identify an overall species such as the human race, but this implies unity and is antithetical to the first usage. Third, race was often used to represent a nation, e.g. the German race, the Norwegian race, but this has fallen into disuse. Fourth, the term 'race' can be used to define a group of people in a society according to physical markers such as skin colour, hair type, facial features and so on. Although the issue is complicated, some writers believe that this use of race equates with racism (van den Berghe 1978).

- *'Race' as signifier.* In discourse analytical terms 'race' is treated as a *signifier*. That is, it is a term, utterance, sound or image-maker that will create a meaning for the person within a known set of discursive rules or codes. For example, within white racist groups the term 'race' would be encoded with meanings of white supremacy and black inferiority. The signifier 'race' is decoded by recipients of the message who know the same set of discursive rules (quotation marks are customary in this perspective).

The final term to be defined is ethnic minority. This is a confusing term because it incorporates two major components, the numerical and the political, which often become mixed up. For example, in simple terms the numerical will refer to a minority group comprising a smaller number than the majority, and the political tends to refer to a disadvantaged, underprivileged and oppressed group. However, we also note that in the UK, as in most countries, we are led by a minority group, known as the elite, who are advantaged and privileged in our society, and it is the insertion of the notion of class that brings this confusion (Wirsing 1981).

Ethnicity and health care

We have seen that 'difference' can cause certain tensions in societies and if we focus on ethnicity we can see that this too can lead to certain forms of prejudice and discrimination (Banton 1994). Prejudice refers to the set of opinions and attitudes that are held by one group in relation to another. Seen in this light it is apparent that there can be few people who are not prejudiced to one degree or another. Of course, this would depend whether these opinions and attitudes are positive or negative, and whether they are based on 'facts' or learnt beliefs. The important point is that they are opinions and attitudes and do not represent behaviours, for if they do, then this brings us to another matter, that of discrimination. Discrimination is active behaviour aimed at social processes that disadvantage certain groups who are socially defined (Collins 1992). Although prejudiced people may not act on those beliefs and attitudes, they may operate at a subconscious level and move their actions into the sphere of discrimination (Whitehead *et al.* 2001). Finally, prejudice and discrimination may exist separately without one being directly related to the other (although there may well be an indirect relationship).

Given our four main characteristics of an ethnic group mentioned above (language, history, religion and dress), we can see that each brings with it a vast array of beliefs, traditions and ideologies. The UK, like many other countries, is now a multicultural society in which many ethnic groups live, work and play together, often harmoniously but sometimes amidst tensions and hostility. Perhaps, with the wealth and diversity of ethnic beliefs, and the ignorance and misunderstanding of cross-cultural traditions, prejudice and discrimination are in some way understandable, even if unacceptable. What are needed, in our view, are mechanisms for breaking down this ignorance and misunderstanding of others' cultures, and development of ways of reflection relating to our own beliefs and prejudices. In terms of health care delivery, all professions need to be aware of cross-cultural issues and an effective service cannot do justice to the health care aims of society unless it addresses these issues. We would now like to explore some issues relating to a few of the areas in which ethnicity and health care interface.

In terms of dental practice it has been argued that ethnicity, or at least the way in which ethnic groups are classified, may well be related to dental health inequalities (Buck *et al.* 2001). These authors are cautious and do not go as far as to say that dental health care is different across ethnic groups, but note that uptake of services may well reflect ethnic differences, and that this may also reflect 'a marker for such factors as social deprivation or the impact of "place" on dental health' (Buck *et al.* 2001: 83). Racial and ethnic differences in health care access and health outcomes for three ethnic groups of adults with type two diabetes were studied (Harris 2001). Although there was little ethnic difference between the groups for access to health care services the author did report some differences between the groups for the way in which self-monitoring of blood glucose and referrals for cholesterol checks were undertaken. This would have a knock-on effect for some of the differences between the ethnic groups' outcomes. Differences in health belief models may account for the differences in self-monitoring.

Chan (2000) studied a Chinese ethnic minority women's group in Manchester in relation to their views regarding health services for them in this city. Their general practitioners and health visitors were then interviewed to elicit their views on the same issues. Unsurprisingly, Chan (2000) reported that a discrepancy existed between the group's views. It became clear that tensions existed between socio-economic factors, demographic profiles, health beliefs and attitudes, and languages spoken. Women were also the focus in Lovejoy *et al.*'s (2001) study of the ethnic differences in dietary intakes, physical activity and energy expenditure in middle-aged pre-menopausal women. They concluded that ethnic differences may be apparent and influence the effect of menopausal transition on obesity in African American women. But, they emphasized that obesity is already highly prevalent in this group. Finally, the stage of readiness to exercise in ethnically diverse women was studied by Bull *et al.* (2001), with significant differences between blacks, American Indians, Alaskan natives, Hispanics and whites reported. However, caution was again expressed, as the differences may be due not to racial features but to cultural 'lifestyle' expectations.

What we see here is a tension between health professionals who, on the one hand, perhaps accept that there are differences between ethnic groups, but, on the other hand, have difficulty identifying whether these differences are due to cultural artefacts or are part of their racial make-up. Furthermore, in terms of take-up of services and access to health care provision confounding factors include the diversity of health belief models (Richman 1987), socio-economic factors (Basu 2001), language barriers (McKeown and Stowell-Smith 1998), perceptions of mental health (Fernando 1991) and religious beliefs (Swinton 2000). Many apparent differences disappear when these variables are controlled for. Finally, it is worth noting that some ethnic minority groups have reported that when they have accessed and taken up health care services they have felt stigmatized and marginalized (Mason *et al.* 2001) and have felt that they have not received the quality of care that other groups have received (Doyle 1991; Cortis 2000; Higgs *et al.* 2001).

Race relations and cross-cultural issues

Within our understanding of race relations there are two basic perspectives that must be dealt with. The first relates to a predominantly theoretical perspective with practical ramifications. In this view *Homo sapiens* is one species and therefore any racial differences are merely physical attributes, as mentioned above. From this perspective studying relations between physical differences of subspecies of humans is tantamount to racism. The argument is then posed that we ought not to be concerned with *race relations* as a distinct form of relations, but instead see the relations between subspecies as merely another form of *social relations*. This position accepts the strength of the theoretical perspective but also agrees that in the real world the lay understanding of race bears some weight. The second perspective relates to a predominantly practical perspective with theoretical ramifications. This recognizes the hollowness of the theoretical concept of race and argues that in the real world people do believe in it. Furthermore, they arrange their beliefs in relation to it, and in some cases operate their behaviour in accordance with those beliefs. Whether or not race exists, if people believe that it does, and it affects their behaviour, then it is a question of *race relations* and ought to be a focus of study, and change. This latter perspective has practical resonance in relation to: the National Health Service as a major employer of, and provider of services to, people from black and ethnic minority communities (Royal College of Midwives 2000); racist comments in nursing classrooms (Sawley 2001); the role of the Department of Health in the promotion of equal opportunities; and multicultural and anti-racial issues in nurse education (Foolchand 2000).

Finally, we can briefly mention cross-cultural issues that are often referred to as practical attempts to overcome many of the problems outlined above. It is an inherent position of our profession to fight racism and discriminatory practices in our health care services, whether these views and practices are our own or belong to others. Creating reflection, raising awareness, informing knowledge, being open and developing acceptance are all laudable enterprises, but it is often the smaller-scale focus that aids these grander schemes. For example, Corless *et al.* (2001) warn us of the many research instruments that may have cultural bias; Davidhizar and Brownson (1999) highlight the fact that there are many discrepancies between reading abilities (in English) and the production of health education and promotion literature; and Krieger (2000) puts forward a view that public health surveillance systems may be viewed differently by different ethnic groups. The picture is clearly complex but all health care professionals, users, managers, planners and administrators of services have a role to play in this area of race relations.

Further reading

Ahmed, W. I. U. (2000) *Ethnicity, Disability and Chronic Illness*. Buckingham: Open University Press.

Sollors, W., Cabot, H. and Cabot, A. (1996) *Theories of Ethnicity: A Classical Reader*. London: Macmillan.

Macbeth, H. and Shetty, P. (2000) *Health and Ethnicity*. London: Routledge.

▌2.12 Employment and leisure

In contemporary society employment is generally viewed as a positive status that carries with it an element of social acceptability and a certain degree of social standing. Leisure is closely related to work, sociologically, and is considered both a payoff for employment and an absorption into the notion of 'being in work'. However, the relations between employment and leisure, at both individual and societal levels, are highly complex, which is one reason why when these relations become fractured they impact on both physical and mental well-being. Types of employment and leisure are social indicators of financial status and social class, and are also markers of educational achievement, psychological make-up and certain cultural dimensions. For example, generally speaking, employment as a barrister as opposed to a bin man conveys different messages in relation to social status, education, finances, class, culture and so on. Similarly, and again generally speaking, differences in leisure activities such as sky diving and dominoes suggest different messages about the person. However, the social picture in relation to health is further complicated by relationships between employment, unemployment, paid work, non-paid work, voluntary work, physical leisure, non-physical leisure, rest and recreation. Some of these relationships can be summed up under the following headings.

- *Financial*. Most people work to provide money for their families to survive and without this salary coping with everyday life becomes a constant worry. Furthermore, without a salary many leisure activities are beyond reach.
- *Social networks*. Work and leisure provide opportunities for the establishment of a circle of friends in which shared activities create bonds between people.
- *Activity*. Both employment and leisure provide a forum for the exercise of skills, competencies and energies. Even when they are routine they structure action and absorb energy, and without this outlet frustration can develop.
- *Temporal rhythm*. Most people's day is structured around the time at work and the time at play. In some work situations the time is mundane, repetitive and slow but none the less it provides structure and direction.
- *Variation*. Employment and leisure offer contrasts, not only with each other but also as alternative contexts to the domestic setting. An often heard comment is 'it's just nice to get out of the house'.
- *Personal identity*. Employment and leisure activities provide the basis for establishing self-esteem, particularly for men who historically have been seen as the main 'breadwinners'.
- *Fulfilment*. Employment and leisure can offer the opportunity for personal fulfilment and give a sense of achievement and self-worth.
- *Social status*. Employment and leisure are close accompaniments to social status and many who are unemployed and cannot, or do not, engage in leisure activities often feel undervalued and have a low self-esteem.

Thus, we can see a complex interrelated picture between employment and leisure and it is not difficult to appreciate how these may impact on a person's physical and mental health.

Employment

When we think of work we tend to have the image of paid employment in which we earn a wage for the work that we do. However, it is a little more complicated than this, as *being* in work is also a statement about making one's own way in life, providing for others and contributing to the wider society. The concept of work is so important in our society that much of our time is concerned with getting a job, keeping a job or in our youth responding to the question 'what will you do when you grow up?' Through industrialization and the development of capitalist societies (2:2) work moved from merely representing survival to having meaning beyond the secular. For example, Weber's (1904) protestant work ethic revealed a relationship between secular capitalism and the aesthetic religion. Hand in hand with employment is, of course, the question of job satisfaction, which is also related to health. There are many studies in which it has been shown that the higher the rate of job satisfaction the less stress, injury and burnout there are. On the other hand, unemployment has been shown to create stress, mental health problems and some degree of physical deterioration through inactivity (Burton and Turrell 2000). We should note, however, that employment may also refer to unpaid work, which is often overlooked. For example, fixing a car, mowing the lawn and doing housework is time consuming effort for which we generally do not receive any financial remuneration. Furthermore, voluntary work for charities or other organizations has an important function in our society. Many people give up their free time willingly and do not seek financial reward, although it is fair to say that such voluntary work is highly rewarding in other ways. This shows that although we tend to have a narrow understanding of employment as referring to being in paid work, the concept of 'work' actually stretches much further.

The health care literature is replete with studies concerning employment, unemployment and retirement in relation to physical and mental well-being. In employment terms it is in everyone's best interest to ensure a healthy productive workforce, and studies to improve health status are common. For example, Dababneh *et al.* (2001) have studied the impact of added rest breaks on the productivity and well-being of workers in a meat processing plant. The subjects identified a preferred rest schedule and, following its implementation, productivity increased, and discomfort and stress levels were reduced. Occupational therapists have, obviously, featured large in studies of employment and health. For example, Tasiemski *et al.* (2000) reported on a study relating to sports, recreation and employment following a spinal cord injury, and highlighted the fact that many patients showed better improvement rates when they felt that they had some level of activity. In a similar vein, Dyck and Jongbloed (2000) examined employment issues for women diagnosed with multiple sclerosis and showed comparable results. Of course, the impact of unemployment is a major concern, as Wadsworth *et al.* (1999: 1491) noted: 'the experience of prolonged unemployment early in the working life of this population of young men looks likely to have a persisting effect on their future health and socio-economic circumstances'. Clearly, rising rates of long-term unemployment are cause for health concerns. Many researchers have also studied the 'natural' state of unemployment, otherwise known as retirement. Problems in adapting to retirement following a lifetime of work have been noted (Hugman 1999), and Jonsson and Andersson (1999) have shown how some opportunities for retirees to engage in some form of occupation following retirement have increased satisfaction rates. Ominously, Whiteford (2000) warns of a new global challenge, that of occupational deprivation.

Leisure

There is a strange relationship between work and leisure, as they are not merely binary oppositions. As we have noted, there is a tremendous pressure to become employed, and then a huge impetus to decrease our work time and increase our time for leisure. As First World countries have become more affluent the importance of leisure time activities has increased accordingly. Most leisure activity is done in the home, approximately 70 per cent for men and 80 per cent for women, but there are significant differences in leisure patterns for gender, life cycles and class divisions (Marsh *et al.* 1996). Although leisure activities can be related to financial resources, there are also cultural differences between certain social groups (Crespo *et al.* 2000). Studying the changing work–leisure relationship throughout the 1990s, Lobo (1998) reported that contrary to expectations there was strong evidence that some people worked longer hours but that non-standard work shifts had allowed for increased leisure time. In a later paper, Lobo (1999) argued that leisure is a complex activity that aids experimentation and risk-taking, and provides the experience for learning how to respond to challenges. Physical activity in leisure time is linked to healthy lifestyles and Lindstrom *et al.* (2001) showed how socio-economic differences in leisure time physical activity shaped health-related behaviour. However, finances are only one variable and psychosocial factors are also important elements in decisions to engage in leisure activities. The social network itself contributes to satisfaction with leisure time.

Increased leisure time with inaction also brings some health-related problems. In an interesting research study Farnworth (1998) produced a paper entitled 'doing, being and boredom', in which it was argued that the experience of boredom was associated with perceptions of victimization and entrapment. Furthermore, the subjects reported that they felt that it was society's responsibility to prevent this boredom. In Farnworth's (1998) study this could explain why young people turned to crime. Crist *et al.* (2000) studied the effects of employment, play/leisure, self-care and rest in relation to mental health. It was reported that 'the type of environmental support needed to function with a mental health problem is an indicator of differences in abilities to perform daily activity patterns' (Crist *et al.* 2000: 27). Leisure time activity is an important factor in health behaviour and should be a priority despite common pressures of 'lack of time' or 'work demands' (Burton and Turrell 2000). The move towards automation, computerized lives, and electronic games has led physical leisure activities to decline. This is likely to have a negative impact on health, and as health care professionals we should be concerned with this trend.

Further reading

Bunton, R., Burrows, R. and Nettleton, S. (1995) *The Sociology of Health Promotion*. London: Routledge.

Grint, K. (1991) *The Sociology of Work: An Introduction*. Cambridge: Polity Press.

2.13 Health and illness

The 'sociology of health and illness' is now the preferred term to the older 'sociology of medicine' label. The main reason for this shift in focus is that the sociology of health and illness reflects the emphasis on the theoretical underpinnings of sociology in relation to the states of health and illness, rather than the professional interests of medicine as a discipline. However, the two terms are probably more closely related than they are disparate, owing to the complex relationship between the power of professional medicine, the society in which medicine operates and its use (and some say abuse) of the concepts of health and illness. We should note that although we may criticize medical power for its dominance, this power is attributed to it by the society in which it is located, and therefore we must take some responsibility for this. The type of health belief system that we hold will determine our relationship with the professionals involved in that system, and we will either accept or reject their power status in terms of efficacy depending on our belief in a particular model of medicine.

Defining states of health and illness is a difficult task, as these states are both relative and contextual. Yet they are defined, at least at a lay level, in order for people to engage in sick role behaviour. As we have seen (2:6), part of becoming sick entails engaging with the appropriate professionals, complying with their instructions, and attempting to 'get better'. This again links into the health belief system that we hold and particularly the belief in the advancement of medical technology. However, when this belief is shaken there may be moves towards more complementary or alternative therapies, which is a growing trend in our society. This causes some tensions between mainstream medicine and these alternative therapies. The limitations of mainstream medicine are becoming increasingly acknowledged, particularly following recent scandals in the UK (Bristol, Alder Hey), and medical errors are being increasingly brought before the courts. This has now raised the profile of health risk and assessment that is based on individual relativity and personal choices of lifestyles. Thus, the sociology of health and illness comes full circle.

Medicalization and the medical model

Medicalization is a process by which some aspect of the human condition becomes designated as an illness, disease or disorder (Conrad and Schneider 1992). While many 'conditions' are appropriately placed under the rubric of medicine, others are less clearly truly medical conditions. For example, the use of certain illicit substances, gambling, domestic violence, road rage and alcoholism are now being referred to as somehow 'medical conditions'. Furthermore, some natural life events have become medicalized and fall prey to the all-encroaching medical machine, such as childbirth, menstruation, menopause and dying (McCrea 1983; Reissman 1983; Scambler and Scambler 1993; Figert 1996). Once they are defined as 'medical' they are subject to control, cure or care. This medicalization process is said to have five key components.

- *Identification.* Some aspect of the human condition or human action must be identified as different. This may be a distinction between abnormality and normality (however they are defined) and may be measured along any number of poles, i.e. tall-short, fat-thin, aggressive-passive, noisy-quiet and so on.
- *Classification.* The 'abnormality' must then be classified according to a particular nosological framework. This may be the sub-divisions of the numerous medical manuals reducing the body into organs, structures, cells and genes, or in mental health it may be the DSM-IV (Diagnostic and Statistical Manual) or the ICD-10 (International Classification of Diseases).
- *Diagnosis.* This is often confused with classification but diagnosis has the added dimension of requiring an aetiological explanation. For the 'abnormality' to become a medical condition its origins and genesis require for it to be understood.
- *Treatment.* The 'abnormality' must be seen to be, or accepted to be, susceptible to some form of medical intervention, even if this is merely palliative.
- *Prognosis.* Medicine must be able to supply a prediction as to what the course and outcome of the 'abnormality' is likely to be.

Once the human abnormality has become medicalized it rarely falls out of the clutches of medicine, but history has shown that this is infrequently possible. For example, prior to the 1960s homosexuality was considered a medical condition and subjected to medical interventions. However, it was declassified by the World Health Organization in the 1960s and is now demedicalized and merely considered an aspect of human sexuality.

The (Western) medical model is the dominant view of disease and disorder and has reigned supreme since the development of germ theory. It is based on cause and effect and considered 'scientific'. It has three fundamental assumptions.

- *Reductionism.* It regards all diseases and disorders as having an aetiological agent, which may be a virus, a parasite, a bacterium, a chemical, a gene and so on.
- *Mechanistic.* It views the body as a sort of logically structured machine and medicine as the science by which its workings can be understood. It

does not see the person in a holistic fashion as a functioning unit in a complex social environment.

- *Restoration.* Restoring the body (and its broken parts as in a machine) to a state of health is considered to require medical technology and scientific advances.

The medical model has been criticized by sociologists (as well as others) on four basic grounds. First, it is a belief system based on the use of medical technology and excludes alternative therapies and procedures. Second, it was born out of a fight against acute infectious diseases and is less responsive to chronic conditions. Third, it clearly does not fit many of the issues involved in mental health. Finally, it is reductionist and sees the patient as an organism rather than a person with social and psychological needs. Challenging the medical model is a hugely difficult task due to its dominance, power and scientificity. However, some theoreticians of medicine have attempted to do just this. Brulde (2001) suggested that a goal model was perhaps more appropriate and identified seven plausible goals within a unified theory. These were to promote functioning, to maintain or restore normal structure and function, to promote quality of life, to save and prolong life, to help the patient to cope well with their condition, to improve the external conditions under which people live and to promote the growth and development of children. Brulde (2001) argues that each of these goals needs to be qualified in some way, but taken together they form the basis of a multidimensional medical enterprise rather than a singularized approach as in the medical model. Black (2001: 293) reported on a middle-aged, working-class man's physical and spiritual journey towards death and stated that, 'just as the medical model of illness breaks down the person into symptoms and parts, the relational model of illness and death in narrative "puts him back together again" by embedding him in a personal and social history'.

Other health care professions have also challenged the dominance of the medical model, mainly in relation to its reductionist approach, and argue for a more holistic perspective. For example, occupational therapists have argued for meaningful and relevant occupation-based activities to facilitate health and wellness as an accompaniment, rather than an alternative, to the medical model (Chisholm *et al.* 2000), but mental health professionals have been outright dismissive in their challenge to it (Wedgeworth 1998). Others have made their challenge by focusing on specific 'conditions' such as maternal death (Anonymous 1999c), complications of diabetes (Payne 2000), user involvement (Munro 1999) and HIV (Gallison 1992). Finally, nurses have featured large in confronting the medical model and have offered other approaches in contrast. For example, we note the management model and issues of power (Tilah 1996), the social model of care (Collins 1996), humanistic approaches (Reed and Watson 1994) and Parse's human becoming theory (Bauman 1997). It is important to understand that, despite the dominance of the medical model, critical challenges to it come from many quarters, and also to recognize that those who have a vested interest in maintaining it will vigorously defend it.

Some tensions within the medical model

Noting the above constructs, and criticisms, of the medical model we can see that in sociological terms certain tensions and conflicts are likely to arise in practice. The first concerns sick role behaviour, as outlined above (2:6). Within the medical model the patient is the passive recipient of medical interventions and within the traditional understanding of the sick role the patient is expected to engage appropriate professionals, comply with their instructions and attempt to get better. However, with globalization and the cross-fertilization of numerous cultures there is an increased awareness of differing definitions of health and illness and differing responses to disease processes. For example, tensions in the medical model will occur when patients do not engage in direct health-related behaviours and even prefer to undertake unhealthy activities (Woller *et al.* 1998). In the promotion of health habits there is a tension created when the person makes the decision to self-manage their own health and illness (Osman 1998). Furthermore, once a person becomes ill the patient may not fully partake of the treatment regime and decide to manage part of their disease process themselves (Chapple *et al.* 1998). Bertero (1998) highlighted how leukaemia patients managed their own transition between health and illness *within a medical regime* and undertook this despite the dominance of the medical model.

The second major tension that we note within the medical model of illness concerns the issue of alternative or complimentary therapies. Although it is fair to say that there is an increase in the number of Western medical health care professionals who accept some alternative therapies there remains a considerable degree of dismissal by the majority. The criticisms levelled against alternative therapies, by traditional Western medical believers, usually involve questions of cause and effect, efficacy, science and logic. Note here that these are the very structural beliefs involved in the Western medical model. Alternative or complementary therapies usually involve a mixture of physical and/or psychological approaches, with the two most common non-Western medical belief systems being ayurvedic medicine (traditional healing) and Chinese folk medicine. Ayurvedic medicine involves the theory of equilibrium between physical and psychological aspects of human nature, imbalances of which are addressed through nutritional and herbal approaches. Chinese folk medicine is also based on the conception of harmony and involves the ingestion of herbs and the use of acupuncture (Richman 1987; Giddens 1989a). However, there are now many variations of these that are used in the Western world as alternative or complementary therapies. Furthermore, many of these have been the focus of research. For example, herbal products were studied for both efficacy and access by Harnack *et al.* (2001) and prayer, over-the-counter medications, herbal teas, vitamins and massage were studied for their use in paediatric asthma (Mazur *et al.* 2001). Murata *et al.* (2001) reported on the effects of Dai-kenchu-to, a herbal medicine, on uterine and intestinal motility, and Roberts (2001) suggested that traditional healing, spiritual preachers and psychiatry were a way forward for mental health. Of course, Western 'scientific' medicine likes to produce research to counter, or explain from their own beliefs in knowledge, the claims for alternative or complementary medicine. Ho *et al.* (2001) argued that a potential new anti-tumour agent had been identified in traditional Chinese medicine by analysing the herbs and combining demethylcantharadin with a platinum moiety. This gave the alternative medicine Western 'scientific' credence. Finally, Joshi and Kaul (2001) analysed four of the most widely used herbal products for chemical, pharmacological, clinical and toxicological profiles, again giving a good helping of 'scientific' credibility at the turn of the millennium for the use of these herbs for 3,000 years.

A third tension involves the belief in medical technology and the advancement of science. Medical technological advancement has been inexorable, although much slower at some times in our history than at others. It has leapt forward with great discoveries, such as penicillin, but at other times it wages a slow war over an extended period, such as in the fight against cancer (Underwood 2000). The developments of surgical techniques, particularly keyhole surgery, and an increase in knowledge about pharmacology have led to huge developments – for some. Fibre optics, body imaging and mapping techniques and the use of computer technology have aided the diagnosis and treatment of many conditions. However, some are now questioning the use, and direction, of such medical technology. For example, the human genome project, cloning and embryo research are causing considerable ethical difficulties for some (see Chapter 6) and there is a suggestion that such medical technology is being abused as a form of colonial power (Baber 2001). Furthermore, the speed of technological advancement that we are currently witnessing is said to change our personal identities, expectations and relationships with medicine (Rogers 2000). Finally, it is said to give us false expectations in the search for eternity (Gendron 1999) and in making end-of-life decisions (Nyman and Sprung 2000).

The fourth tension concerns medical errors. The belief in the medical model and the growth in medical technology are accompanied by higher expectations and increasing demands (Scambler and Higgs 1998). Many medical interventions bring side-effects and cause iatoagenesis, and it is often a question of cost–benefit decisions as to whether we accept them or not. However, it is the area of actual error that brings the greatest conflict. The great scandals apart, such as the Bristol children's heart operations, for the individuals involved errors are usually life-changing and in some cases fatal. For example, Hughes and McGuire (2001) reported a case of delayed diagnosis of a woman with disseminated strongyloidiasis who, thankfully, survived, but was critically ill for an extended period. Bhagat *et al.* (2000) described a less fortunate woman with ascites who died because of delayed diagnosis. Human errors in a multidisciplinary intensive care unit over a one-year period were studied by Bracco *et al.* (2001), who classified errors into: (a) technical failure; (b) patients' underlying conditions; and (c) human errors. The human errors were subclassified as caused by poor planning, execution or surveillance. These authors reported that there were 241 (31 per cent) human errors in 161 patients evenly distributed among planning

($n = 75$), execution ($n = 88$), and surveillance ($n = 78$). Nursing errors are also common and usually involve the administration of medication (Cohen 2001), but can involve other procedures such as the giving of injections (Adams 2001) and changing dressings (Karch and Karch 2001).

The final tension to be mentioned here concerns the notion of health risk and assessment. The medical model emphasizes not only diagnosis but also prognosis and, as mentioned above, expectations of, and demands on, medicine have increased. Through increased litigation and compensation following medical errors there is now an increased medical surveillance, and identification, of risk factors. In mental health circles this has been attempted by examining, for example, such aspects as longitudinal predictors of behavioural adjustment in pre-adolescent children (Prior *et al.* 2001) and family and parenting interventions in children and adolescents with conduct disorders (Woolfenden *et al.* 2001). In non-mental health arenas examples include Vundule *et al.* (2001), who attempted to identify risk factors for teenage pregnancy among sexually active black adolescents, and Brunswick *et al.* (2001), who argued that there was a public awareness of the warning signs for cancer caused through the medical research on this disease. The search for predictors of health risks is likely to continue, but caution must be given about the possibility of spurious relationships, as once given medical credence they will affect human lives to one degree or another.

Further reading

Annandale, E. (2002) *Feminist Theory and the Sociology of Health and Illness.* London: Routledge.
Friedson, E. (1970) *Profession of Medicine: A Study of the Sociology of Applied Knowledge.* Chicago: University of Chicago Press.
Illich, I. (1978) *Limits to Medicine.* London: Caldar and Boyars.

2.14 Conclusions

We have seen a complex world with various ways of understanding society and its structures: not only in terms of the wider society at large and the theoretical perspectives that are employed to create knowledge, but also in terms of being a health care professional attempting to work amidst the numerous definitions of health and illness. Sociological theories are extremely useful perspectives in understanding our world and its complexities, and we urge the discerning student to do two things: first, to continue their reading of the sociological literature through either the further readings offered throughout this chapter or their own exploration; second, to apply the theories to their own practice to analyse and understand the social situations in their health care setting. This is important for a number of reasons: First, health and illness are complex states in all societies and it is understood that they also differ across many and varied cultures. Second, the structure of health services, and the delivery of health care, are undertaken according to the values and norms of the society in which they are located. Third, health care professionals are no different from other members of society and can operate from positions of power that can lead to the abuse of others. Finally, it is important because it sees the patient not in isolation, but as part of a community, and we hope that the community of which we are a part cares.

Thinking psychology

3.1 Introduction

There are many definitions of psychology and most are constructed according to the method that each branch of psychology adopts or in relation to the field of study that is undertaken. However, Drever (1964) provides a generalized and comprehensive definition to incorporate aspects of the original and historical meaning of the word. He states that psychology is 'the branch of biological science which studies the phenomena of conscious life, in their origin, development, and manifestations, and employing such methods as are available and applicable to the particular field of study or particular problem with which the individual scientist is engaged' (Drever 1964: 232). We can see from this definition that psychology is the scientific study of the mind, but that this may differ according to the particular science that is preferred, and adopted, by the individual scientist. There are many branches of psychology and these include abnormal psychology, animal psychology, child psychology, genetic psychology, industrial psychology, educational psychology and social psychology, with each branch defining the term from its own specific perspective.

The importance of studying psychology in nursing pivots on two factors relating to the human mind. The first is that the human mind is considered to have an internal working mechanism, as well as internal drives that operate it. Second, it is also considered to be responsive to external forces that affect its operation. Thus, at this interface between the internal and external forces lies each and everyone's individual personality. Nursing (as well as medicine) is much more than the robotic actions of, say, changing a dressing or administering a drug, it is also about the human interaction in undertaking these practices. This is traditionally understood in the concept of the 'bedside manner'. This chapter outlines the general theoretical constructs of psychology and relates them to the nature of nursing in health care settings.

PART ONE: THEORY

3.2 Human development

From the moment of conception we are in a constant state of development towards our ultimate decline, and this is a journey that billions before us have taken and, we hope, billions will take in the future. From this moment of conception external factors (as well as internal genetic ones) will influence our development. For example, whether our mothers smoke or drink alcohol in pregnancy may influence our growth, and whether we are going to be born into, say, a family of child abusers or religious fanatics will also influence how we develop (4:5). So, it is as we grow that external physical factors as well as social ones will have an impact on us as individual human beings, and they will have an influence on the development of our thinking, emotions and relationships.

Human development of cognition, emotion and relationships

Cognition

Thinking, also known as cognition, is very difficult to define, as it includes many processes of the human mind, such as attending to information that is received, representing it in our minds, reasoning about it employing judgements on it and making decisions regarding it. In human developmental terms cognition requires certain building blocks. The first are termed concepts. These are categories of objects, events or activities, or even abstractions of future possibilities, and much of our early teaching of children concerns the categories of colours, numbers, animals, plants and so on (2:7). These concepts grow to become highly complex as we begin to store different levels of information. For example, Rathus (2002) gives us the example of the category of objects that store information, which includes newspapers, school newsletters, textbooks, novels, merchandise catalogues and now floppy disks and DVDs. An important point in the development of cognition concerns how we learn to understand and manipulate the relationships between the items in the categories and also the relationships between them.

The second type of building block is the prototype. In building the categories, or concepts, we use prototypes to match the essential features of the item into the concept. For example, originally we may learn to fit 'dog' and 'elephant' into the category of 'animals on land with four legs', but later this is refined into distinct categories of the dog family and the African or Indian elephant (2:7).

The third building block is the ability to solve problems. The development of thinking in human history has been central to our survival and dominance, and problem-solving has been one of the main keys. Problem-solving is a large and complex area of psychology and involves many features. An example is the ability to understand the problem, which includes: (a) that the elements of our mental representation of the problem relate to one another in a meaningful way; (b) that the elements of our mental representation of the problem correspond to the problem that we are faced with; and (c) that we have a stock of knowledge that we can apply to the problem (2:7). We learn certain strategies to solve problems and these can be summed up in the following way.

- *Algorithms*. These are specific procedures, or formulas, that if chosen appropriately and applied correctly will produce the correct solution. Examples of algorithm approaches include the Pythagorean theorem concerning problems regarding triangles with right angles. Another example is systematic random search algorithms, in which possible solutions are tested in relation to sets of rules, as in solving an anagram by systematically matching each letter with the others to provide all possible words of sense.

- *Heuristics*. These strategies are shortcuts, or rules of thumb, and involve an element of creativity, say, as in solving an anagram by attempting some words beginning with each letter. An example of a heuristic device is the means–end analysis in which we evaluate the current situation in relation to our desired goal.

Emotions

Emotions are said to be states of feeling that have physiological, cognitive and behavioural components (Carlson and Hatfield 1992). Physiologically, strong emotional feelings arouse the autonomic nervous system, and the more intense the feeling the greater is the arousal (LeDoux 1997). Cognitively, interpretation of events can create emotional reactions such as fear or anger. Behaviourally, we can often evoke emotional reactions in response to taking some action, such as sorrow or regret when we have hurt someone. Rinn (1991) suggested that many emotional expressions may be universal – that is, found in all cultures – for example, smiling to show friendliness or approval. It is the facial expression that we learn in childhood that accompanies each particular emotion. Many researchers have shown that facial expressions indicate the same emotions across all cultures (Ekman 1980; Izard 1994). However, it is not only the facial expression that gives an indication of a person's emotional state, as the voice, posture and certain gestures also provide clues (Azar 2000). This is important, because facial expressions can sometimes be faked, or produced without the usual accompanying emotion. There have been many theories of emotion, but three central ones lie at the heart of contemporary psychology.

- *James–Lange theory*. These authors suggest that certain external stimuli will trigger specific arousal patterns. The emotions are a result of our appraisal of our body reactions, e.g. we become angry because we are acting in an aggressive way.
- *Cannon–Bard theory*. This theory argues that an external stimuli can simultaneously trigger bodily responses and the feelings of an emotion, e.g. we experience something that makes us act aggressively and become angry at the same time.
- *Theory of cognitive appraisal*. In this theory external stimuli and our state of arousal are appraised, followed by the interpretation of our arousal in relation to the situation; this then leads to the experience of the emotion.

Relationships

Relationships are central to most people, most of the time. They are crucial in childhood as our survival may depend on them, and in adult life they contribute to our happiness and satisfaction. There are numerous aspects that influence the formation of relationships and these include psychosocial development, attachment theories, styles of parenting, the effects of significant others and the presence or absence of child abuse. We discuss the first three in this section and first briefly outline Erikson's stages of psychosocial development. Erikson (1963) argued that there were eight stages of psychosocial development from infancy through to late adulthood and the first four stages are important to us in this section. The first stage (from birth to 1 year old) is *trust versus mistrust*, in which the child learns to trust the mother and the environment, which produces pleasant feelings in the child. The second stage (from 1 to 3 years) *is autonomy versus shame and guilt*, in which the child learns to make choices and develops self-control in order to make those choices. The third stage (from 4 to 5 years) is *initiative versus guilt*, in which the child begins to plan and be more forceful in their choice making. The fourth stage (from 6 to 12 years) is *industry versus inferiority*, in which they become absorbed in skills, tasks and productivity. Erikson believed that there was a tension between the development towards autonomy (6:2), the feelings of shame regarding this and the formation of relationships with others.

Attachment, according to Ainsworth *et al.* (1978), has one secure and two insecure forms. The secure attachment is where there may be mild protestation at the mother's departure and the child seeks interaction on her return, and is quickly comforted. The first insecure form is avoidant attachment, where the child is not distressed by the mother's absence, plays happily without the mother and ignores her on her return. The second insecure form is ambivalent/resistant attachment, where the child shows severe distress at mother's absence but becomes ambivalent towards her when she returns by clinging to her and then pushing her away. Parenting styles also influence relationship formation. Baumrind (1973) focused on four aspects of parenting in her research: (a) strictness; (b) demands for the child to reach intellectual, emotional and social maturity; (c) communication skills; and (d) warmth and involvement with the child. She outlined three types of parenting styles: authoritative, authoritarian and permissive.

Major theorists: Freud, Piaget, Bowlby

There are now numerous interpretations, and extensions, of the major theories of human development and here we restrict ourselves to the basic principles of the three leading theorists, Freud, Piaget and Bowlby. Freud's theory of psychosexual development was based on a five-stage approach. The first stage, the *oral stage*, runs from birth to approximately 1 year of age. In this period the child derives much pleasure and relief from sucking for food as well as non-nutritional sucking and mouthing of objects. Later in this stage biting and chewing help to relieve the discomfort from erupting teeth and hardening gums. In the second stage, the *anal stage* (1 to 3 years), the main sources of pleasure are the anal cavity and sphincter muscles. As the child is potty trained it encounters the first restrictions on where and when they should have their bowels opened. By producing the contents of their bowels appropriately the child can please the parents, or by withholding them or producing the contents inappropriately the child can show the parents their disobedience. The third stage, between 3 and 5 or 6 years of age, is known as the *phallic stage*. Pleasure and sensitivity is now focused on the genitals, and the child becomes aware of differences between the sexes. In this stage conflicting emotions in relation to same-sex and different-sex parents can arise, which may lead to Oedipus and Electra complexes. The penultimate stage, the *latency period*, continues from 5 or 6 years of age through to puberty. In this period the earlier sexual preoccupations are repressed, allowing the child to learn new skills and develop new knowledge of the world. The final stage is the *genital stage*, which covers the period from puberty to maturity. In this stage the sexual desires now come to the fore. Freud's theory of psychosexual development has both its supporters and its critics.

Jean Piaget's (1963) cognitive-developmental theory also adopts a staged approach to human growth, although Piaget saw the stages not as discontinuous but as gradual and developmental. Piaget's theory has been hugely influential in our understanding of child development. The first stage is the *sensorimotor stage* (from birth to 2 years), which incorporates several other conceptualizations. In *assimilation*, the child incorporates new experiences into their existing, but primitive, schemes of knowledge; for example, a new toy would be placed in the mouth to see where it would fit in the child's sucking scheme of things. *Accommodation* concerns the way in which the child transforms their existing schemes to incorporate these new experiences. In the earlier sensorimotor stage the child is responding instinctively but later in this period they begin to act purposefully. They learn object permanence, which refers to the concept whereby when a child is shown an object, and then it is hidden from view, the child knows that it still exists.

The second stage is the *preoperational stage* (from 2 to 7 years), which is characterized by the use of words and symbols to represent actual objects and relationships between them. In this stage children are egocentric and cannot understand why others cannot see the world the way that they see it. The third stage is the *concrete operational stage* (7 to 11 years), in which children learn to be able to focus on two dimensions of a problem, which is termed *decentration*. They become subjective in their moral judgements, and they develop the awareness of reversibility; that is, that one thing can change into a different shape and back again. Finally, there is the *formal operational stage* (11 years onwards). In this stage the child begins to manipulate ideas or propositions. They can think hypothetically.

Finally, Bowlby (1969, 1973) argued that new-born children were genetically programmed to behave in ways that ensured their survival, and attachment to a female figure was a major part of this. This is achieved through sucking, cuddling, eye contact, smiling and crying that results in being comforted. Bowlby believed that the child is attached to the mother, whereas she is bonded to her baby, and he argued that there was a critical period during which the synchrony between mother and child results in attachment. He believed that mothering, if delayed about two and a half to three years, was ineffective in terms of attachment or bonding. Bowlby felt that there was a strong innate tendency for a child to become attached to an adult female, which he termed *monotropy*. A lack of this led to maternal deprivation.

Further reading

Durkin, K. (1995) *Developmental Social Psychology: From Infancy to Old Age.* Oxford: Blackwell.
Erikson, E. (1963) *Childhood and Society.* New York: W. W. Norton.

3.3 Personality

The concept of personality is both simple and complex. It is complex because psychologists, and others, have long attempted to unravel the nature of this aspect of the human condition, and indeed continue to do so today, but there remains little agreement as to its constituent parts. There are voluminous works on personality, with many theoretical perspectives being multifaceted and complicated, and here we merely subcategorize the main divisions within the overall schemata. It is worth noting that Arthur Reber (1985: 533), writing in *The Dictionary of Psychology*, states that personality 'is a term so resistant to definition and so broad in usage that no coherent simple statement about it can be made – hence the wise author uses it as the title of a chapter and then writes freely about it'. We are happy to take Reber's advice and recommend to the reader that they will simplistically know what personality refers to in common parlance even though they may not be able to define it in a sophisticated manner. Yet, despite this, as we note above, it has been a quest of psychological scientists, as well as others throughout the ages, to attempt to understand it and to identify its constitution. We can fit most theories of personality into one of six broad categories, but it should be remembered that an element of overlap may be evident in some cases.

Categories of personality

Type theories

Personality has long been attributed to physical aspects of the body. The ancient Chinese believed that there are four instinctive elements of a person – happiness, anger, sorrow and fear – and that they are dependent, respectively, on the health of the heart, liver, lungs and kidneys (Carlson and Hatfield 1992). However, we now know that there is no evidence for this. Hippocrates hypothesized four basic temperaments – choleric, sanguine, melancholic and phlegmatic – with the idea being that each individual represents a unique balance between these basic elements. The bodily humours were considered controlling aspects of one's psyche. Kretschmer (1888–1964) attempted to relate body types to a propensity for certain personal attributes, particularly mental disorders. He outlined the *pyknic* (stocky body build) as being prone to manic depression, the *asthenic* (slender body type) as being prone to schizophrenia and the *athletic* (muscular build) as being more prone to sanity than insanity. A much more elegant, but no less unconvincing, typology of body types was that of Sheldon (1898–1970), who outlined three fundamental constitutional types as being related to personality. He suggested three primary components in physique: *endomorphy* (heavy but with poor muscular development), *mesomorphy* (strong, well developed musculature) and *ectomorphy* (thin, with light bones and muscles). He also outlined three component parts of the temperament: *viscerotonia* (loving, easy going, sociable), *somatotonia* (outgoing, vigorous, physical) and *cerebrotonia* (restrained, self-conscious, timid). Sheldon then attempted to establish correlations between these types. As we say, this was an elegant attempt, but a failure in practice.

Trait theories

Many psychologists have focused on trait theory in an attempt to understand personality constructs. A trait refers to an enduring characteristic of a person that can be said to account for regularities and consistencies in their behaviour, and that can be observed. As with personality, we tend to know a person's trait when asked about it, but it is difficult to explain exactly what it is when asked to do so. We usually use adjectives such as 'shy', 'outspoken', 'ebullient' and so on. Understanding personality as a series of traits requires a discussion as to whether these traits are permanent or whether they are changeable. Furthermore, we may ask the question: are the traits unique to each individual or are they general to the whole population, so that it is merely a question of the degree to which each person has a particular trait? The former is called an *idiographic* approach and the latter is termed a *nomothetic* approach.

A major author in this area is Hans Eysenck (1916–97). He began with two personality trait dimensions: introversion–extraversion and stability–instability. He then catalogued various personality traits and located them along these polarizations. For example, an anxious trait would be located high on the introversion and neuroticism dimension; that is, the person would rate high for being preoccupied with their own thoughts and for being emotionally unstable (emotional instability is also known as neuroticism). Many personality traits were identified by Eysenck, such as quiet, unsociable, reserved, touchy, restless. Interestingly, Eysenck noted that his scheme was similar to that outlined by Hippocrates above, i.e. choleric equated with extraverted and unstable, sanguine equated with extraverted and stable, phlegmatic equated with intraverted and stable and melancholic equated with introverted and unstable. Another major author in this area is Raymond Cattell, who identified three sources of data, which he considered were relevant to understanding personality: life (L) data, questionnaire (Q) data and test (T) data. Cattell believed, much more than Eysenck, that behaviour, and therefore traits, fluctuated in relation to situational factors. In short, a leopard could change its spots according to the situation it found itself in.

Psychodynamic and psychoanalytic theories

There are now several theories of psychodynamic or psychoanalytic structures to personality, all of which owe their origins to Sigmund Freud. Although there are subtle differences between these theories they all share common principles. For example, each theory argues that conflict lies at the heart of the personality and this conflict is underpinned by a constant struggle. Although to begin with the conflict is external – that is, the drives of sex, aggression and dominance come into conflict with social rules, laws and moral codes – at some point in child development these regulatory forces, of rules, laws and codes, are internalized and brought within the constructs of the personality. Following this internalization the conflict rages within us and our behaviour, actions and decisions are a result of this inner contest.

The first theorist, and leading figure, in this perspective was Freud. We have noted his influential thinking in a number of key areas (2:5, 2:6, 3:2, 4:4), and his structure of the personality is yet another of his major offerings. Freud's approach was to view the human mind as having certain psychic structures, and although we cannot see these, nor measure them in any direct way, we can see the result of their operations through behaviour, verbalized thoughts and expressed emotions. These psychic structures are known as the:

- *Id*. Primitive, present at birth, representing physical drives and unconscious. It follows the *pleasure principle* and it demands instant gratification of its urges.
- *Ego*. A developmental psychic structure that begins at about 1 year of age. It is based on reasonable action, good sense and appropriate ways of coping with needs and frustrations. It curbs the rampant appetite of the id and conforms to social norms and rules. The ego is guided by the *reality principle*.
- *Superego*. Develops throughout childhood and tends to adopt customs, standards and practices of parents and peers through the process of identification. It acts as a conscience and holds up the ideals of moral actions. It is guided by the *moral principle*. It establishes right and wrong and floods the ego with guilt and shame when it is negative.

Thus, it is easy to see the conflict element in psychodynamic and psychoanalytic theories, and to protect the mind from the ravages of this turmoil we have *defence mechanisms*: denial, repression, sublimation etc.

Two other psychodynamic theorists, who were at one time followers of Freud but later developed slightly differing ways of viewing the psyche, were Carl Jung (1875–1961) and Alfred Adler (1870–1937). Jung was, like Freud, fascinated by unconscious processes of the mind, and believed that not only do we possess an individual, or personal, unconscious but also we have a collective unconscious (2:2). For Jung, the collective unconscious possesses primitive images, which Jung called archetypes, that are representative of our history as a species. Although there may be cross-cultural variations, universal themes run through the collective unconscious: the all-powerful God, the young hero, the nurturing mother, the sage, the jealous brother, the underdog, the prodigal son and so on. These are often seen in fairy stories and legends. Jung believed that they remain unconscious but nevertheless influence our thoughts and emotions. Adler, like Jung, felt that Freud had placed too much emphasis on sexual impulses. For Adler, it was the inferiority complex that motivated people, and he located this in the smallness of children in their developing years. He claimed that this gave rise to a drive for superiority and that it was self-awareness that played a major role in the development of personality.

Behavioural theories

Although strictly speaking there are no direct behavioural theories of personality, it is worth outlining the major thinking in this perspective in relation to the age-old debate regarding nature versus nurture. In behavioural science (behaviour modification) there is little use of conscious or unconscious processes; instead, there is a focus on actual observed responses, and on how the person becomes conditioned to behave in a certain way. A leading proponent of this science was B. F. Skinner, an American psychologist. Skinner used operant conditioning, which is a simple form of learning in which an organism learns to engage in certain behaviours because of the effect (reward) of so doing. A dog fetches a ball because of the reward of attention. The training of behaviours, whether animal or human, is undertaken by the use of reinforcers. Reinforcers can be of several types.

- *Positive reinforcer.* This increases the probability that a behaviour will occur when it is applied. A pay packet serves as a positive reinforcer for working.

- *Negative reinforcer.* This increases the probability that a behaviour will occur when it is removed. Removal of food for misbehaving at the table acts as a negative reinforcer.

- *Immediate versus delayed reinforcer.* Immediate reinforcers are more potent than delayed reinforcers. Eating chips is an immediate reinforcer, dieting is a delayed reinforcer.

- *Primary and secondary reinforcers.* The former are effective because of the biological make-up of the organism, and include water, food and warmth. The latter are valued because we have become conditioned to them, and include money, attention and social approval.

Behaviourist approaches come and go in popularity, but many find the reduction of the human condition to a set of behavioural responses according to certain reinforcers uncomfortable in terms of choice and freewill (6:5).

Social learning theories

As we have just seen, the problem of personality is ever-present when we attempt to separate out the factors that both constitute it and influence it, whatever 'it' may be. In social learning theories personality is treated as those aspects of behaviour that are acquired in a social context. The leading worker in this field is Albert Bandura. Bandura, and others, have attempted to objectify Freud's psychoanalytic theory in terms of classical and operant conditioning theory. In this, the focus is on the idea of imitation; that is, how children imitate adult behaviours in relation to the extent that adults are rewarded or punished for their actions. In one experiment Bandura showed a film of an adult behaving aggressively (hitting and punching) towards a bobo doll to three groups of children. Group A saw the film only, group B saw the film plus the adult being rewarded for his behaviour and group C saw the film and then the adult being punished (chastised) for his behaviour. All the children then played in a room of toys including a bobo doll and a mallet. The results were that while group C showed significantly fewer aggressive acts than either A or B, there was no difference between these latter groups. The conclusion that Bandura drew was that vicarious punishment is more powerful than vicarious reinforcement. Later the children were requested to reproduce the adult's behaviour as best as they could and were rewarded for doing so. All three groups showed the same high levels of imitative aggressive behaviour. The conclusion here is that all three groups had originally learnt the behaviour from the film but had not reproduced it until they were rewarded for doing so.

Phenomenological/humanistic theories

These approaches have their roots in phenomenological and existential philosophies. They are characterized by experiences that are distinctly and uniquely human, i.e. uniqueness, being, freedom and choice. We are all human beings and have first hand experience of this, and thus much of this approach to personality revolves around the self concept. Carl Rogers (1902–87) rejected the deterministic approaches of both psychoanalytic theory and behaviourism, and saw human behaviour as a response to our individual perception, and interpretation, of external stimuli. Rogers focuses on the self, which he views as an organized, consistent set of perceptions and beliefs about oneself. We understand what we are and we evaluate experiences in relation to maintaining a consistency between our self-image and our actions. However, discrepancies can, and do, occur between our self-image and our actual behaviour, which leads to what Rogers termed incongruence. This incongruence can be threatening and painful to us and *defence mechanisms* may block our awareness and subsequent ability to grow and change. Rogers believed that much of what we have learnt in childhood is based on conditional positive regard and leads to problems in later life. The antidote, for the therapist, is to view the client with unconditional positive regard.

Very briefly, we will mention the work of George Kelly (1905–66), who offered us the *personal construct theory*. According to Kelly we are all scientists putting our own theories and interpretations on the world, and from these we produce hypotheses (predictions). Kelly suggested that we all see the world through our own, irremovable, 'goggles' and we cannot match it to others' views to see if it is 'real', but only match it in relation to others' interpretations. Although we cannot remove these 'goggles' we are constantly engaged in testing, checking, modifying and revising our view of the world. Hence, this is a phenomenological perspective (2:7).

In conclusion, personality can be seen in two 'lights', first, as an internal entity with a causal role, which represents a legitimate theoretical construct with some explanatory power of our behaviour; or, second, as a secondary factor, inferred from human actions, which are a result of external influences and have little explanatory power. In short, personality is a question of internal nature versus external nurture.

Further reading

Carver, C. S. and Scheier, M. F. (1992) *Perspectives on Personality*, 2nd edn. Boston: Allyn and Bacon.

Pawlik, K. and Rosenzweig, M. R. (2000) *The International Handbook of Psychology*. London: Sage.

3.4 Intelligence, thought, language

Intelligence can be defined as the relating activity of the mind in which the individual is aware of the relevance of his of her behaviour to an objective, has the capacity to meet novel situations by new adaptive responses and has the ability to perform tasks involving the grasping of relationships between concepts. Thought can be defined as all of the mental activity associated with concept formation, problem-solving, intellectual functioning, creativity, complex learning, memory etc. Language can be defined as the medium through which we code our feelings, thoughts, ideas and experiences (Reber 1985). Thus, there appears to be a close relationship between the three concepts, and some have suggested that one cannot exist without the others (Watson 1913). However, in attempting to define these three concepts we are struck, once again, that at a simple level we all 'know' what the terms mean to us but the moment we attempt to deconstruct them into any number of parts, or structures, they disappear into the chimera of semantics.

Relationship between intelligence, thought and language

Let us look a little more closely at this relationship between intelligence, thought and language. Intelligence is not a 'thing' that exists, it is not a noun, it is a process, a verb. Intelligence must have multifactorial aspects to it and some of these aspects must be contextual in nature. Moreover, some people will have distinctive skills in one area, while others may be more competent in other areas. This was noted by Gardner (1985) in his model of multiple intelligences. Gardner claimed that intelligence is not a single thing but has seven entirely different categories, with each having a distinct biological source in the brain. The seven categories are:

- *Linguistic intelligence*, which refers to the intelligence we use when we are reading, writing or understanding speech.
- *Musical intelligence*, which refers to the intelligence we use when we appreciate, compose or perform music.
- *Mathematical–logical intelligence*, being the intelligence that we use in arithmetic, numerical calculations and logical reasoning.
- *Spatial intelligence*, concerning the arrangement of objects spatially, visual art and the ability to find one's way around.
- *Bodily–kinaesthetic intelligence*, which we use in sport, dancing, everyday movement and the dexterity of fine movement.
- *Intrapersonal intelligence*, which refers to understanding and predicting one's own behaviour, and identifying aspects of the self and one's own personality in relation to others.

We can see that intelligence may relate to many aspects of human behaviour and although Gardner outlined these seven categories there is nothing to suggest in real life that they are quite so distinct; they may overlap and interrelate considerably with each other.

We noted above that thought (thinking) (3:2) was another word for cognition and there have been many theories that have linked thought to intelligence. The fact that we think is indisputable, but we need to ask ourselves certain questions regarding this. For example, how do we do it? What are the processes by which it functions? What do we use in order to think? Finally, the link to language is said to have four possibilities. The first is that thought is dependent on, or caused by, language. A number of disciplines, such as psychology, sociology, linguistics and anthropology, have proponents of this view. Second, language is dependent on, and reflects, thought. For example, Piaget considered that language reflects the individual's level of cognitive development. Third, thought and language are initially quite separate activities but join as one entity at a later stage. Fourth, language and thought are one and the same. This last theory is considered extreme and is associated with early behaviourism.

Intelligence

As intelligence can mean different things to different people, we can now begin to categorize these ideas into a schema. Sternberg (1985) proposed the triarchic theory of intelligence, in which there are three distinct aspects that work together to form what we know as intelligence. The first aspect, or subtheory, is termed contextual intelligence, which refers to intelligence within a socio-cultural setting. This refers to purposive behaviour that helps the individual to select, shape or adapt to events in their world. Thus, the young Western person entering the stock exchange alone for the first time may be just as intelligent as the young African person entering the bush in the Kalahari Desert for the first time. The second subtheory concerns experiential intelligence, which refers to how past experiences can influence how someone tackles a current problem or situation. This involves two processes: first, the ability to deal with the current situation, the novel task and the demands; second, the ability to automate the processing of information to create a smaller cognitive demand for the individual. This will, of course, depend on the extent to which the person has previous experiences of new and novel problems to overcome, and this has a resonance with the 'stock of knowledge' in phenomenology (2:7). The third subtheory is that of componential intelligence, which refers to the cognitive mechanisms by which we achieve intelligent behaviour. This final subtheory has, in turn, three elements: meta-components, being higher order processes of planning, decision-making etc; performance components, which are mental processes for actually carrying out the task; and knowledge-acquisition components, being the mental processes involved in learning new information (Sternberg 1977).

There are many theories of intelligence, in fact too many for us to mention all; but we discuss two here, Spearman's two factor theory and Thurstone's primary mental abilities. Spearman (1927) employed factor analysis, which is a statistical technique, in which he took large samples of children's scores on certain tests to ascertain whether they correlated to other tests. From this he concluded that intellectual activity involves two factors, a general (*g*) factor and a specific (*s*) factor. Spearman claimed that differences between people are largely attributable to differences in their *g*. The *g* refers to neogenesis, which is the ability to identify the relations in logical assumptions; for example, 'hand is to glove as foot is to . . .?' Spearman suggested that this *g* factor accounted for the finding that if people perform well on these tests they usually perform well on the other types.

Thurstone (1935), in his research, found that not all mental tests correlate equally and suggested that they form seven distinct factors or groups. He referred to these as primary mental abilities (PMA).

- *Spatial* (S): the ability to recognize spatial relationships.
- *Perceptual speed* (P): the ability to detect visual detail quickly and accurately.
- *Numerical reasoning* (N): the ability to perform arithmetical operations quickly and accurately.
- *Verbal meaning* (V): the ability to understand the meaning of words and verbal concepts.
- *Word fluency* (W): the ability to recognize single and isolated words quickly.
- *Memory* (M): the ability to recall a list of words, numbers or other material accurately.
- *Inductive reasoning* (I): the ability to generate a rule or relationships that describe a set of observations.

As we note above, there are many theories of intelligence, and many tests employed in an attempt to measure it. The discerning student may wish to read up on some of the theories and tests outlined in Box 3.1. Measures of intelligence quotient should be taken with caution, as many psychologists assert that the tests measure many things, but not intelligence.

Box 3.1 Theories of intelligence and tests

Some theories of intelligence	Some intelligence tests
Vernon's (1950) hierarchical model	Stanford–Binet test
Guilford's (1967) structural model	Wechsler Scales
Horn and Cattell (1967) fluid and crystallized intelligence	Army Alpha and Beta tests
	British Ability Scale (BAS)

Thought and language

Once you have read this sentence sit back a moment and think about think-ing, and ask yourself whether when you think you are thinking in a lan-guage. Watson (1913) rejected the notion of mind and claimed that thought was silent speech, or put another way, thought is talking to oneself very quietly. Watson's theory, known as *peripheralism*, sees thinking as occurring peripherally in the larynx, rather than centrally in the brain. This extreme view was supported by the fact that movements do occur in the larynx when thought is taking place, but this merely suggests that these movements accompany thought and does not necessarily indicate that they *are* thought. This theory was later discounted by Smith *et al.* (1947), who had himself injected with curare, a drug that paralyses all skeletal muscles, while being assisted to breathe artificially, and once the drug had worn off he reported on his thought processes. However, despite Watson's radical views we are left, today, with many questions regarding the relationship between thought and language.

There have been a number of major theorists working in this field and we will briefly mention four perspectives. Bruner (1983) argued that language was essential if we, as humans, were to develop beyond learn-ing through mere actions or images. Bruner suggested that there were three modes, or forms, of knowledge – enactive, iconic and symbolic – which develop in that order. The enactive mode of knowledge is con-cerned with learning through actions, and many basic aspects of life, such as bicycle riding, tying knots and driving a car, appear to be represented in our muscles, so to speak, once we have learnt the operation. These actions are difficult to describe in language. The iconic mode of knowledge is concerned with how we build up representations, as mental images, of our experiences. These images usually comprise past encounters with similar experiences and resonate with phenomenology (2:7). The symbolic mode refers to the development when language becomes an influence on thought and the person can move from the immediate context to the symbolic.

Vygotsky (1934) believed that we do not learn to think in a social vacuum but that the development of inner speech, or verbal thought, is the result of a fundamental social process. For Vygotsky cognitive development involves an internalization of problem-solving processes that occurs as the child interacts with others. Vygotsky's theory is a culturally based approach to thinking and he argued that the child is not merely the passive recipient of knowledge but part and parcel of their own intellectualization. Another perspective is the Sapir–Whorf linguistic relativity hypothesis (LRH). In this view language determines *how* we think about our world and even *what* we think. If our language does not possess a certain idea or concept then that does not exist for those of that community. For example, Inuit have many more words for snow conditions than we do in Western society and each word relates to a particular concept or idea of the type of snow it is. We, in our world, according to Sapir and Whorf, cannot think about those concepts (snow conditions) until we have the language to link into them (Sapir 1929; Whorf 1956).

Finally, more recent approaches talk of information-processing (IP) perspectives rather than a single distinct theory. Information-processing theorists believe that there are psychological structures of the human mind, which can explain behaviour, and are independent of social relationships, cultural practices and environmental influences (Meadows 1995). Information-processing theorists employ the computer analogy and suggest that the child becomes better and more efficient at thinking, rather than undergoing a reorganization of major mental structures (Bee 2000). They use task analysis to study such approaches and claim that children develop better strategies for remembering, organizing and encoding more aspects of a particular problem.

In conclusion, we note different theories of intelligence, thought and language and, again, some believe that there are inherent structures within the mind that exist independently of external forces, while others believe that the internal mechanisms are influenced by social and cultural processes. Whichever view dominates will tend to have an impact on our society, particularly in relation to the education of our children.

Further reading

Carroll, J. B. (1956) *Language, Thought and Reality: Selected Writings of Benjamin Lee Whorf*. Cambridge, MA: MIT Press.
Sternberg, R. J. and Grigorenko, E. (1997) *Intelligence, Heredity and Environment*. New York: Cambridge University Press.

3.5 Communication

Broadly speaking communication is the transmission of something – which can be a message, a signal, a meaning, a sign etc. – from one location to another. In these broad terms effective communication must involve the transmission and the receiver, both of which must share a common code in order that the meaning, or information contained within the message, can be understood without fault. This general, and basic, understanding of communication has been extremely helpful in various fields of psychology, such as language development, interpersonal skills, memory processing, information theory, certain physiological functions and coding/decoding operations. The importance of communication in health care settings is obvious. Good communication can lead to effective health care delivery and improved patient care, whereas bad communication can lead to catastrophic scenarios. Communication between wards, departments and units, and between disciplines, groups and individuals, are clearly of central importance. Communication can take place via a number of media in health care: verbally, in writing, by telephone, by e-mail etc. However, there are more subtle forms by which we communicate, including the use of body posture, proxemics, dress, emblems and adornments, to name but a few.

Verbal communication

The evolution of language in the human species is clearly a significant step forward in developmental terms. Although we know that animals communicate with one another, it is our ability as humans to manipulate meanings in many ways, through verbal speech, that gives us an advantage over the rest of the animal kingdom. There are numerous theories of how human speech developed and we will briefly outline two. The first is the operant conditioning theory of the behaviourist Skinner. Skinner (1957) argued that although a baby's cooing and babbling is probably inborn it is the fact that certain forms of sounds come to represent items and situations, and are selectively reinforced, that distinguishes primitive sounds from developed speech, in any given community. Skinner believed that imitation plays a significant role and he termed this *echoic responses.* As the child attempts to imitate the adult's sounds the mother and father reinforce the child by excited and happy responses. Language is then further reinforced by the connection of certain verbal labels to items, which meets with parental approval.

The second theory is that of Chomsky (1957, 1965, 1968). Chomsky believed that although language cannot develop without some element of environmental prompting, this alone could never fully explain the development of human language. Chomsky suggested that children are born already programmed to formulate and understand many forms of sentences despite the fact that they have never heard them before. This he called a *language acquisition device* (LAD), and central to this theory are *phrase-structured rules*. These rules specify what utterances are acceptable, or not, in any given language. Chomsky argued that a baby born of English parents who was taken to China and adopted by Chinese parents would learn to speak Chinese just as easily as a Chinese baby. This, it was proposed, could only take place if everyone was born with the LAD.

Another way of looking at language is to see its development in relation to what language is used for. Bruner (1983) suggested that language involves not only the rules of grammar but also knowledge of how to realize our intentions through it by its appropriate use. Language, for Bruner, meant a social discourse as well as a verbal one. We learn a language through interacting with our parents and we come to understand what language means through this process. Thus, we learn the grammatical rules as well as the meaning and the intent. Bruner called this the *language acquisition support system* (LASS) model. Within this perspective there is debate as to the extent to which the mother is seen as being the prime influence, or the baby is seen as the more active partner (Gauker 1990).

Non-verbal communication

Non-verbal communication refers to any aspect of communication that does not use the spoken language. We all employ both verbal and non-verbal communication when we are interacting with others, and the situation will usually dictate which one dominates. For example, in a noisy environment we will tend to gesticulate with our hands, arms and facial expressions to get our message across. In fact, non-verbal behaviour and verbal communication are not usually employed separately, but tend to be used complementarily to each other. However, we must take care, as non-verbal communication may also enhance, replace or contradict verbal messages. We make judgements about each other all the time based on non-verbal communication, and frequently we are wrong regarding those judgements. Despite this, we do continue to make judgements regarding non-verbal behaviour and 'we usually base our decisions about meaning on what we would *expect* the behaviour to mean, given the particular cultural and situational context in which it occurred' (Kagan *et al.* 1986: 45).

Although non-verbal behaviour can be meaningful, unfortunately much of it can also be based on habit. Non-verbal habitual behaviour will be interpreted by others and meaning will be ascribed to it, despite the fact that we may not mean anything by it ourselves. Furthermore, non-verbal habitual behaviour is difficult to change, as it has usually been built up over a long period of time. Of course, non-verbal behaviour is also useful in encounter regulation, in which it helps to govern the rules of social interaction. For example, it helps to govern when we want someone to speak or to remain quiet while we are speaking. It also assists in the conveyance of dominance or subordination and can make someone feel at ease or feel uncomfortable. Non-verbal communicative strategies are numerous, and Box 3.2 highlights a few.

Persuasive communication

Communication is important when one is attempting to persuade someone to do something, or not to do something, as the case may be. This is just as important in everyday life as it is in health care settings where nurses, and others, are often called upon to persuade someone to take a course of action concerning an illness, a wound or a course of treatment. The best way of undertaking an effective persuasive appeal is to plan it thoroughly. An effective persuasive appeal has several component parts, which should be thought through carefully. The first concerns the *source* of the persuasive appeal. The source refers to the authority for the message, and this will affect how readily it is absorbed and heeded. So, if a junior nurse suggests that a particular treatment should be undertaken this will have less impact than the same message from a consultant physician. Therefore, the authority carries some weight but this is dependent upon the credibility, the trustworthiness and the popularity of the persuader. Hence, top sports personalities and pop stars advertise products in an attempt to persuade us to buy them. The

Box 3.2 Some non-verbal behaviours

Facial expressions	Physical gestures	Proximity/ touch	Eyes	Body posture	Vocal	Artefacts
Eyebrows	Hands	Social space	Eye contact/ avoidance	Position of limbs/head	Tone	Dress
Forehead	Arms	Pointing (jabbing finger)	Staring	Body position	Pitch	Hair
Eye area	Head	Self touching (twiddling with hair/ring etc.)	Gaze duration	Walking speed	Clarity	Cosmetics
Mouth area	Body	Etc.	Etc.	Regular movements	Volume	Bags
Lips	Foot tapping			Etc.	Amount	Jewellery
Cheeks	Vocal sounds				Sighs	Spectacles
Eyeballs	Facial				Mouth sounds	Badges
Tongue	Etc.				Hesitations	Uniforms
Etc.					Speed	Type of car
					Silence	Hairstyle
					Laughs	Etc.
					Etc.	

second element to an effective persuasive appeal is *the nature of the communication*, and this involves both the message itself and the medium by which it is expressed. The message may be emotional, fear producing, humorous, entertaining, informative and so on. It may recommend a course of action (immunization) or a course of inaction (drink driving). The essence of the message may come at the beginning, middle or end of a total persuasive appeal. The message may arrive via a leaflet, letter, video, song, play, story, picture etc. The important point to note in deciding on the nature of the communication is to understand those it is aimed at. Thus, the third element is *the nature of the audience*. The audience should be carefully considered, as they react differently in different situations. For example, individuals react differently to groups, so a group audience may require a different persuasive appeal. People with low self-esteem are more susceptible to persuasion than people with high self-esteem. Those who have undergone previous attempts at being persuaded on a particular issue may be 'inoculated' against the message to some degree. So, in short, undertaking a persuasive appeal involves taking 'account of who says what to whom via what medium and with what effect' (Kagan *et al.* 1986: 183). This brings us to the final element of a persuasive appeal, and that is *the situation or context* in which the appeal is being delivered. For example, the persuasion may be more or less successful depending on whether the situation is formal or informal, and whether it is a real life context or a 'laboratory' setting (Laswell 1948).

Privileged communication

This simply refers to any communication that is not open for public inspection. In health care settings this is important because of medical confidentiality (6:9). It may refer to what is written in medical notes or what is verbally said between the doctor (and others) and the patient. There is no need to dwell further on this at this point other than to advise the reader to take great care regarding the notion of confidentiality.

In conclusion communication is central to the effective delivery of health care and it is wise to think carefully about the elements that go to make up both an effective communication and an effective persuasive appeal.

Further reading

Ajen, I. (1988) *Attitudes, Personality and Behaviour*. Milton Keynes: Open University Press.

Zimbardo, P. G. and Leippe, M. R. (1991) *The Psychology of Attitude Change and Social Influence*. New York: McGraw-Hill.

3.6 Learning and memory

Learning is a very difficult concept to define, as most of us see it as an end-product; that is, something that has *been* learnt, in the past tense. However, in psychology the main focus is usually on the present tense and the study of *how* the learning takes place. Simply stated, we can say that learning is the process of acquiring knowledge or the actual possession of such knowledge (Reber 1985). Alternatively, a more complex definition might be that learning is 'a relatively permanent change in response potentiality which occurs as a result of reinforced practice' (Reber 1985: 395). Whereas the former definition indicates the two elements of process and content, the latter establishes the four constructs of (a) relative permanence, (b) response potentiality, (c) reinforcement and (d) practice, all of which are central to our understanding of learning, and discussed below. Learning is inextricably linked to memory, which can, for our purposes, be defined in three ways. Memory can refer to the mental capacity to hold information about ideas, images, events, situations, stimuli etc.; or it may refer to the hypothetical 'storage system' that is believed to be in the brain that contains such information; or it may refer to the actual information itself that is being stored. In any event, both learning and memory should be perceived as hypothetical constructs that cannot be observed directly but only inferred from observations (Gross 2001).

Learning

Behaviourist approaches

Behaviourist approaches dominated learning theory in the first half of the past century and we can identify a traditional distinction between classical conditioning and operant conditioning.

CLASSICAL CONDITIONING

Classical conditioning is associated with Ivan Pavlov (1927), who was studying the digestion of dogs at the turn of the past century. He observed that the dogs would start to salivate *before* the food arrived, either at the sight of the bucket containing the food or at the sound of the approaching laboratory assistants who fed them. Pavlov observed that 'a stimulus (such as a bell), which wouldn't normally produce a particular response (such as salivation), eventually comes to do so by being paired with another stimulus (such as food) which *does* normally produce the response' (Gross 2001: 146, emphasis in the original). The main characteristics of this type of conditioning are:

1   Before the conditioning takes place the food causes salivation, so the food is termed the *unconditional stimulus* (UCS) and the salivation is called the *unconditioned response* (UCR).

2   During conditioning the sound of a bell is paired with the food, the

sound is called a *conditioned stimulus* (CS) and it produces salivation (UCR) only because it has been paired with the food (UCS).

3 Once conditioning has taken place the dog will salivate at the sound of the bell alone and *before* the food has been given, and the salivation is now called a *conditioned response* (CR).

Classical conditioning developed into a complex theory and went some way in explaining how such things as phobias might develop as a conditioned stimulus. However, although the principles generally hold true when conditioning animals, very young children and people with severe learning difficulties, when dealing with older children and adults, differences in responses occur.

OPERANT CONDITIONING

Operant conditioning is a type of conditioning in which behaviours are not as much elicited by a stimulus as reinforced by it. Skinner was interested in how animals operate in their environments and how this operant behaviour was reinforced, and would determine the probability of it being repeated. He used a puzzle box, which became known as a Skinner box, to analyse the behaviour of animals, which were set certain tasks (for example, pressing a lever). If the animal touched or pressed the lever, even randomly to begin with, Skinner delivered a reward (food pellet) or a punishment (mild electric shock) depending upon what behaviours he wanted to reinforce in the animal. If he wanted to *strengthen* the behaviour associated with pressing the lever he would deliver a *positive reinforcer* (food pellet) and if he wanted to *weaken* the behaviour associated with the lever and encourage the animal to avoid touching it he delivered a *negative reinforcer* (electric shock). This developed into Skinner's ABC of operant conditioning (see Box 3.3).

Reinforcers and reinforcement is a complex area, particularly in relation to the notions of rewards and punishments. We can only decide, Skinner suggested, whether something is a reward or a punishment *after* it has been made contingent on a specific behaviour and consistently over a number of occasions. For example, food may be a reward for someone who is hungry but also may be perceived as a punishment for someone with anorexia. There are *primary reinforcers* such as food, water and sex, as they are in themselves natural reinforcers, and *secondary reinforcers* such as money,

---

Box 3.3 Skinner's ABC of operant conditioning

A Antecedents – understanding the stimulus, i.e. the lever, the bell, the assistant's footsteps.

B Behaviour – these refer to the operations of the animal/human, i.e. pressing the lever.

C Consequences – this is the result of the behaviour, i.e. reward or punishment.

praise and tokens, which have to be learnt first through classical conditioning.

Cognitive approaches

Cognitive approaches to learning suggest that there are higher order processes being undertaken as well as the mere stimulus and response of
behavioural operations. Tolman (1948) produced a theory of *place learning*,
or *sign learning*, in which rats in a maze showed expectations as to which
part of the maze was followed by the next part. Tolman referred to these
expectations as *cognitive maps*. These are characteristics of a type of spatial
relationships that we learn, say of a road map of the way to go to work.
Cognitive maps can only be inferred but seem to have some credibility given
that most of us learn to traverse our houses, streets, areas etc. *Insight learning* is a cognitive approach that originates from the Gestalt school of psychology and stands diametrically opposed to the behaviourist school. Insight
learning is considered to be a type of *perceptual restructuring* of the components of a particular problem, and when a particular element is supplied
all the components are seen in relation to each other and thus the whole is
seen in a more meaningful way.

   In the usual developmental way, Harlow (1949) later argued that the
behaviourist stimulus–response approach to learning, and the theory of
insight learning, were just two elements of the same continuum. Harlow
argued that we learn to learn and that the *learning set* was a process between
stimulus–response and insight learning. The greater number of sets we have,
the greater is our ability to adapt to new challenges. This, it was suggested,
was a trial and error approach. Finally, Koestler (1970) believed that it was a
person's, or animal's, *ripeness* to solve a problem that was the central issue.
By this, Koestler meant that the ability to learn, make a discovery or solve a
problem was based on relevant knowledge, skills and previous experience.
He believed that traditional experiments with animals were undertaken
ill-advisedly, as they were set tasks to which they were biologically ill-fitted.

Memory

It would be a strange life indeed, and possibly an unacceptable one, without
memory. We would merely be reflex organisms responding to life events,
while being trapped in the ever-passing moment. Memory, like learning,
remains a hypothetical construct, which appears to have three aspects to it,
but with interrelationships between them. The first aspect is *registration* or
encoding, and this refers to the way in which we enter information into our
memory. The sensory data, such as sound and vision, is transformed into a
type that allows us to place it in our memory. This encoding is analogous to
a computer requiring data to be formatted in the correct style before it can
be placed on the hard drive. The second aspect concerns *storage* of information. While a computer stores data by means of changes in the electrical
circuitry, the changes in the brain that allow information to be stored are

unclear. Whatever the mechanisms that are involved we have the capacity for holding, or retaining, information in our memory. The third aspect refers to *retrieval*. This means the process by which we recall information from the unconscious into our conscious thoughts. These processes also remain unclear, but again we tend to have the ability to extract or recover information that perhaps we had not thought about for many years.

We have to be clear that these aspects are interrelated, as when someone states that they cannot remember something it may be that it was not registered in the first instance (a problem of availability) or that we cannot retrieve it (a problem of accessibility). Furthermore, in the multi-store model (Atkinson and Shiffrin 1968, 1971) there is a distinction made between short-term memory (STM) and long-term memory (LTM). However, strictly speaking these refer to experimental procedures for investigating STM and LTM *storage*. The STM is analysed in relation to: (a) *capacity*, which refers to how much information can be stored; (b) *duration*, which concerns the length of time we can hold information in storage; and (c) *coding*, referring to how sensory information is represented by the memory. The LTM is believed to have an unlimited capacity for storage and there are numerous models produced to represent ways of structuring the information that is stored there, too numerous to mention here.

Forgetting

We are all aware that the main problem with memory is forgetting. To understand why we forget we must focus on the distinction we drew above between availability and accessibility of stored information. We assume that STM information passes into LTM for permanent storage. Therefore, availability is mainly concerned with the transformation from STM to LTM, and the functioning of the STM itself, while accessibility is mainly concerned with LTM. Thus, forgetting can occur at the encoding, storage or retrieval stages of memory functioning. Two theories will be briefly mentioned. The first is the *decay theory*. In decay theory it is suggested that metabolic processes occur over time, which cause the structural changes assumed to occur during learning to break down. This results in the memory becoming unavailable. When learning is taking place it is thought that neurochemical and neuroanatomical changes occur to form what is known as an *engram*, and unless this engram is reinforced by repetition it is very delicate and easily disrupted by the passage of time (Hebb 1949). The second theory is called the *displacement theory*. As the STM is a limited capacity system and can only hold a relatively short number of items in it at any one time, when the system is 'full' the newest material is retained and the oldest material is 'pushed out' (displaced).

In conclusion, learning and memory are inextricably linked and one cannot, generally, operate without the other. Problems can equally occur with the process of learning as with the functioning of the memory. In the course of your professional careers you will probably meet many people who will have problems in one or both of these areas.

Further reading

Anderson, J. R. (1995) *Learning and Memory: An Integrated Approach*. New York: John Wiley and Sons.

Baddeley, A. (1999) *Essential of Human Memory*. Hove: Psychology Press.

Walker, S. (1984) *Learning Theory and Behaviour Modification*. London: Methuen.

3.7 Sensation and perception

It is often thought that sensation and perception are one and the same. However, in psychology there is a clear distinction drawn between them, although they are interlinked. Sensations are what we experience as a result of stimulation from the external world. We have sensory receptors in our eyes, ears, skin and throughout our entire body that pick up the sensations from the world around us. Perception, on the other hand, refers to our internal organization and interpretation of the sensations that we feel, which forms inner representations of, and provides meaning to, the external world. The interplay between sensation and perception gives us the ability to navigate, and make sense of our world, and our place in it – that is, when they are working correctly!

Basic constructs

Gestalt psychologists (3:6) argue that a pattern, or whole, is greater than the sum of the individual parts. For example, four equal lines joined together may form a square, but above and beyond this it has a 'squareness', which is a qualitative coherent perceptual experience. *Form perception* requires us to establish the figure and ground; that is, an object and its surroundings. We are probably all familiar with the picture of the vase, which, when figure and ground are interchanged, becomes two silhouetted faces facing each other. The principle of camouflage is based on ensuring that we cannot distinguish between figure and ground. *Depth perception* is vital to the animal kingdom, as it allows hunters and prey to gauge the distance between each other. Our retinas pick up two-dimensional images and organize for us three-dimensional perceptions, which gives us a prediction of distance. We, as human beings, like most predators have our eyes on the front of our heads, and this influences the way we perceive the world. There are four non-pictorial primary cues that influence this: (a) retinal disparity (difference between two images); (b) stereopsis (the combining of the two images); (c) accommodation (focusing on an object); and (d) convergence (process whereby the eyes point inwards the closer an object gets). There are also pictorial secondary cues that influence our perception of the world, and these refer to the visual field itself rather than our eyes. At greater distances depth is appreciated by pictorial cues such as relative size, relative brightness, superimposition, linear perspective, aerial perspective, height in the horizontal plane, light and shadow, texture gradient and motion parallax.

Once we perceive something for depth we must be able to maintain our perception of it irrespective of whether it changes shape, size, location, brightness and colour. This is called *perceptual constancy*. Obviously this is a survival mechanism for visual animals.

- *Shape*. The angle at which we view an object does not actually alter its shape.
- *Size*. We need to know that when someone, or something, moves away from us they are not actually getting smaller, and vice versa.
- *Location*. Moving our heads around does not portray a spinning world.
- *Brightness*. We see objects as having more or less constant brightness in relation to each other irrespective of the amount of illumination.
- *Colour*. Familiar objects will retain their colour under different lighting conditions.

Our perceptions of the world are usually quite accurate but there are occasions when all is not what it seems and in these cases we may refer to them as *illusions*. When our perception of a real physical object does not marry up to its true physical properties we have experienced an illusion. One of the best known illusions is the appearance of a bent stick when placed in water, which is actually straight when taken out. According to Gregory (1983) there are four types of perceptual illusion:

- *Distortions (geometric illusions)*. In these cases lines appear longer or shorter, or converge or separate in relation to other lines that perceptually distort the picture.
- *Ambiguous (reversible) figures*. In these cases two figures tend to interchange, as in the vase–faces, young woman–old woman, pictures.
- *Paradoxical figures (impossible objects)*. These tend to look normal at first but on closer inspection they are impossible; for example, Escher's falling water flowing back up hill only to fall again.
- *Fictions*. In these cases there appear shapes without the presence of physical contours.

The five senses

There are commonly known to be five senses: sight (visual), hearing (auditory), taste (gustatory), smell (olfactory) and touch. However, within these five areas there are a number of interrelated senses, which we mention below. Before we do, take note of the measures of absolute thresholds for the five senses as indicated by Rathus (2002: 79).

- For vision, the equivalent of a candle flame viewed from a distance of approximately 30 miles on a clear dark night.
- For hearing, the equivalent of the ticking of a watch from about 20 feet away in a quiet room.

- For taste, the equivalent of about one teaspoon of sugar dissolved in two gallons of water.
- For smell, the equivalent of about one drop of perfume diffused throughout a small house (one part in 500 million).
- For touch, the equivalent of the pressure of the wing of a fly falling on a cheek from a distance of about 0.4 inch.

Although there are clearly individual differences in these thresholds, some of these averages are quite remarkable. We do not wish to outline the anatomy and physiology of the senses, as these are more than adequately covered in numerous textbooks. Instead we will give a brief outline of the relationship between the external sensory information, which leads to the internal process of perception.

Vision

Light is one part of a spectrum of electromagnetic energy. This light passes through the transparent cornea of the eye and the amount is controlled by the muscles of the iris opening or closing the pupil. Once past the iris the light encounters the lens, which accommodates to the image by changing its thickness. This projects a clear image on to the retina, which consists of cells called photoreceptors that are sensitive to light. There are two types of photoreceptors called rods and cones. The rods are sensitive only to light intensity and let us see things in black and white, while the cones transmit sensations of colour. The rods and cones are stimulated by the light, and nerve impulses take the message to the brain for interpretation.

Hearing

Sound is caused by changes in air pressure as a result of vibrations, and needs a medium such as air or water to pass through. A vibration is a cycle of compression and expansion, with a single cycle being one wave of sound. The human ear is sensitive to sound waves of frequencies between 20 and 20,000 cycles per second. The ear captures the sound waves, vibrates and transmits them through the work of the eardrum, via the three small bones of the middle ear, and on to the fluid filled cochlea of the inner ear. Here the vibrations are passed to the organ of corti, which has thousands of receptor cells that transmit the neural impulse to the brain via the auditory nerve.

Taste

There are four primary taste senses: sweet, sour, salty and bitter. Flavour depends on odour, texture, taste and temperature. Taste cells are receptor neurons located on the taste buds, of which there are approximately 10,000, and these specialize for sensitivity to certain chemicals. These stimulate nerve cells, which then transmit the impulses to the brain.

Smell

Smell is the sense that senses odours. Odours are detected by receptor neurons in the olfactory membrane in each nostril. Gaseous molecules of the substance we smell trigger the receptor neurons, which transmit information to the brain via the olfactory nerve.

Touch

The skin senses include not only touch, but also pressure, warmth, cold and pain. These senses rely on different receptors that lie on or beneath the skin and hair follicles. The receptors transmit signals to the brain for interpretation.

Three other types of senses are worth mentioning here in relation to how we perceive them in the brain. The first is *kinesthesis*, which is the sense that keeps us informed of the movement of the body and the position of the limbs. Sensory cells in the joints, tendons and muscles feed information to the brain and we are able to perceive where our limbs are, and the movement of them, even with our eyes closed. The second is the *vestibular* sense, which tells us when we are upright. Sensory cells in the semicircular canals, as well as other places in the ears, inform the brain of body motion and position in relation to gravity. Finally, *phantom limb pain* is worthy of mention. In phantom limb, pain is felt in the amputated part. It is real pain and not simply imagined. It may be due to nerve endings in the stump, but may be reflex activation of other neural circuits that have 'memories' of the amputated limb.

Organization, recognition and selective attention

As we have noted above, senses and perception are not the same thing. Once we have received the information our brains must analyse and interpret the data. The organization of visual perception is the area of research that has received most attention and the Gestalt psychologists were most interested in this. They identified three basic processes by which we organize information into meaningful units.

- The principle of similarity. If we have a number of stimuli that are similar we will tend to group these together.
- The principle of proximity. Stimuli that appear close to each other will tend to be perceived as a group.
- The principle of closure. We tend to search for complete shapes and mentally 'fill' in any gaps if the association to the shape is suggested.

Recognition is important even at a very early stage in life, as it is basic to survival. Recognition is also important to establish who are friends and who are strangers, and to assist us in navigating social interactions. However, the process by which we do this is controversial. Some research suggests that when we are observing a known face we tend to focus on internal structures such as mouth, eyes and nose. However, when we are looking at strangers we will tend to focus on their outline and hair (Banyard and Hayes 1994). A possible explanation has been put forward for this, which suggests that we have face recognition units for those who are familiar to us based on our experience of them. Thus, we are relying on a mental description of what we know of people.

Selective attention refers to the fact that we can be in a crowded room, chatting away, and suddenly become aware that someone has mentioned our name (known as the cocktail party phenomenon). Early explanations for this suggested that we adopt basic filtering strategies by attending only to information with particular characteristics. Later explanations, however, suggested that filtering out did not occur, but instead the signal is attenuated. Information that is meaningful is strengthened, and information that is not is weakened. Therefore, our name, which is highly meaningful to us, is strengthened and it reaches our conscious attention.

Further reading

Groome, D. (1999) *Cognitive Psychology: Processes and Disorders*. London: Psychology Press.

3.8 Attitudes and group behaviour

Attitudes are an intensely well researched area in psychology and we associate them here with group behaviour because belonging to a group usually means adopting at least some of the beliefs of that group. Attitudes have been defined in many ways but probably the most appropriate for our purposes are the following two. 'The term attitude should be used to refer to a general, enduring positive or negative feeling about some person, object, or issue' (Petty and Cacioppo 1981: 4). 'An attitude is an evaluative disposition towards some object. It's an evaluation of something or someone along a continuum of like-to-dislike or favourable-to-unfavourable' (Zimbardo and Leippe 1991: 8). The interesting thing here is that both definitions employ a binary polarization from positive to negative, and this clearly leads us into the area of prejudice and group behaviour, which we discuss below.

Attitudes

It is fair to say that we are not born with attitudes, but that they come along later in life and, therefore, we must learn our attitudes to politics, religions, people and many other areas of our lives. Some believe that we are conditioned into our attitudes by parents and teachers who reinforce, either positively or negatively, children who express similar views to their own.

Certainly, in experimental conditions, it has been shown that attitudes can be influenced by associating the target of the attitude with either positive or negative words (Lohr and Staats 1973). For example, if a national group is associated with words such as clever, kind or happy then attitudes are positively reinforced towards that group, and vice versa for negative words. Another approach to understanding how attitudes are formed, in a less mechanical way than conditioning, is what is termed *cognitive appraisal*. According to Wood (2000) the main reason why attitudes are formed is that people are motivated to make sense of the world, to form understanding, to help to make predictions and to have some control over events. Attitudes can be formed or changed based on the evaluation of new information that is received. This, of course, is the fundamental basis of advertising, or at least the hope that it is, in which new information changes our attitude to a product, which we then purchase.

Attitudes are often held in high esteem and sometimes two attitudes that a person holds may be in conflict with each other, and a state of *cognitive dissonance* occurs. This is a negative psychological state, creating discomfort and tension, and provides an impetus for resolution, or at least reduction in the tension. Leon Festinger (1957) argued that people are driven to create realistic mental maps of the world and when two attitudes are at odds with each other, or when there is a discrepancy between an attitude and a behaviour, there is a drive to reduce the discrepancy. One example will be noted. Festinger *et al.* (1956) described a cult group in the United States who believed that a flood would destroy the northern hemisphere on a particular day. They sold all their possessions and climbed a high hill on the night before the prophesized flood to pray to be spared. When the flood did not occur they managed their cognitive dissonance by claiming that their prayers had been heeded and that they had been spared and saved the northern hemisphere from the flood.

We now need to address the relationship between attitudes and behaviour. Rosenberg and Hovland (1960) argued that attitudes were predispositions of response to some class of stimuli. They suggested that these responses could be grouped into: (a) affective, what a person believes about the object of the attitude; (b) cognitive, what a person believes about the object; and (c) behavioural, how a person actually responds to the attitude object. This is called the three-component model, and in this format there is an assumption that the behavioural aspect of the response is highly correlated to the affective and cognitive aspects, but this is not always the case. People can behave differently from their expressed attitude. Attitudes, perhaps, ought to predict behaviour; for example, a positive attitude towards a particular political party would suggest that the person would vote for them in an election. When this does not occur we would question their attitude (Gross 2001). Of course, the compatibility between attitudes and behaviour is not that simple, as Ajzen and Fishbein (1977) point out. Behaviour involves four specific elements: a specific action, performed with respect to a given target, in a given context and at a given point in time. Modern approaches, however, do not focus on a single instance of behaviour (voting) as indicating an attitude, and instead sample many instances of related behaviours (attending meetings, joining the party etc.).

Group behaviour

We all like to think that we are individuals, and indeed we are. However, we all belong to a number of groups at one level or another, and belonging to a group requires the fulfilment of certain conditions. For example, there may be some form of acceptance or initiation rite (4:3, 4:9), there may be a need to pass through the 'stranger' role as an outsider until one is accepted or there may be a need to express certain views that the group adheres to in order to be accepted. *Social influence* is a powerful medium, which can exert huge pressures to conform to certain practices. For example, few of us would be comfortable at a funeral dressed in party clothes or attending a wedding in shorts and T-shirt, unless it conformed to everyone else's dress, and this is due to the social pressures to dress in a certain way while being a part of that group, albeit temporarily. *Conformity* lies at the heart of this social group dynamic, and conformity is just as responsible for many historically positive group behaviours as it is for negative group reactions, e.g. the Holocaust and Bosnian rape camps. Let us look at conformity in a little more detail.

Obedience to authority is demanded in many institutions and organizations around the world. Outside of the traditional services such as the armed forces and the police, there is an ever-increasing demand that workers conform to a set of employer regulations. But what do we do when we feel that the pressure to conform is so great that we will transgress a moral code to do so? Milgram (1974) showed how ordinary everyday human beings would deliver an electric shock, which could severely injure or even kill someone, in an experimental situation. Of course, in Milgram's experiment no real electricity was applied but the subjects did not know that. The subject delivered what they thought was an electric shock when the trainee (an assistant to Milgram) failed to complete a set task. The subjects delivered more and more electricity. Another study on conformity was Asch's (1952) research, in which seven stooges were employed with one true subject. The experiment is ostensibly on visual discrimination. All eight were seated in a row with the subject seated seventh. The experimenter had two cards at the front and asked everyone which two lines on the cards were the same length (the true answer was number two). The first stooge said three, the second said three, the third said three and so on up to number seven, the real subject. In Asch's study the social pressure to conform was such that the real subject also said three, although he later reported that he thought the true answer was two.

Groups have certain processes that are important to our understanding of human behaviour, as they override individual preferences. In many walks of life groups are used to make decisions, such as in committees or juries, and this is based on the belief that group decision-making is more accurate. Stasser (1999) outlined a number of social 'rules', or schemes, that govern group decision-making.

- *The majority-wins scheme*. In this scheme it appears that the group arrives at the decision that was supported by the majority. This usually applies where there is no conclusively correct decision.

- *The truth-wins scheme*. In this scheme the more information that is received and discussed, the more the group recognizes that one decision is objectively correct.

- *The two-thirds majority scheme*. In this scheme a majority of two-thirds tends to be sufficient to make a decision, e.g. juries.

- *The first-shift scheme*. In this scheme the group tends to make the decision based on the first shift in the argument, as one person 'shifts' their decision.

Another group process worthy of a mention here is the concept of *groupthink* (Janis 1982). In this situation group members tend to be more influenced by such group processes as cohesiveness, overall objectives and a dynamic leader than by the realities of the situation (Esser 1998). This is particularly so when the group is under threat and stress levels are raised, and in these conditions the group tends not to consider all the options but relies on the dynamism of the group leader. Another group process is the concept of *deindividuation*, which is closely associated with 'mob' behaviour. When we act as individuals we are responsible for our actions, fear negative consequences and tend to restrict ourselves to appropriate social behaviours. However, in deindividuation, as in a 'mob', there is reduced self-awareness, a low concern for social evaluation, a belief in anonymity, a diffusion of responsibility, a heightened state of arousal and an awareness of the mob's group norms and beliefs rather than one's own values (Baron and Byrne 2000).

Finally, mention can be made of prejudice as a relation between attitude and behaviour. Prejudice is an extreme attitude, but has the basic components of all attitudes: cognitive, affective and behavioural. Prejudice can be defined as 'a learned attitude towards a target object that typically involves negative affect, dislike or fear, a set of negative beliefs that support the attitude and behavioural intention to avoid, or to control or dominate, those in that target group' (Zimbardo and Leippe 1991: 84). Although this definition, as is the case with most definitions of prejudice, locates it within the individual, some prefer to see prejudice as a case of inter-group conflict (Vivian and Brown 1995). A number of theories have been put forward to account for prejudice, the most well known being the *authoritarian personality* (Adorno *et al.* 1950). The authoritarian personality is typically hostile to people considered to be of an inferior status, contemptuous of weakness but servile to those of a higher status. They tend to be rigid in their thinking, inflexible and intolerant and unwilling to introspect feelings, and prefer to uphold conventional values. As Gross (2001: 369) puts it, 'this belief in convention and intolerance of ambiguity combine to make minorities "them" and the authoritarian's membership group "us"; "they" are by definition "bad" and "we" are by definition "good" '.

Further reading

Brown, R. (1995) *Prejudice: It's Social Psychology*. Oxford: Blackwell.
Turner, J. C. (1991) *Social Influence*. Milton Keynes: Open University Press.

3.9 Social interaction

As we have seen, human beings are, in effect, social animals and most of us enjoy being with others, at least for some of the time. We need others to socialize with and to form relationships of friendship, courtship and partnership. Again, there are 'rules' to forming these relationships, which we learn throughout our childhood and adolescence, and there are also 'rules' governing how we should operate in social situations, as mentioned above. The effectiveness of social interaction is based on our interpersonal skills, and these in turn are learnt as we grow. Interpersonal skills 'refer to those interpersonal aspects of communication and social skills that people (need to) use in direct person-to-person contact' (Kagan *et al.* 1986: 1). As nursing is primarily a social action, interpersonal skills are of paramount importance, and we all tend to 'know' when we meet someone with poor interpersonal skills, although it may be difficult to define.

Self-awareness

This is central to our interpersonal skills and will influence how we plan our part in any social interaction. We need to have self-awareness, particularly in relation to our past experiences, in order to know how to respond to others. Self-awareness will affect what we notice of others' behaviour and how we will interpret it. Self-awareness is said to comprise the following.

- *Personal identity*: questioning who we are.
- *Internal events*: such as thoughts, values, attitudes, beliefs, emotions.
- *External events*: such as our social environment, membership of clubs, general behaviours.
- *Agency*: our sense of self as an 'agent', the extent of control we believe we have over things that happen to us.

Self-awareness involves a mature approach to creating a sense of a relatively objective but open and accepting appraisal of one's true personal nature. Clearly, this is difficult for some to achieve but only through this can we respond to interpreting and helping others in a mutually interactive way. Whether we are attempting to form a helping relationship with others as part of our professional duty, or forming a relationship of one description or another in our private lives, self-awareness is a fundamental building block.

Psychologists talk about *affiliation* as the basic human need for the company of others. Indeed, the need to affiliate with, and be accepted by, others is one of Maslow's basic survival needs (Maslow 1968, 1970). Furthermore, affiliation is a major motivation for establishing conformity. When we want to affiliate with others we must be able to assess our values, beliefs and norms in relation to others, especially in ambiguous unstructured situations (Gross 2001). Duck (1988) suggested that we are more likely to seek the company of others in different situations; for example, when we are anxious, have recently left a close relationship ('rebound' phenomena) or moved house or job. For Duck (1988) the underpinning motivation for affiliation is anxiety. Furthermore, Schachter (1959) had earlier shown, albeit in an ethically dubious study by today's standard, that anxious people prefer the company of other anxious people. His results would suggest that *social comparison* is the main motivation for affiliation rather than anxiety.

Relationship formation

Psychologists have made a distinction between liking and loving. This may not be surprising given the fact that we can do this reasonably comfortably for ourselves. However, what psychologists have done is to delineate the component aspects that differentiate between them. Rubin (1973) suggested that whereas liking is a case of positively evaluating another person, loving is qualitatively different and has three aspects.

- *Attachment*: the desire for the physical presence of the other and the need for emotional support.

- *Caring*: including the important aspects of concern for the other and a responsibility for them.

- *Intimacy*: the need to feel close and confidential with the other, a desire to communicate with them, and to share personal thoughts and emotions.

There are cultural differences in how relationships are formed and maintained and wide variations are noted. While in Western cultures the emphasis is on romanticism and dyadic (two-person) relationships, in most non-Western cultures the emphasis is on family ties and responsibilities within the relationship (Segall *et al.* 1990). A further cultural difference was noted by Moghaddam *et al.* (1993), who argued that Western cultures tend to be individualistic, voluntary and temporary, while non-Western cultures tend to be collectivist, involuntary and permanent.

A number of theories have been put forward to account for the development of relationships and we will mention two here. The first is the *filter model*, in which it is suggested that our choice of friends, the social network that we belong to and our type of employment will restrict the likelihood of meeting certain individuals in the first instance. Kerckhoff and Davis (1962) argued that it is the similarity of sociological variables that was most influential in providing the opportunities for meeting individuals. In short, we are most likely to meet others who are in our own ethnic, racial, religious, educational and social class group. The second filter to occur involves agreement on basic values. When values coincide between individuals the relationship is more likely to last than when they conflict. The final filter is the complementarity of emotional needs. Long-term relationships are said to be more reliant on this need than on the similarity of values (Kerckhoff 1974). The second theory is termed the *stimulus–value–role theory* (Murstein 1976, 1987). According to Murstein, intimate relationships proceed through stages. The first is based on a stimulus stage in which the emphasis is upon physical attributes. The relationship then moves through a value stage in which the emphasis is upon the similarity of values and beliefs. Finally, there is the role stage, which is based on establishing the successful performance of anticipated roles.

Territoriality, personal space and altruism

The concept of territoriality in humans derives from early studies of animal behaviour, from which it was wrongly deduced that human action, such as aggression or putting up fences as boundaries, was a sign of inherent territoriality. Later it was proffered that human beings have three types of territoriality. The first, and most important, are primary territories such as homes or offices, in which the occupants feel some degree of ownership and permanence. Unwelcome entry into these territories is a serious matter. Secondary territories are such spaces as classrooms or football grounds, where the occupants feel a qualified sharing with a number of other occupants. Third are public territories such as the beach, where defending a space is difficult and occupants see themselves as just one of many possible users (Altman 1975).

Another closely related concept concerns *proxemics*, or personal space, which refers to how closely we interact with other people in physical terms. This personal space is highly complex and there are cultural and individual differences that can lead to confusion and misunderstanding. Personal space is sometimes imagined as a series of 'bubbles' around the person, which governs the social interaction depending on who the other person is and whether we want them in our particular space or not. Hall (1963) suggested four zones of proximity: (a) intimate distance, for kissing, cuddling and comforting, and in some sports celebrations; (b) personal distance, for social contacts with friends and colleagues; (c) social distance, for impersonal contacts such as meetings; and (d) public distance, for formal contact between person and public, such as at conferences. Each 'space' can be defended to different degrees.

Finally, there is altruism, which is an act that benefits someone, but not the person performing it. Altruism is difficult to pin down psychologically and a number of ideas have been suggested to account for its existence. Piliavin *et al.* (1981) suggested the *arousal–cost–reward model* of helping, in which helping is determined by (a) the level of the person's arousal, such as distress at the victim's plight, and (b) the cost–reward assessment of the consequences of helping or not helping. Another theory is the *social impact theory*, which suggests that the greater the number of potential helpers present, the less pressure there is on a single individual to help. Third, there is a theoretical orientation based on sociobiology. This position argues that altruism is a type of kin selection in which one helps related others to survive in order to perpetuate their genes. Yet this does not adequately explain non-related altruistic behaviour. Finally, some have suggested that altruism is a form of social 'glue', which binds a society together. One voluntarily helps another because in turn one may need help oneself in the future. This is the basis on which blood is donated. Whatever the nature of altruism, it seems apposite to conclude this theoretical section on psychology with the problem of understanding the helping relationship, as it forms the cornerstone of health care delivery.

Further reading

Brehm, S. S. (1992) *Intimate Relationships*, 2nd edn. New York: McGraw-Hill.
Duck, S. (1999) *Relating to Others*, 2nd edn. Buckingham: Open University Press.

3.10 Health psychology and stress and coping

As the science of psychology progresses and the knowledge base expands there is an impetus for some psychologists to specialize in specific areas of human behaviour. Health psychology is one such specialized area, and most psychology textbooks tend to deal with the issues of stress and coping within the concept of health. Health psychology has been defined as 'a sub-discipline of psychology which addresses the relationship between psychological processes and behaviour on the one hand and health and illness on the other hand' (Maes and van Elderen 1998: 8). These authors go on to state that health psychologists are more concerned with 'normal' human behaviour and 'normal' psychological functioning in relation to health than with psychopathology or abnormal behaviour. Definitions of stress tend to fall into three categories: as a stimulus, as a response or as an interaction between a person and the environment (Goetsch and Fuller 1995). Gross (2001) sums up the concept of stress in terms of the difference between three models: 'the engineering model is mainly concerned with the question "what causes stress?", and the physiological model with the question "what are the effects of stress?" The transactional model is concerned with both these questions, plus "how do we cope with stress?" '.

Health psychology

Health psychologists are principally concerned with why people engage, or do not engage, in health behaviour. Numerous models have been produced by health psychologists in an attempt to explain this relationship between thoughts about health and actual behaviour related to it. Most health belief models fall into the category of *expectancy-value* (Stroebe 2000), and assume that decisions about alternative choices of action are based on two types of thinking. The first concerns subjective probabilities, which assume that a particular behaviour will lead to a set of anticipated outcomes, and the second refers to an evaluation of behavioural outcomes. The basic premise is that people will choose behaviour, or a course of action, from a range of options, that is likely to produce the most positive outcomes, while avoiding negative ones (Gross 2001). However, the early work on health belief models was initiated because psychologists wanted to know why people did not take up screening tests and disease prevention strategies. This continues to be a problem today, as does non-compliance with medication, which is a similar scenario. There is an assumption that a person evaluates the extent to which they consider themselves to be susceptible to a particular disease or illness and makes an assessment of the consequences of that disease. These evaluations amount to a measure of the perceived threat that people consider themselves to be under.

Health belief models are only one way of understanding healthy behaviour and health psychologists have drawn on the work of social psychologists who have attempted to predict human behaviour through the theory of reasoned action (TRA). This theory is based on the assumption that human behaviour is a function of human intention to act in a certain way. The behavioural intention is determined by two main factors: first, their attitude in relation to the behaviour based on their beliefs about outcomes; an assessment of expected outcomes; second, the person's subjective norms. Another way of understanding healthy behaviour uses a modification of the TRA, which is known as the theory of planned behaviour (TPB). This draws on the concept of self-efficacy, which refers to the idea that we can have some control over certain events that have an effect on our lives. This is crucial for health psychologists, as, for example, if someone thinks that they cannot lose weight then they are unlikely to try.

Stress and coping

What is stressful to one person may not be stressful to another; therefore, stress is a subjective interpretation of a particular event. It is well recognized that too much stress can cause ill-health, yet it is difficult to outline the relationship between a particular stressor and an outcome of ill-health because of this subjectivity. For example, in a study on nurses working night shifts Hawkins and Armstrong-Esther (1978) found that performance was significantly impaired on the first night but this gradually improved throughout the week. They also found that there were significant differences between individual nurses, with some showing little stress to working nights, while others reported constant disruption to their body system and personal lives. This study was undertaken because of the long established view that shift work is stressful, with reported associated problems including digestive problems, insomnia, depression, tiredness and irritability. Other disruptions that are reported to cause stress are changes in the circadian rhythm, jet lag, life changes, the problems of everyday life and occupational factors.

The effects of stress cause the body to defend itself, and this has been termed the general adaptation syndrome (GAS) (Selye 1956), which comprises three stages: (a) the alarm reaction stage, (b) the resistance stage and (c) the exhaustion stage. In the alarm reaction stage there is an initial phase of shock, followed by a counter-shock period in which the body fights back. There is a series of chemical changes involving adrenaline and noradrenaline and the autonomic nervous system. In the resistance stage, unless the stressor is removed, there are further complex chemical changes, which lead to the final stage of exhaustion. In coping with stress there are a series of moderator and mediator variables. The moderator variables include personality, ethnic background and gender, which affect how we deal with the stress in order to affect the health outcome. The mediator variables, such as appraisal and evaluation, intervene to assist with this relationship between stress and health outcome. Coping with stress has been studied by Cohen and Lazarus (1979), who identified five main categories.

- *Direct action response*: the person directly responds to the stress by manipulating their relationship to the stressor.
- *Information-seeking*: the person gathers information about the situation that they find themselves in and make predictions about the future.
- *Inhibition of action*: the person does nothing.
- *Intrapsychic or palliative coping*: the person reappraises the situation and employs mental defence mechanisms or alters the 'internal environment' with drugs, alcohol etc.
- *Use of others*: the person turns to others for help and support.

Further reading

Bartlett, D. (1998) *Perspectives and Processes*. Buckingham: Open University Press.
Crossley, M. C. (2000) *Rethinking Health Psychology*. Buckingham: Open University Press.
Lee, C. and Owens, R. G. (2002) *The Psychology of Men's Health*. Buckingham: Open University Press.

PART TWO: APPLICATION TO PRACTICE

3.11 Attitudes to nurses and nursing, and attitudes of nurses

We saw above that an attitude is an evaluative disposition towards something or someone (3:8) that can have an impact on the way that we behave towards that person or object. Furthermore, when these attitudes are held by large groups of people they are even more entrenched and difficult to change than when held by individuals alone. Nurses and nursing are no different from other professional services and service personnel, in that just as others hold views about our profession we, as nurses, hold specific attitudes to other professional groups, as well as to patients (as members of the public).

Attitudes to nurses and nursing

Attitudes to nurses can be viewed as either positive or negative. Positive attitudes refers to those that enhance the quality and dignity of the nurse and the profession, while negative attitudes denigrate and belittle them both. However, within this basic division of positive and negative, it can be argued that even the positive attitudes towards the nurse, and towards nursing, may have negative connotations. We may view positive attitudes as those that represent the nurse and nursing as highly skilled, which involves a caring and nurturing attitude towards others. However, as we all know, nurses are often referred to as 'angels' or 'martyrs' who have a dedication to a cause, and this dedication is viewed as sufficient reward for undertaking the task. The term vocation is often used as a requirement for the profession (Downe 2000), and martyrdom is said to be part of our nursing heritage (Shaddox 1999). Although many nurses appear to be reasonably comfortable about the application of these labels to them, and may even feel a sense of reward from their attachment, they may be applied as a substitute social reward in the place of other forms of remuneration. Positive attitudes towards nurses and nursing ought to be viewed with a cautionary note. Positive attitudes towards the nursing profession have undergone a subtle shift with the expansion of private facilities. Public attitudes differ towards nurses when they move from the NHS (Payne 2000), and can differ again when they move from hospital care to private nursing home care (Ghusn *et al.* 1998). However, although this shift from positive to negative attitude occurs towards the overall nursing profession it does not seem to occur towards individual nurses in the private facilities (Ghusn *et al.* 1998).

To some degree negative attitudes to nurses and nursing are more easily dealt with, as they are more explicit – at least for all but those who adhere to them. The first point to note is the fact that some individual nurses have been involved in negative behaviour, which justifiably warrants the evoking of negative attitudes in others. In the extreme, there are a few nurses who have been involved in the murder of patients, and clearly this is accompanied by negative attitudes towards them. Furthermore, some nurses have been found guilty of abuse and mistreatment of patients, as evidenced in a number of public inquiries. However, negative attitudes towards nurses, and nursing, can occur in the absence of any behaviour that warrants them. Female nurses are often viewed as sexual objects, and this is noted in numerous pornographic materials, which depict females scantily dressed in nurses' uniform in provocative poses. Male nurses are frequently sexualized as gay. In terms of the psychological impact that this may have, we are reminded of the process of deindividuation mentioned above (3:8). Nurses may become the focus of lewd commentary and antagonistic sexual behaviour while on duty, particularly when those concerned are intoxicated. Although this type of reaction can occur when the person is alone, it is more common when individuals are acting as in a 'mob' (Baron and Byrne 2000). The negative aspect of being viewed as an 'angel' or a sexual object involves the devaluing of the skill of the profession. This means that nurses may be viewed as 'cheap' and treated accordingly.

Nurses' attitudes to . . .

In terms of the psychology of health care, nurses too have both positive and negative attitudes to a wide array of issues. As professionals we are expected to bracket out and shelve our own personal views regarding many personal and professional matters. However successful we are at undertaking this in our everyday working practice, research has shown that nurses can, and do, hold both negative and positive attitudes, as do other health care professionals. Moreover, as we have already noted that attitudes can impact on behaviour, then we must assume that these attitudes may also have an effect on the delivery of health care services. This was supported by a study of nursing attitudes to automated medication dispensing systems (AMDS). This study concluded not that the attitudes were positive or negative but merely that the 'attitude of nursing staff towards AMDS can be an important factor in influencing whether or not the technology will be successfully implemented' (Novek *et al.* 2000: 1).

There are many aspects of health care that nurses have positive attitudes towards, which influences both how the message is delivered and its impact on uptake. For example, breastfeeding is generally viewed as positive by nurses, with one study reporting a nearly unanimous verdict that 'breast is best' (Hellings and Howe 2000). However, as in many cases, attitudes change with the amount of knowledge one receives regarding an issue and also with the amount of experience in the job. This finds some resonance in a study by Register *et al.* (2000), who reported that when nurses held incorrect information regarding breastfeeding they also tended to have negative attitudes towards it. Another major issue in which nurses' attitudes carry an influence is with patients with HIV and AIDS. Although nurses, overall, held attitudes to people with these conditions that ranged from neutral to positive, this varied according to personal circumstances. As Suominen *et al.* (2000: 184) note, 'nurses who knew people with AIDS showed a more positive attitude than those who did not'. Thus, personal knowledge and experience of nursing AIDS patients were said to account for a more positive attitude. Even within the area of nursing education it was noted that managers had a positive attitude towards theory-based nursing if they had sufficient knowledge to inform their decision (Beynon and Laschinger 1993). Positive nursing attitudes have also had an influence on how issues such as homelessness (Kee *et al.* 1999), patient advocacy (Mallik 1998) and substance abuse (Eliason and Gerken 1999) are viewed.

Not surprisingly, nurses, as well as other health care workers, hold a range of negative attitudes concerning many aspects of health care, although they tend to keep their own council on these views and only reveal them through the privacy and confidentiality of the research process. For example, medical students were reported to have significant homophobic attitudes to male homosexuality, and this was exacerbated for those with strong religious beliefs (Parker and Bhugra 2000). Furthermore, this was linked into greater fear of treating HIV/AIDS patients – thus emphasizing again the link between attitudes and behaviour. Physicians' knowledge of and attitudes to the use of analgesic pain relief for cancer were studied by Ger *et al.* (2000). These authors found that physicians displayed significantly inadequate knowledge and negative attitudes towards optimal use of analgesics. Again, we see the linkage between the theoretical constructs of attitude development, as mentioned above (3:8), and the practical ramifications of health care delivery. In terms of nurses, and other health care staff, Biley (1995) reported that negative attitudes towards physically disabled patients, especially those attending the wards in wheelchairs, was very apparent, and Mashazi and Roos (2000) observed negative attitudes of nurses towards a community-based midwifery obstetric unit. Finally, McIntosh *et al.* (1999), studying the attitudes towards patients with dementia, reported that nurses had negative attitudes towards them, but that GPs were even more negative. There are many more examples that can be given but these suffice to illuminate here the relationship between attitudes, knowledge and behaviour in practical health care settings.

Further reading

Jolley, M. and Brykczynska, G. (1993) *Nursing: Its Hidden Agendas*. London: Edward Arnold.
Kenworthy, N., Snowley, G. and Gilling, C. (2002) *Common Foundation Studies in Nursing*. Edinburgh: Churchill Livingstone.

▌3.12 Nature and nursing knowledge

In psychology, and other disciplines such as philosophy and sociology, there is a healthy debate, often called a controversy, regarding nature versus nurture. This is sometimes referred to as the heredity–environment controversy. By this, psychologists are referring to the relative contribution of a person's experience (nurture, environment, learning) and what they inherit (nature, genetic material, heredity) to the overall make-up of the person. There are some who would argue that we are born with psychological mechanisms and structures that have the major influence on what we are, and there are those who would argue that we learn through experience, which creates us as personalities. However, most thinkers today tend to see the influence and importance of both views. The importance of this perspective for us here concerns the relationship between nature and nursing knowledge. Here, nature refers to the processes of health and illness as seen in the conditions of sickness and disease, and nursing knowledge concerns the nurturing process underscored by a theoretical framework. In short, it is about the theory and practice of nursing – not as separate entities, which are adequately covered in numerous textbooks, but as a relationship between the two, and, more specifically, how this middle ground is constructed.

Disorder, disease, illness

Living in the world informs us that certain events occur to us that may be considered natural, although undesirable. We know that accidents happen and the human body may be injured, we know that illnesses are acquired and the integrity of the person is threatened and we know that as we progress through our lives tissues become diseased, organs become disordered and degeneracy and decay of our body are inevitable. This richness of life is part and parcel of nature. However, natural accidents, natural bacteria and viruses, and natural degeneracy are one thing, but when we begin to question whether these triggers of disorder are truly natural or whether some form of responsibility for them can be identified, then we question how natural they really are. If 'accidents' occur because of poor industrialized working conditions in a capitalist society, or radiation poisoning occurs through working with nuclear reactors, or brain damage becomes rampant through the use of mobile phones, then to what degree can these be seen as natural life events? To emphasize the point, what if the bacterial infection is the result of supermarkets incorrectly storing foodstuffs or the virus infection is the result of biological warfare? Are these deemed natural? Clearly they are not. One might argue that to the sufferer of any of these unnatural ailments it is merely an academic point and the immediacy of the suffering is what matters most. However, this misses, in our view, a fundamental aspect of sickness, which is rooted in the age-old question: 'why me?' Locating a rationale for a sickness is a fundamental psychological mechanism that helps us to adjust to what may be a negative life event. Yet this adjustment is dependent upon to whom the responsibility can be attributed. For some, if it is God, an act of God, nature's way or fate then it is more readily accepted. However, if it is deemed the fault of a government policy, a county council, a corporate organization or even another individual then full acceptance is less likely. This leads us into the realms of how disease, disorder, illness etc. is *constructed*.

Socially constructed disease

As we note above, the body, and mind, of humans (not to mention animals) can be injured, diseased or disordered due to what might be viewed as natural processes. However, once we begin to attach a particular rationale for such a condition (God, sin, justice, fate) then we create a set of images that surround and penetrate the illness state, in a social sense. Social constructionism and social representation theory refer to the ways in which we come to understand our social world through the images and symbols that we share in our cultural group. According to Potter (1996), we use these images and symbols as a type of map that allows us to become familiar with, and to 'understand', difficult and new social experiences. From this we are able to provide assessments of the situation, which helps us conclude whether they are, in our view, good or bad. We saw in the previous section (3:10) how attitudes can influence behaviour towards patients, and those attitudes are formed from, and rely on, images created in our minds. From a social constructionist perspective we have long known that those with a mental illness may be perceived as associated with personal sin and demonic possession (Gray 2001). Obese people may be attributed with factors such as laziness, gluttony and lack of will power (Packman and Kirk 2000) and people with HIV/AIDS may be viewed as homosexual, sexually promiscuous and deserving of the condition (Williams and Semanchuk 2000). Finally, Susan Sontag (1983) clearly showed the social constructionist nature of cancer, which has the imagery of the 'crab', creeping sideways, stealthily stalking its victim and then powerfully grasping them in its claws. Even today we tend to avoid using the word, or at least delaying its use for as long as possible, because of the impact that the word brings to the individual and their social sphere.

Feminist psychology

Much of what we have written so far in this section concerns what some may call 'natural' conditions, coupled to the socially constructed images that are created around them. Feminist psychologists have long been concerned with attempting to identify the illusory images of these generally accepted social realities, as they specifically relate to women. Through this they hope to challenge the male-dominated medical positivist assumption that its science is value-free and unbiased. They argue that it is not, in fact, and they are at pains to point out that it is clearly biased towards the pathologization of women (Nicolson 1995). This pathologization of women, and women's bodies, has occurred over centuries, with such things as childbirth, menstruation and female infertility becoming increasingly the domain of predominantly male doctors. The majority of gynaecologists and obstetricians are men. The fact that cosmetic surgery is undergone, by and large, by women who are coerced into a stereotypical male image of what constitutes beauty, and what the parameters of normality are, has not been overlooked by feminist psychologists. The socially constructed image of beauty as 'thinness' has its medicalized poles of anorexia and bulimia. Feminist psychologists, and other feminist 'voices', have had, and continue to have, a big impact on how we understand the patriarchal system of Western society, Western medicine and in particular our own health care system.

Nursing knowledge

We hope that you will be able to see, from the foregoing, that knowledge is not always a question of absolute fact, but is often socially constructed according to a set of values, beliefs and biases. In this respect we must view nursing knowledge in the same vein – not as absolute truth but as constructed out of the values and beliefs of the nursing profession. This may be based on the quest for scientificity, credibility, objectivity etc., but this may well be just another biased ideology. Notwithstanding this, the quest for nursing knowledge continues, and here we outline a few of the attempts that highlight the relationship between disease, illness and disorder, and the construction of nursing knowledge.

In an interesting attempt to structure nursing knowledge in order to maintain computerized information, Harris *et al.* (2000) discussed three domains: (a) scientific reasoning, (b) expertise and (c) standardized nursing languages. They argued that nursing knowledge, and presumably any other area of knowledge, could be set into areas or domains, which represents clinical information as science, a set of skills or procedures as expertise and a lexicon of nursing terms as a distinct language. This approach to delineating nursing knowledge is set within the world of information technology models and reference terminology as a requirement for capturing such knowledge electronically. A particular disease or illness will evoke specific domains of nursing knowledge.

Another attempt to structure nursing knowledge was undertaken by Liaschenko and Fisher (1999). These authors proposed a classification of nursing knowledge that they referred to as case, patient and person. Case knowledge is concerned with general knowledge of pathophysiology, disease processes, pharmacology and all other concrete therapeutic protocols. Patient knowledge concerns the relevant information that defines the patient as a recipient within the health care system and that enables nurses to move the individual through the system. Person knowledge is that which the individual brings as a subject with a personal biography, a personal social space and a set of desires, wishes and intentions. The authors argue that this is a particularly useful way of understanding the illness/disorder, the person and the health care system in which they are located. What this model shows to us is the construction of knowledge that emerges from the context of illness, person and medical system as a unified entity and not as a set of distinct parts.

Finally, Kim (1998) outlined a typology of nursing knowledge that was based on four domains: (a) the client domain; (b) the domain of environment; (c) the client–nurse domain; and (d) the practice domain. The rationale for this was that 'assuming that nursing is actively involved in delineating the sphere of nursing phenomena, it is important to develop a typology that can be used to systematize research and ever cumulating knowledge in nursing' (Kim 1998: 367). What is important in all these attempts to structure nursing knowledge is that they are rooted in practice. That is, nursing as a practice actually occurs and knowledge emerges from that. These three attempts to delineate structures of nursing knowledge are three among many. The wealth of nursing models (over 100 at the last count) are testimony to the impetus of the profession, which seeks to understand the uniqueness of the nature of nursing (whether this is a 'Holy Grail' remains to be seen).

Further reading

Riehl, J. P. and Roy, C. (eds) (1980) *Conceptual Models for Nursing Practice.* Norwalk, CT: Appleton-Century-Croft.

Payne, S. and Walker, J. (1995) *Psychology for Nurses and the Caring Professions.* Buckingham: Open University Press.

3.13 Nursing as social action and nursing as therapy

We noted above (3:5) that communication between people and the ability to interact socially (3:9) with them are reliant upon a number of factors, including our self-awareness, what we say, how we act and how we manage personal space with others. Furthermore, effective social interaction also relies upon how we treat others in the relationship structure. In nursing practice we engage the patient (as well as family and friends etc.) in a temporary helping relationship in which there is an implicit assumption that the nurse wishes to assist and the patient desires the assistance. This is not always the case, however, as some patients may decide that they do not want any help and others may be irrational, intoxicated or unconscious. In the case of this latter group, we make the assumption that if they were not irrational, intoxicated or unconscious, they would wish our help. Many procedures in nursing employ practical skills to varying degrees of technicality, with some merely requiring basic expertise and others needing more sophisticated mastery. However, while all patients would probably desire that the practical nursing procedure being performed upon them was undertaken skilfully and adeptly we also know that, if given the choice, some patients would choose one nurse in favour of another to undertake the procedure. This preference is, in large part, concerned with the nature of nursing as a social action, and will be as much to do with the quality of the interaction within the helping relationship as it is with the effectiveness of the procedure. Thus, nursing can be viewed as a social action and also as a form of therapy in itself.

Nursing as social action

There are many areas of life where we temporarily engage in a social interaction that is superficial, yet meaningful, for the time that we spend within it. The relationships that are formed at the local pub may be helpful, friendly and amiable, as are some of the relationships that we may have with our working colleagues. However, what differs in the nurse–patient relationship, among other things, is the fact that the helping relationship is a fundamental part of the nurse's role, to be enacted professionally and in confidence, and the patient is to some extent vulnerable and has some form of need deficit. Therefore, in all areas of nursing there is a focus on constructing the delivery of nursing care that is geared towards facilitating the patient to maintain as much autonomous action as is feasible, while fulfilling the tasks set by the demands of nursing care requirements. Let us now look at a few of the practical attempts to highlight the complexity of nursing as a social action from a variety of clinical areas.

Strydom *et al.* (2000) were concerned with establishing guidelines for implementation in an education-learning situation with patients diagnosed with tuberculosis. They wished to promote the nurses' knowledge and skills in a wide range of areas that could be seen to form a part of nursing as a social action. These areas included, among many others, interpersonal relations, subject knowledge, motivation of the nurse, stimulation of the patient's motivation, recovery from the patient's chest centredness and the acceptance of responsibility for their own health. We can see in this research that nurses have multifaceted constructs to their role and if any of these factors is going to be successfully completed then they are going to require a social forum in which they can be managed. This forum is the helping relationship set within nursing action.

Although many aspects of social interaction are based on the social skills that we learn in childhood and develop throughout our adolescence, there are other interactional skills that we can learn as adults, which will enable us to perform nursing more effectively as a social action. Kuiper (2000) argued that the quest to improve nursing practitioners for the future has led to a focus on the metacognitive control of critical thinking abilities. The modern nurse, it is proposed, is 'a self-regulated individual [who] requires a dependable experiential knowledge base, uses cognitive critical thinking strategies in a reflective manner, and is affected by social and cultural influences' (Kuiper 2000: 116). The self-regulation model pivots on: (a) metacognitive self-regulation, which involves critical thinking and information processing; (b) behavioural self-regulation based on reflective practice; and (c) environmental self-regulation in terms of nursing social interaction in the clinical context.

Social interaction may be more difficult when the patient has a contagious disease and requires barrier nursing, or when the patient has some form of communication deficit. It can also be difficult when the patient is disfigured in some way. Clarke (1998: 13), discussing facial disfigurement, noted that 'problems arise principally in the area of social interaction, with intrusions such as staring and comments commonplace. The resulting social anxiety and poor self esteem can often lead to outright avoidance of social situations.' It is in these difficult social situations that such important aspects as reflective practice and cognitive critical skills come to the fore. Understanding one's own embarrassment, disgust, sadness and shame is equalled only by empathizing with the patient's feelings in these situations. Managing these social situations is a skill, and it is reliant to a large degree on managing the feelings of oneself and the feelings of the patient (Clarke 1998).

Nursing as therapy

If it is accepted that the social interaction that nurses engage in may be viewed as inextricably linked to the helping relationship, then it is a relatively short conceptual step to understanding nursing itself as a therapeutic activity. It has long been accepted that many of the practical skills of nursing procedures can contribute to the overall therapeutic endeavour. For example, Pomeroy *et al.* (2001) described current nursing and therapy interventions for the prevention and treatment of pain following a stroke. However, it is in relation to the psychological impact that nursing as a therapy can have on the patient well-being, rather than the mere practical aspect of, say, dressing a wound, that we are concerned. Cowan *et al.* (2001) researched the impact of psychosocial nursing therapy following sudden cardiac arrest. They attempted to describe the efficacy of psychosocial therapy in sudden cardiac arrest survivors at the two-year stage and following discharge from hospital. The psychosocial interventions they used indicated three components: (a) physiological relaxation with biofeedback training focused on altering autonomic tone; (b) cognitive behavioural therapy aimed at self-management and coping strategies for depression, anxiety and anger; and (c) cardiovascular health education. They concluded that 'psychosocial therapy significantly reduced the risk of cardiovascular death in sudden cardiac arrest' (Cowan *et al.* 2001: 68). This is not, by far, the only study that highlights the psychological relationship between nursing therapy and physical relief. Day (2000) made a case for relaxation therapy in the management of cardiac chest pain and suggested that 'nurses caring for patients with chest pain need to look beyond medical management and begin to challenge nursing practice to help patients deal effectively with chest pain in a way that meets individual needs' (Day 2000: 40).

Obviously the psychological impact of nursing therapy is more explicit in psychiatric nursing, where models are in abundance (Wilshaw 1997) and the practical applications are well noted (Sullivan and Rogers 1997). However, it should be remembered that the structure of the nurse–patient relationship in general nursing is little different from that in psychiatric nursing. One difference is that the social interaction and the application of nursing interventions in mental health settings may be more formalized, with varying aspects of the interaction being set out and evaluated more formally. However, this can also take place in general nursing. For example, Corner (1997), working with nursing therapy for cancer patients, argued that nursing therapy has the potential to operate on four levels: (a) fundamental knowledge or theory generation; (b) therapeutic interventions for individuals; (c) developing and changing health systems; and (d) critique and reconstruction of care from a social perspective. Nursing therapy, Corner argues, is a therapeutic enterprise in its own right. Finally, in an interesting paper that sets the issue of nursing therapy in a new light, Bailey (1995) suggested that lung cancer provided a new insight for nursing as therapy. Breathlessness, which accompanies many disorders of the lungs, has traditionally been treated by addressing the underlying causes with pharmacological approaches. However, breathlessness is a frightening and powerful experience that symbolizes a basic threat to life. Bailey (1995) argued that nursing therapy is aimed at alleviating the loss of lung function and easing the psychological burden that restricts the sufferer. So, in this sense, nursing therapy is not only the application of a set of practices but also the provision of psychological support that is aimed at relieving suffering.

Further reading

Hinchliff, S., Norman, S. and Schober, J. (1998) *Nursing Practice and Health Care: A Foundation Text*. London: Arnold.

Hogston, R. and Simpson, P. M. (1999) *Foundations of Nursing Practice*. London: Macmillan.

3.14 Pain and suffering

Pain and suffering lie at the heart of the human condition and are usually perceived as pre-states towards death. Certainly pain is usually seen as a warning sign of the body informing us that something is wrong. Before we begin to look at the differences between pain and suffering in human terms let us spend a moment on the relationship between pain and suffering and the health care professional. If it is accepted that pain and suffering create an inherent fear in us and that we associate pain and suffering as conditions that lead towards death then those who are considered to have the knowledge, skill and power to relieve the pain may also be viewed as having the ability to stave off death. This puts doctors, nurses and other health care workers in a perceived powerful position of (falsely) having the power over life and death (Richman 1987; Turner 1987), and perhaps more importantly having the power to provide a pain-free death. The relief of pain, and the fear attached to its production, is clearly seen in the young toddler who falls, hurts themselves, cries and seeks the mother's reassurance, rubbing the injured part (to release endorphins for pain relief), cuddling and patching up (plaster, bandage, cream and/or tender loving care). Thus, the relief of pain and suffering involves physical, psychological and emotional aspects, which suggest that pain and suffering can also hurt in physical, psychological and emotional ways.

Differences in pain and suffering

Any definition of pain must include numerous factors that contribute towards the overall experience of it. For example, it has a subjective element that involves sensory feeling such as shooting, stabbing, throbbing, burning and aching pain, and an emotional aspect such as frightening, annoying, frustrating and sickening pain. It also has a fear/anxiety aspect, which can worsen or heighten the pain, and a depressive element that takes away the will to live (L. A. Bradley 1995). Although we understand pain as primarily a physical phenomenon, which is concerned with the removal or avoidance of a noxious stimulus, this does not explain the experience of pain in all its ramifications. For example, we know that people have different tolerances for pain, with some having a low pain threshold and others having a high pain threshold. Furthermore, some people are able to tolerate the intense pain of torture, while others react emotionally to a relatively slight pain. Another aspect of pain was suggested by O'Connell (2000), who argued that pain is never perceived as an isolated sensation in a 'pure' sense, but is always accompanied by emotion and meaning. This meaning structure makes the sensation of pain unique to each individual. Finally, in terms of aspects of pain, we should note the cultural component. Rollman (1998) suggested that the expression and management of pain had biological, psychological and social elements that interacted in an extremely complex way. It was argued that much of this was culturally learnt and that differing cultures assumed different attitudes to pain, which were learnt from birth and extended throughout life. Two elements of the attitude to pain were described by Zborowski (1952).

- Pain expectancy, which is concerned with the anticipation of pain that is to some extent unavoidable.

- Pain acceptance, which is the willingness to experience pain as an inevitable part of a cultural experience.

Suffering is usually identified with pain but may be better understood as a continual, highly noxious, emotional state, which can be associated with pain or other forms of distress. Suffering may vary according to the meaning associated with it and it usually has a temporal dimension, which often extends into the future. It can be related to a personal or religious dimension, which often overlaps with the physical or medical meaning of suffering. In an extremely interesting study Baines and Norlander (2000) set out to research the relationship between pain and suffering as viewed from the patients' perspective in a hospice setting. A sample of 92 patients were asked to score both their feelings of pain and feelings of suffering. Pain scores and suffering scores were categorized into four areas: (a) no pain or no suffering; (b) mild pain or mild suffering; (c) moderate pain or moderate suffering; and (d) severe pain or severe suffering. Interestingly, more patients experienced suffering than pain, and the only statistically significant correlation was between severe pain and severe suffering 'in the categories of loss of enjoyment of life, unfinished business, and concern for loved ones' (Baines and Norlander 2000: 319). They concluded that the data clearly indicated that patients view pain and suffering as separate entities. Thus, suffering may be accompanied by physical pain but it may also be more concerned with psychological, emotional, personal and religious aspects of the patient's condition that may be causing distress. Let us now take a brief look at some of the practice and research areas that have been investigated in relation to pain and suffering.

Practice and research areas of pain and suffering

Following on from the previous section, some interesting approaches to understanding pain and suffering, from a research perspective, in practice areas will now be mentioned. In an attempt to promote the use of evidence-based practice in relation to the management of pain and suffering, Dooks (2001) argued that outdated approaches were still amazingly evident. This author explored Rogers's diffusion of innovation theory to examine how changes diffuse through a social system over a period of time and can expose some of the barriers and facilitators to this process. The basis of this argument is that evidence-based approaches to pain management will relieve more suffering than traditional approaches. However, this may depend on what constitutes evidence-based practice, as some advances, particularly technological ones, have been questioned in this area. Tinnelly *et al.* (2000), although at pains to point out that technological advances have been remarkably helpful in alleviating the pain and suffering of some terminally ill patients, have outlined some reservations. They argued that, for some, the use of technology appears to have augmented the distress, and have suggested that some believe technology is an invasive procedure that can overrule decision-making, and the manner in which it is sometimes employed is seen as a replacement for other types of care. Furthermore, when technology is considered to be a cheaper option than, say, the provision of a nurse, the cost considerations can outweigh the quality issue of palliative care.

A number of studies have focused on the use, or development, of a pain assessment instrument, which is reflective of the 'scientific' drive to objectify pain and suffering. For example, Tayler and McLeod (2001) outlined the development and implementation of a pain assessment and treatment flow sheet (PATF) to enhance patient care in this area. This tool is used to assess pain and suffering, to provide information for decision-making and to provide documentary evidence of pain management. It is used, the authors state, by multidisciplinary members of the palliative care team. Another set of tools for the systematic assessment of pain and its management are the pain assessment tool (PAT) and the pain flow sheet (PFS), as outlined by Faries *et al.* (1991). These authors researched the use of these tools against the standard charting of pain as indicated in nurses' narrative reports. The research group concluded that the use of the PAT and PFS resulted in a significantly lower average of pain intensity ratings on a three-day follow-up. They suggested that the use of systematic pain records can improve pain management and relieve suffering. In a review of pain assessment tools by Baillie (1993) it was argued that a number of pain assessment tools have been developed and implemented in clinical settings, which has led to improvements in the assessment and management of pain. Each of these tools, it was proposed, have specific attributes that aid communication, remove subjectivity of assessment and promote a systematic approach. This was earlier borne out by Dalton (1989), who concluded from research that pain assessments were influenced by, among other things, *the characteristics of the nurse*. By this it was meant that pain assessment was dependent upon how the nurse viewed the patient's pathology, the patient's character and their concern about addictive behaviour. None the less, this clearly showed the subjective nature of nursing pain assessment at that time.

It is difficult to discuss the treatment and management of pain and suffering without dealing with the issue of terminal care, and this has implications for the right to life (6:11), the right to death (6:12) and the issue of euthanasia (6:15). As we cover these issues in Chapter 6 we restrict ourselves here to one excellent article that deals with the ethical implications of terminal sedation in different situations for pain and suffering. Hallenbeck (2000) outlined two hypothetical cases. The first concerns terminal sedation for severe distress in a patient close to death who has ceased eating and drinking, and the second is a patient with a non-terminally ill spinal cord injury who requests terminal sedation because of psychic distress. Hallenbeck supports sedation in the first case but not in the second one. The guiding principles are set out as follows.

- *Respect for autonomy* (6:2). While this is important, there is no obligation to provide sedation in all circumstances.
- *Physician intent*. The main intent for a physician to prescribe sedation should be to alleviate suffering.
- *Inferences of intent and physician action*. Reasonable inferences can be made between intent and action to safeguard proper care by titrating sedation to observable signs of distress.
- *Proximity to death*. This is a more useful concept than terminality in deciding the benefits and burdens of sedation.
- *Physician action and the nature of suffering*. Not all suffering is appropriately treated with sedation, and other interventions should be considered.
- *Hastening death*. In patients who are close to death and who have already ceased eating and drinking, sedation cannot be said to hasten death through either dehydration or starvation.
- *Informed consent*. If dehydration may in fact hasten death and terminal sedation is otherwise appropriate, ethical concerns may be addressed through informed consent. If hydration is refused, then terminal sedation cannot be considered synonymous with euthanasia.

Although these views by Hallenbeck may well be taken issue with, and international laws vary, they serve to highlight the complex area of relieving pain and suffering as prioritized in the Hippocratic oath.

Further reading

Cassell, E. (1991) *The Nature of Suffering and the Goals of Medicine*. New York: Oxford University Press.

Hawthorn, J. and Redmond, K. (1998) *Pain: Causes and Management*. Oxford: Blackwell.

3.15 Death and dying

The one certainty in life is that we are all going to die, and in fact, we can view death as a natural process. However, we also view death in relation to a set of culturally determined norms and standards. For example, we may see death as 'peaceful' following a long life and we may consider 'passing away naturally' in one's sleep as a 'good' way of dying. Alternatively, the younger one dies the more it can be viewed as unnatural or unjust. In purely physical terms it is merely the cessation of adequate function of the organs and cells of the body, yet few of us would see death or dying in these terms. As we will see, the psychological impact of death and dying is hugely important both for the person who is in the process of dying and for those close to them who, following the event, will be left behind. It is also important for health care professionals to understand the psychological impact of death and dying, as we are often involved with people who have terminal conditions and their family and friends. The grieving process, for all concerned, will be affected by health care professionals' attitude and behaviour during contact with those involved and will determine how the entire process will be reflected upon long after the event has passed. We now outline the three most influential theories of death and dying, but we cover these from a practical perspective in relation to the psychological impact of the process.

Death, dying and grief

In 1970 Dr Elisabeth Kubler-Ross, a psychiatrist, published her work on the psychological stages and process of death and dying, which has become a landmark theory in this field. Her theory was based on her work as a psychiatrist with over 200 dying patients. In short, she was particularly interested in how people come to terms with their own death (anticipatory grief) and how they overcome the natural fear associated with it. Kubler-Ross (1970) outlined five stages that, it was argued, most people go through once they have received the news of a terminal illness.

- *Denial*. In this, the first stage, the dying person employs the psychological strategy of denial, which is a temporary defence against the overwhelming news. It is characterized by the phrase 'No, not me, it can't be', and the person often asks for double-checking of results to be undertaken.
- *Anger*. In the second stage the person loses the denial and becomes angry and resentful. It is characterized by the phrase 'It's not fair, why me?', and is a difficult stage for family, friends and health professionals to deal with, as the anger is often displaced in all directions.
- *Bargaining*. This third stage involves a quest to extend life in some way as a type of reward for something. It is characterized by such phrases as 'Please God let me . . .' or 'If only I could . . . one last time'. They are promises that are usually kept secret and only revealed to close loved

ones or religious ministers, but when the 'deal' involves the hospital it may also involve health professionals.

- *Depression.* Once it is realized that the negotiation will not work the fourth stage of depression may set in. It is usually based in the realization of the loss that they anticipate and common phrases such as 'How can I leave all this behind?' and 'What will happen to . . .?' are often heard.

- *Acceptance.* In this final stage the dying person is almost devoid of feeling and will often be tired for long periods. They will express their acceptance of their fate with statements such as 'Leave me alone' and 'I am ready to die'. Acceptance is not a happy state, it is more of an end to the struggle.

Kubler-Ross's theory is clearly a stage approach, and it should be noted that not every dying patient will go through each phase and that for those who do there may well be different durations in each stage. Another stage theory is that of Bowlby (1980). Bowlby argued that adult grief was a similar state to the separation loss that is seen in children when there is a disruption to the attachment bond. He saw the grief of dying as a preparation for the inevitable separation and identified four phases.

- *Numbing.* In this phase the person feels numb and is in a state of disbelief. It may last for up to a week and may be punctuated by sudden outbursts of anger and resentment.

- *Yearning and searching.* This phase may well last for months and involves the person feeling restless and unsatisfied. They are constantly wanting and wishing for something and may well not know exactly what. This phase may also be punctuated by anger and resentment, as in phase one.

- *Disorganization.* This phase involves feelings of depression and despair and the person feels that they have little control over what have been regular patterns of behaviour. They may become apathetic and lethargic.

- *Reorganization.* In this phase the grieving person becomes more reorganized and has a general acceptance of what has occurred. They may not fully reorganize but they lose the despair felt in phase three.

In Bowlby's theory of grief the four phases are interlinked to some degree and, although they are set out as distinct states, Bowlby believed that the boundaries are, in reality, blurred and some people may move in and out of the phases. The stage and phase theories have been criticized as being not universal processes that everyone goes through but merely individual experiences (Archer 1999). Later workers who have undertaken research in this area now prefer to talk about the components of grief, some of which may come early in the grieving process and others later. For example, Ramsay and de Groot (1977) outline nine components of grief.

- *Shock.* This is most often described as numbness but can include apathy, pain and feelings of *depersonalization.*

- *Disorganization.* This may involve the inability to undertake even the most basic of tasks, or there may be periods of organization followed by sudden collapse.

- *Denial.* This component usually comes in the early part of the grieving but can occur at any time. The person denies the death and waits for them to come home or sets them places at meal times.

- *Depression.* As denial evaporates a depression can emerge, but it can also appear at any time throughout the process.

- *Guilt.* This can be for not saying or doing something for the deceased before they died or for having negative thoughts about them when they are dead.

- *Anxiety.* This can involve concerns about finances, family and friends but may also be about oneself.

- *Aggression.* Angry feelings may emerge, which may be directed at the person who has died or God, fate, doctors and nurses.

- *Resolution.* There is an acceptance of the death and a feeling that life must go on.

- *Reintegration.* The grieving person moves on and reorganizes their life without the loved one.

In all these components we can see a type of 'natural' reaction that the person is undergoing in response to the loss of a loved one. However, once they have been experienced many of the components may well reappear at different times, particularly in relation to birthdays or anniversaries.

Nursing and the afterlife

Dying is, of course, a deeply moving, personal and subjective event and for many people is also a profound religious experience. There are many different religions that deal with issues of death, dying and the afterlife in culturally diverse ways. In Jewish culture the expression of grief following a bereavement is considered to be therapeutic and an outpouring of emotion is expected, particularly in the few days following death. On the other hand, in Muslim and Buddhist religions less outpouring of grief is expected in relation to weeping but wailing is more common (Dickenson and Johnson 1993). Japanese culture allows a woman to accept her husband's death quietly and with composure and their strong belief in the afterlife indicates a long ancestral history, which provides help and support for the deceased. In British culture some outpouring of grief is expected but this should be done quietly. An understanding of the different religious beliefs and their impact on death, dying and grieving is important for health workers, as they can assist the process through appropriate action (King *et al.* 1994; Flatt 1998).

It is common for nursing staff to be present at the dying person's bedside, and family and friends are often in attendance. Therefore, the nurse's role is critical at this stage. Nursing staff may feel anxious and helpless at the impending death of a patient and may convey this to both the patient and their family (Martins *et al.* 1999). The expectation that health care workers have the power over life and death is not only an issue for the dying person but can also create a tension for many staff (Locsin 2001). This was researched by Arblaster *et al.* (1990: 34) and it was found that 'patients desired responsive nursing care that enabled them and their families to bring their own resources to the dying process, rather than having imposed upon them care which nurses deemed appropriate'. This shows the complexity of the dynamic that concerns all those who are involved in the death of a person, and the need for nurses to be aware of their own emotions (Wong *et al.* 2001).

Further reading

Archer, J. (1999) *The Nature of Grief: The Evolution and Psychology of Reactions to Loss.* London: Routledge.

Seymour, J. E. (2001) *Critical Moments: Death and Dying in Intensive Care.* Buckingham: Open University Press.

Cobb, M. (2001) *The Dying Soul: Spiritual Care at the End of Life.* Buckingham: Open University Press.

3.16 Violence

Violence is important to us in health care settings for a number of reasons. First, many patients attend hospital and health care centres because they have been the victim of some form of violence, and many of these patients may be considered vulnerable; for example, children, women and the elderly. Second, some patients, and their relatives and friends, may become perpetrators of violence while attending hospital, although this may not be the reason for the attendance. Third, health care professionals may become victims of assault from patients, for many reasons. Finally, some patient groups are more prone to violence than others; for example, those intoxicated with alcohol or illegal drugs. Given the central role that violence plays in our society it is not surprising that there has been a voluminous amount of work published in this area. This has led to the establishment of a wide array of theories, with a different definition emanating from each one. Therefore, for the purposes of our project we define violence as 'the harmful and unlawful use of force or strength; of or caused by physical assault' (Mason and Chandley 1999: 6).

It is popularly held that violence is on the increase in our society and, although this has been challenged by some (Marsh 1986), it is generally viewed that there is a greater risk of violence today than at any other time in our history. What is not at issue is the fact that health care professionals are the victims of violence more today than previously. This may be due to the fact that some violence is medicalized as a condition and health care staff are expected to intervene, it may be due to the increased use of intoxicating drugs or it may be due to a breakdown of certain value systems in society. Whatever the cause, it is likely to be complex, and it is certainly unacceptable.

Theories of violence

As we note above, the theories of violence are numerous and here we briefly give a flavour of how they are grouped.

- *Evolutionary*: for example, Lorenz's (1966) instinct theory.
- *Psychoanalytic*: for example, Freud's (1920) psychic conflict.
- *Behavioural*: for example, Zillman's (1979) instrumental aggression.
- *Sociological*: for example, Wolfgang and Ferracutti's (1967) subculture of violence.
- *Social cognitive*: Bandura's (1982) reinforcing contingencies.

Whatever theories are propounded for the use of violence, it would appear to us that it is the practical issues that are more relevant to us in the immediacy of the health care setting. This is not to dismiss the relevancy of theoretical expositions *per se*, as they can serve to provide information that may be useful for us to understand violence in relation to distal or proximal causative factors (Blackburn 1993). Distal causative factors are those that can be considered to be occurring at some considerable time before the violence (e.g. environmental upbringing). Proximal causative factors are those life events or situational factors that occur directly before the violence (e.g. alcohol). Clearly we have more control over proximal factors than we do over the distal ones, but many proximal factors themselves are also not subject to immediate remedial action. For example, if long waiting times at an accident and emergency (A&E) department are a proximal causative factor to a violent encounter then reducing these waiting times is not always feasible given the restrictions on resources. However, given that some situations are remediable, we need to be aware of how best to approach these situations. Mason and Chandley (1999) outline a useful contributory factor analysis framework that can be employed when violence appears to be occurring.

- *Physical factors*, such as pain, tiredness, discomfort, withdrawal, medication side effects.
- *Social factors*, such as loneliness, requiring attention, unable to communicate, frustration.
- *Environmental factors*, such as heat, cold, noise, space, overcrowding.
- *Contextual factors*, including time, restrictions, resources, lack of staff availability.

- *Clinical factors*, such as mental state, change in psychopathology, behavioural changes.
- *Other factors*, such as threat from peers, pressure from family, stress from staff.

Clearly these are merely a few of the many contributing factors to violence that could be mentioned. However, the framework is useful when a situation is appearing to deteriorate towards violence and a preventative action is necessary, or following a violent scene when an analysis is required.

Anticipating violence

We are all reasonably accomplished at anticipating violence if we are given cues regarding it. However, in the absence of these cues we are unlikely to anticipate its occurrence. We have all learnt to watch for the signs of impending violence from the school playground and the local park of our childhood and the clubs and bars of our adolescence. Even merely walking down the street is an area of life in which we watch for the cues of potential violence. In the health care setting we watch for the signs of violence from others in four main areas.

- *Posture*. We note how the person is sitting or standing, if they are gripping something tightly, whether their hands are on their hips, or they are leaning forward threateningly.
- *Speech*. We check if they are speaking calmly or shouting, speaking through clenched teeth, and any signs of verbal threat.
- *Motor activity*. This area is often overlooked but we need to check for pacing or inability to sit still, fidgeting or tapping fingers or feet.
- *Past history*. This includes not only any previous knowledge of the person, but also whether they actually state that they have been violent in the past.

Managing violence

There are numerous techniques that are available to health care workers in managing violent encounters. The first concerns the talk-over techniques in which we first make an assessment of the mental state of the person concerned. If they are considered to be clearly rational and lucid, although extremely angry, open discussion may be the most appropriate way forward (Farrell and Gray 1992). This requires some degree of skill on the part of the professional and a degree of willingness on the part of the person to engage. However, if the person is irrational and disorientated then conversation that is distracting may be more usefully employed (Mason and Chandley 1999). The second set of techniques can be summed up as averting approaches and involves discussions with the person through a series of questions. Time is given for the person to think and for them to review the situation. It is important not to rush them for answers and to ensure that you listen to their story in full. Ask how the person is feeling rather than telling them that you know, and ask how they think the situation can be resolved. Avoid making any retaliatory comments and reassure them that you accept that they are angry. Finally, when a conciliatory gesture is made make sure that you respond accordingly (Jambunathen and Bellaire 1996).

A third set of techniques involves what are known as slow-down approaches (Mason and Chandley 1999). When a person is about to become violent their minds are racing and they are usually over-stimulated, which means that they are making decisions rapidly. Slow-down approaches help the person to reduce the speed of decision-making. In practice, it involves slowing the speech down and talking in a slightly lower tone. Calming gestures should be made to slow the pace of the situation down. Ask slowing questions such as 'Let's think about this for a minute' and 'What do you think should happen?' The fourth set of techniques is what are known as verbal de-escalation approaches (Mason and Chandley 1999). They are based on the individual's social skills, confidence and professional authority. No single approach can be outlined as they are employed according to each situation that is developing. However, Mason and Chandley (1999) have provided a set of practice principles, which are reproduced here in Box 3.4.

All the techniques mentioned here are useful in the situation directly before an actual assault occurs. They are based on interpersonal skills and the use of psychological principles, and are very much dependent upon each person's personality and character. If an actual assault takes place then there are further sets of skills that can be used to manage the situation

---

Box 3.4   De-escalation techniques: practice principles

1   Maintain the patient's self-esteem and dignity.
2   Maintain calmness (your own and the patient's).
3   Assess the patient and the situation.
4   Identify stressors and stress indicators.
5   Respond as early as possible.
6   Use a calm, clear tone of voice.
7   Invest time.
8   Remain honest.
9   Establish what the patient considers to be his or her need.
10   Be goal-orientated.
11   Maintain a large personal space.
12   Avoid verbal struggles.
13   Give several options.
14   Make clear the options.
15   Utilize a non-aggressive posture.
16   Use genuineness and empathy.
17   Attempt to be confidently aware.
18   Use verbal, non-verbal and communication skills.
19   Be assertive (not aggressive).
20   Assess for personal safety.

physically. These will not be mentioned here as they can be dangerous without specific training. We strongly recommend attendance on recognized training courses that are available for health care workers.

Violence and 'silent' victims

We finish this section with a brief look at violence and some specific patient populations. Of course, not all violence actually occurs in the health care setting in which we may become involved. Patients who attend the hospital or the health care setting may well be the victims of violence by others, with injuries clearly attributable to an act of violence. These may well be fractures, bruises, lacerations, stab wounds etc., and there may be a clearly identifiable perpetrator as indicated by the victim's, or other witnesses', accounts. However, there are certain groups of patients in which it is unclear whether their injuries are the result of violence, and the victim is 'silent', for one reason or another, about the real cause of the injury. We can briefly mention three such groups.

In domestic violence, on both men and women, there may be some reluctance on the part of the victim to reveal the true cause of the injuries. These injuries may well include both physical and mental health conditions. Piesik (1998) argued that some women want to protect their partners and that some may fear them, and stated that 'triage nurses and primary care practitioners should learn the signs of abuse and how to elicit the necessary information quickly and discreetly' (Piesik 1998: 18). However, confidentiality issues are paramount and it is a question of complying with the victim's wishes. The second group to be mentioned are children who present with injuries that are suspected of being non-accidental. Clearly, great care must be taken to ensure that false allegations should not be made but multi-professional and multi-agency systems must be initiated to protect the child. Finally, elderly confused patients may present with non-accidental injuries but be unable to recall, or give an account of, how the violence took place. Again, multiprofessional and multi-agency systems should be initiated to protect the person.

Further reading

Green, R. G. and Donnerstein, E. D. (1998) *Human Aggression: Theories, Research, and Implications for Social Policy*. London: Harcourt Publishers.
Mason, T. and Chandley, M. (1999) *Managing Violence and Aggression: A Manual for Nurses and Health Care Workers*. Edinburgh: Churchill Livingstone.

▌ 3.17 Conclusion

We have seen throughout this chapter that, as in other sciences, the psychological theories have an important part to play in the understanding of the nature of the human condition. We have also seen that it is often the case that theory and practice are not easily separated as distinct forms, and in fact on the contrary they can appear as being inextricably entwined. Human action is a complex affair and when set in terms of ill-health and disease it embroils many threatening aspects of the human condition, such as fear, pain, anger and helplessness. Furthermore, there is an intense pressure on the physical integrity of the body as well as psychological pressure on the mind. Understanding this is central to our role as nurses so that we can assist the patient in their health career, alleviate suffering and keep in touch with our own emotions in the, often, stressful practice of caring.

4 Thinking anthropology

4.1 Introduction

At first sight the relationship between nursing and anthropology may not be self-evident and the reader may be forgiven for questioning the relevance of this. However, we will show that the scientific discipline of anthropology not only has a long history in relation to nursing but also is as relevant to contemporary nursing practice as, say, psychology or sociology. The first issue to be dealt with concerns the old, and familiar, related concept of sociology *in* as opposed to sociology *of* medicine (Strauss 1957). In these terms Holden and Littlewood (1991) outline the relationship of this discipline as anthropology *for* nurses as opposed to anthropology *of* nurses. The former application, anthropology *for* nurses, involves the use of anthropological methods, employed by nurses, to explore, examine and investigate aspects of patients lives. The latter, anthropology *of* nurses, concerns the study of nursing traditions, myths, taboos, hierarchies and cultures using anthropological approaches. We take the view here that both perspectives are important for nursing and that employing anthropological understanding, of both our patients and our profession, will equip us with skills and knowledge to deliver more appropriate nursing practice. The second issue we deal with concerns the anthropological understanding of the difference between nursing and medicine. Biomedicine's central concern is not holistic, it is not general well-being or individual persons' status, it is their bodies in disease. 'Medicine is primarily (and properly) concerned with disease, its etiology, pathophysiology, and treatment' (Dougherty and Tripp-Reiner 1985: 220). Nursing, on the other hand, is holistic and concerned with individual responses to health-related matters. This distinction outlines a crucial domain for nursing, which 'uses the model of illness and the model of disease and mediates the two' (Dougherty and Tripp-Reiner 1985: 220).

When groups of people come together to undertake a common goal, over a period of time, and when that objective is passed down over many generations, those involved will usually form strategies of human behaviour that are highly complex and deeply profound. This complexity and profundity is due to the cognitive processes, or ways of thinking, that underscore human knowledge. Human knowledge, as we know, is developmental. That is, it constantly grows, changes, is supported or falsified and most importantly differs across time and between people. The contention between what constitutes truth and belief is apparent around the world in the many conflicts of, and diversity in, ideologies and cultures. Although differences of opinion and belief exist between these ideologies, in themselves they have a logic, meaning and structure that are subject to anthropological interpretation. In the first part of the chapter we outline some of the main anthropological structures that are relevant to us in health care settings.

PART ONE: THEORY

4.2 Myths

The first anthropological structure that we discuss is the myth, and as we will see, myths are both complex and varied. At one level we can understand a myth to be a fictitious story that usually employs supernatural or popularized persons, and the function of the story is to explain natural or social phenomena. However, this is too simplistic and does not do justice to the functional importance of myths. Another element to include in attempting to define a myth is the *conscience collective*. Durkheim believed that the moral attitude was essentially social in character, external to the individual, and coerced people into behaving and thinking in certain ways. Thus, a myth can be seen as a narrative explanation of phenomena that are extraordinary, transcendent and sacred, and represent the control of human behaviour through the conscience collective. Although this is more satisfactory for definitional purposes, there is another element to our understanding of myths, which involves the relationship between the content of the myth and the individual's explanatory framework. This was best summed up by Lévi-Strauss: 'the notion of myth is a category of our thought which we use arbitrarily in order to bring together under one word attempts to explain natural phenomena, products of oral literature, philosophical speculations, and cases where linguistic processes emerged to full consciousness' (Lévi-Strauss 1962: 10). Myths, then, appear to be discursive frameworks of meaningful statements that are constructed by human beings to explain binary oppositions, such as conscious–unconscious, divine–secular, real–abstract. We now discuss these in more detail in relation to three important authors in the area of myth.

Malinowski

Bronislaw Kaspar Malinoski (1884–1942) was a social anthropologist who was born in Kraków, Poland. Although his PhD was in physics and mathematics, he soon began to study language and folklore, and was greatly influenced by the Finnish anthropologist Edward Westermarch, who studied sexual taboos and marriage, particularly in relation to incest. Malinowski's approach was to study what was then termed primitive cultures through a systematic method of fieldwork and experimentation that secured his position as a professional anthropologist and an influential academic. He lived among the people he studied and, as an adept linguist, quickly learnt to speak their language, which enabled him to adopt another level of enquiry. He studied people from their perspective, attempting to grasp the native's point of view of *his* vision of *his* world. For Malinowski myths functioned in society to provide a legitimation of the social arrangements of that society. The abstract, divine, contents of myths serve to reinforce the real, secular issues of that society, thus dealing with the binary opposition of the practicalities of everyday life and the philosophical speculations of the meaning of existence. This, in Malinowski's study of the Trobriand Islanders' myths, was reflected in the society's system of exchange of goods and gifts known as *kula* and their belief in magic as a way of dealing with the chaos of everyday facts. At the time of Malinowski's work Freudian psychoanalytical theory was developing and he was greatly interested in this. Anthropology and psychoanalysis are closely related, as both are based on the interpretation of human behaviour and language (3:2). Malinowski's main work on myths was the aptly titled *Myths in Primitive Psychology* (1926).

Lévi-Strauss

Born in Belgium, Claude Lévi-Strauss (1908–) was a social anthropologist whose long academic career enabled him to conduct several expeditions to Brazil. His main legacy was to develop structuralist (2:4) approaches to the analysis of cultural forms, and he was also influential in the area of structural linguistics. Lévi-Strauss always emphasizes the structural basis of social life, which is founded on organized sets of rules and certain binary oppositions. In short, he believed that mythical thought is derived from primitive thought and used his structural method to analyse hundreds of myths from Amerindian societies to show that 'the structures of myths could be traced back to the structures of human thought' (D'Anglure 1996: 171). Myths are used, he claimed, to unify certain tensions that exist between binary oppositions, such as group–individual, nature–culture, edible–inedible, raw–cooked. Myths are also used by different clans to establish their *totem*, to manage their clan identity and to manage relations between them. Lévi-Strauss gives us the example of the *Tikopia* society, which is 'composed of four patrilineal but not necessarily exogamous groups called *Kainanga*, each headed by a chief who stands in a special relationship to the *Atua* (gods, ancestral spirits, souls of former chiefs)' (Lévi-Strauss 1962: 24). If we view modern health care systems as structured according to clan divisions (hospitals, wards, units, medics, nursing, psychologists) we are now in a position to reflect on the mythical structures that abound in such settings and to understand better the function of such health care myths.

Myths are often viewed as 'childish', but this belies their importance in explaining some aspect of the social world. Lévi-Strauss gives us an example of the Australian Aboriginal myth concerning the Wombat and the Kangaroo. The myth is that these two animals were once friends and the Wombat decided to make a 'house' for himself (a wombat lives in a burrow under the ground). The Kangaroo made fun of him until one day it began to rain and the Wombat refused to offer him shelter. The Kangaroo struck the Wombat on the head with a large stone, thus flattening his skull, and the Wombat threw a spear in revenge, which stuck in the base of the Kangaroo's spine. This myth is a 'just-so' story to explain the differences between these two marsupial species in Australia. Lévi-Strauss sums this up: 'the resemblances and differences of animal species are translated into terms of friendship and conflict, solidarity and opposition. In other words the world of animal life is represented in terms of social relations, similar to those of human society' (Lévi-Strauss 1962: 87). In this myth, as in many others, the pairing up of these animals is based on a chosen common characteristic, i.e. both are marsupials, which allows them to be compared and differences explained. Again, we can note this structural form in our modern day society as well as throughout the hierarchy of health care.

For Lévi-Strauss myths do not legitimate social affairs or explain social arrangements, they are essentially cognitive processes employed to account for conceptual categories of the mind. For example, the Oedipus myth is simply a variation on a theme whose elements are mother/son, wife/husband and father/son organized in relation to love–hatred and dominance–submission.

Barthes

Roland Barthes (1915–80) was a French cultural critic whose main areas of work included cultural studies, literary criticism, semiotics and structuralism (2:4). Although he wrote on many topics, above all his main focus was on applying the techniques of semiology (2:4), which is the study of signs and signifying systems. In an imaginative way Barthes showed how cultural objects (texts or discourses) produced meaning and how these texts could be read in many different ways. Treating myths as a system of communication, Barthes analysed the language of the words used, the images that were produced and the sounds that were made. His method was to expose the 'falsely obvious' of both myths and modern mass communication. He used such mythical images of a man wearing a beret on a bicycle with a string of onions around his neck to indicate how this reflects 'Frenchness', or a basket of tomatoes and spaghetti to 'Italianize' an image. Barthes claimed that there was no such thing as an innocent image or myth and the cultural process involved in the production of meaning was political and politicized. This makes images and myths 'messages' rather than concepts, objects or ideas, and if Barthes's view is accepted then deciphering or decoding primitive, or modern, myths is an important function of anthropology, and, more specifically for us in health care settings, medical anthropology.

Myths, then, appear to function in order to give meaning to our contemporary practices through a reference to beliefs regarding higher order rationales, i.e. traditions, histories, ideologies, deities or simply god-like instructions. Often, not too dissimilar to religious instruction, knowledge in health care is handed down as an indoctrinated ideology.

Further reading

Barthes, R. (1993) *Mythologies*. London: Vintage.
Lévi-Strauss, C. (1962) *Totemism*. London: Merlin Press.

4.3 Rites and rituals

Rites and rituals can have both a positive and a negative connotation. When seen in relation to the ceremonial procedures of marriages, christenings or even burials they can be viewed as positive forms of human action that are undertaken for a particular reason. However, when this form of behaviour is taken to an extreme it can be seen as negative. For example, in some forms of psychiatric disorders ritualistic behaviour can be quite incapacitating, and ritualistic murders employing human sacrifice are clearly abhorrent. As we will see below, rites and rituals have a complex social and psychological make-up and, while most of us will be familiar with some of the elements of religious ceremonies, few of us will be able to explain the full meaning of all their intricacies. However, it should be noted that not all rites and rituals are religious, as many of them are concerned with everyday aspects of social life; for example, the rites of hospitality in certain cultures where it is appropriate to offer visitors food and shelter, or the conjugal, or nuptial, rites that refer to sexual intercourse between husband and wife.

Rites are commonly understood as forms of procedures, or required actions, while rituals add the element of set patterns and an order of events. Taken together, rites and rituals can be seen as sets of forward action, which expresses a symbolic meaning through shared signs. Although we may not all share the understanding of these signs each cultural group will learn its own system of signification. In health care settings this can be understood in terms of the different nursing emblems (badges, belts, caps) that are used as signs of hierarchy, and while we may know the relevance of our own hospital's signification, we may be ignorant of another's system. Rites and rituals, then, are structured action designed to serve a particular purpose, and we now need to take a closer look at the constituent parts of their structure.

Structure of rites and rituals

Much of everyday life is structured along patterned lines of behaviour, which we give little thought to, from showering in the morning to driving the car to work. This type of behaviour is broken down into component parts at the point of learning, which once regularized into normal behaviour is performed without strict attention to it. However, this is not behaviour performed as a rite or ritual, as defined above, because the elements of the patterned behaviour do not carry with them higher levels of meaning, nor are they accompanied by shared values. In certain cleansing, or washing, rites the elements of the procedure do carry these higher levels of meaning and can thus be called rites. Washing one's hands can be undertaken simply to clean them, but we can also see that employing a cleansing rite by washing our hands performs a higher level of symbolic meaning, which could refer to the washing away of sins. We have already mentioned manifest and latent functions of social behaviour (2:3) and we can employ these terms to provide a structure to the operation of rites and rituals. The manifest components of rites and rituals are those that individuals will know, and are intended by the participants in the ceremonial activity. On the other hand the latent functions will be those that the participants will be directly unaware of.

We may also structure rites and rituals along procedural lines. That is, it is the progression from one element of the behaviour to the next in a recognized sequence of action. The fulfilment of each behavioural component is required before moving to the next component. In this sense, the order of events is as important as the event itself. Although this is clearly seen in religious and royal ceremonies it is also apparent in some of the regular patterns of human interaction, such as the routine method of starting a conversation with 'how do you do', or 'how are you'. The order of events need to be gone through before progressing to the main conversation.

Meaning of rites and rituals

Rites and rituals have an element of stress that can be seen in relation to their performance as outlined above. If they are not performed according to the recognized order there is an increase in stress and tension. The release of stress is a pleasant and satisfying feeling. Ritual learning refers to the special type of learning that takes place in many tribal initiations, cult formations, techniques of 'thought reform' and intensive religious persuasion (Bock 1980). Little is known about this type of learning but Wallace (1966: 239) argued that it is 'the rapid reorganisation of experience under conditions of stress, resulting in far-reaching cognitive and emotional changes'. However, others have argued that 'becoming a nuclear physicist, a communist, or a

Freudian involves a similar reorganisation of experience under stress' (Bock 1980: 190). Despite our difficulties in understanding the extreme forms of rites and rituals, we do have some knowledge of religious symbolism.

Rites and rituals within religious ceremonies may include engaging in some form of behaviour, such as praying, chanting or singing, or it may include not engaging in a prescribed action, such as fasting or avoiding certain foods. Religion and magic are not too dissimilar, in that invoking a blessing for a safe journey from either a priest or a shaman involves similar practices. Totemism and animism are two forms of religion found in smaller cultures (Giddens 1989a). Totemism refers to specific plants or animals that are believed to have supernatural powers, with each clan or group having its own totem. Although originating in the North American Indian tribal system, it has similarities to sports teams adopting a mascot, or an English county a flower. Animism is the belief in spirits that inhabit the world of humans. They can be either benign or malevolent, and may 'possess' a particular person.

Durkheim believed that religions could be defined according to a distinction between the sacred and the profane. Sacred objects, icons and symbols are held to be apart from the routine aspects of existence (the profane) and such objects are sacred because they represent the values of that group. For Durkheim the reverence that people hold for a sacred object is derived from the respect they have for their central social values. He argued that religion was not just a matter of belief but that all religions employed regular, ordered, ceremonial and ritual activities based on groups of believers coming together to join in a collective action. Thus, the rites and rituals produce a sense of group solidarity and, in short, the higher forces, totems, sacred objects or gods are the expression of the group over the individual. Although Durkheim's work on religion has been criticized (Stanmer 1975), it is a useful starting point for understanding the relationship between rites and rituals and everyday human action.

Rites and rituals as controlling mechanisms

Rites and rituals can also be viewed as forms of controlling mechanisms to maintain social stability. For example, we will all be familiar (at least from the television) with the rites and rituals of the courts of law, with their procedures, wigs, gowns and gavels. The symbol of the scales of justice reflects the power of the court to adjudicate on matters, mete out fines, imprison someone or, in some countries, pass the sentence of death. Durkheim believed that it was the rituals of punishment that reinforced the moral message of that society, and that this emphasis on the *moral* maintained social order. For Durkheim, although punishment had only a limited effect on criminal activity, there were symbolic and emotional elements to it. These elements made the ritual of punishment politically and socially functional. Historically, punishments handed out by courts were undertaken in public, as they are in some countries today, and the spectacle of their enactment served to strengthen and heighten the collective conscience. To a large extent punishments sentenced by the courts in the UK are now a private matter.

Further reading

 Durkheim, E. (1912) *The Elementary Forms of the Religious Life*. London: Allen & Unwin (1976 edn).

4.4 Taboos

At one level we will all be familiar with the concept of taboo, as it is a commonly used word in the English language. However, as with the rites and rituals above there are higher levels of meaning within the concept of taboo, which makes definitions difficult. Reber (1985: 757) in a succinct fashion defined taboo as 'any banned or prohibited act, object or behaviour'. But this succinctness does not do justice to the complex meaning of taboo, as behaviour such as speeding in a car may be prohibited but it does not carry the weight of a taboo. Taboo is a term that is derived from the Polynesian word *tabu*, which refers to something sacred or inviolable, and this clearly adds another dimension to it. In Polynesian culture the *tabu* may be concerned with anything sacred, such as food, place or activity, that is forbidden, and is closely related to their clan totem. As mentioned above, the rites and rituals surrounding such totems are in turn closely related to the values that are preciously held by that particular clan or group. Thus, breaking a *tabu* is considered immoral and reprehensible and, in effect, breaks the binding force that holds the culture together. In short, it is considered a very serious matter.

Taboos as communication

We have seen above that a central figure in sociology is Émile Durkheim and it is to this author that we turn in attempting to understand the meaning of taboo. The ways in which individuals are free to act in society may well be viewed as being reliant on the extent of our free will (6:5) and in response to our own volition. Yet to a large extent our choices are made for us through our behaviour being learnt in childhood. If we were born in another age and in another culture then our behaviour would be different from what it is today, according to Durkheim. He believed that the achievement of social life, through social order and social solidarity, was undertaken by agreed collective standards and normative behaviour. These values are taught to us in childhood, in school and in church, and in this sense a taboo is a communicative strategy to reinforce a social value and increase our social cohesion. The breaking of a taboo is seen as behaviour that goes beyond the mere realms of right and wrong, and communicates a message of extreme prohibition. Common taboos in childhood are taught through various expressions of shock at what might be called 'taboo behaviour', such as telling lies to parents or breaking the Brownies promise. A double message is applied, which informs the child that even though telling lies and breaking promises are wrong, telling lies to *parents* and breaking the *Brownies* promise are somehow *beyond* that, and located in the realm of taboo.

The meaning of taboo

Another major writer on taboo was Sigmund Freud. While we, strictly speaking, regard Freud as the father of psychoanalysis, we must remember that he also studied art, literature, history and anthropology, and was well versed in the theoretical constructs of his time. Bock (1980: 28) highlighted the fact that 'in the Freudian view, culture is to society as neurosis is to the individual. If we accept this proposition it follows that institutions may be analysed to reveal their latent content and the conflicts that they at once mask and are meant to resolve.' In accepting this, Freud was then in a position to employ his knowledge of neuroses to interpret cultural institutions. In his book *Totem and Taboo* (1913), Freud suggested that some individuals with neuroses establish for themselves certain taboo prohibitions that they adhere to with the same veracity as primitive people obey the communal taboos of their tribal society. Freud warns us, though, that the similarity between a neurotic's individual prohibition, say to touch something or to avoid it as in the case of an obsessive–compulsive disorder, and the social taboo may only be superficial. He claims that a 'touching phobia' is derived from parental prohibition of the young child's desire to touch his or her own genitals. However, because of the child's love of their parents, although the parental taboo is accepted, the prohibition does not abolish the desire, it merely represses the instinct into the unconscious. The principal characteristic underlying this person's later psychological make-up is ambivalence; that is, the coexistence of antithetic emotions, attitudes or ideas. Freud's search for a clearer understanding of taboo led him to analyse numerous cultures and thematically identify three broad types.

- *Taboos and treatment of the enemy*. In many tribal people there are sets of rules regarding the treatment of the slain enemy. While the dead person is offered gifts and prayers until they are considered 'appeased', the victor is placed within a framework of taboos. In this he may be socially isolated and cannot touch or be touched, and certain food taboos may apply, until the appeasement is complete or the victor is 'purified'. Freud suggests that there is emotional ambivalence towards the enemy involving hostility and admiration, which requires appeasement of the 'ghost' and prohibition of the killer.

- *Taboos and surrounding rulers*. Freud suggested that many tribal people consider their rulers to have far-reaching powers over nature and hold such rulers in high esteem, but on the other hand also impose many unpleasant restrictions on their lives. The taboo rituals apply excessive solitude, which Freud believed represented an unconscious hostility towards the rulers. He argued that their importance was elevated so that they could be blamed for any disappointments.

- *Taboos and the surrounding dead.* Freud noted the extensive use of taboos regarding the bodily contact of the dead, and the use of purification ceremonies if the taboo had been transgressed. He also noted the taboos regarding the use of the deceased person's name to increase the fear of the dead. Positing the question of why it was that a loved one in life should become such a fearful spirit in death, Freud suggested that it was the projection of hostility on to the dead person, which was rooted in ambivalent feelings towards them. This is seen in our own taboo of 'not speaking ill of the dead'.

There are many taboos in our society that have these elements in them. These taboo elements were neatly elucidated in a linear fashion by Bock (1980), who claimed there were *taboo prohibitions*, which when violated resulted in *pollution or contagion*, which then required *purification or renunciation*. In our society the crossing of a picket line was considered a taboo, which when broken polluted and contaminated the person, resulting in him being termed a 'scab'. Purification of this contagion required social isolation, in some cases considered to be a permanent state. Similarly, there are many taboos throughout the professional cultures in health care settings and we would name 'whistle-blowing' as one example. Despite, at one level, the contemporary move to encourage workers in the health care professions to bring to light bad practices, with some success, at another level the breaking of this taboo continues to carry some pollution. This is evidenced by those 'whistle-blowers' who have had great difficulty gaining employment following their allegations, even to the extent that some have had to move to another country. Thus, taboos are deeply entrenched in history, ideology and tradition.

Further reading

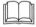

Freud, S. (1913) *Totem and Taboo*. New York: Norton (1950 edn).

4.5 Cultures

For us, the importance of understanding culture is set in the everyday use of the term as it is applied to the medical culture, the nursing culture, the hospital culture, the theatre culture, the psychiatric culture and so on. Like so many concepts popularized by common parlance, we 'know' what they mean and the manner in which we use them. However, as we have seen, they also tend to have higher, or, if preferred, deeper, levels of meaning, which, we would argue, if understood provide us with the potential for creating change.

There are numerous ways of defining what a culture is, but it should be noted that there is little agreement among sociologists and anthropologists.

Giddens (1989a: 18) suggested that when the term is used in everyday practice it usually refers to the 'higher things of the mind – art, literature, music and painting'. However, he goes on to explain that when employed by sociologists it includes a lot more: 'culture refers to the ways of life of the members of a society, or of groups within a society. It includes how they dress, their marriage customs and family life, their patterns of work, religious ceremonies and leisure pursuits' (Giddens 1989a: 18). Here we begin to see the all-encompassing nature of the concept of culture. From a founding figure in social anthropology, Sir Edward Tylor, we have an even wider catchment: 'culture . . . taken in its wide ethnographic sense is that complex whole which includes knowledge, belief, art, morals, law, custom, and any other capabilities and habits acquired by man as a member of society' (Tylor, 1871: 1). This interesting definition produces, at least some, agreement by anthropologists: first, that the definition implies that culture is learnt rather than being inherited genetically; and, second, that it is social in nature rather than being the property of the individual. So, in putting the problem of definition of culture to one side, we would finish with a particularly apt statement from Peacock (1986: 2): '[culture is] an enduring way of thinking and of ordering our lives that survives the struggle to survive. Whatever culture is, "it's real". At least something is, which we can conveniently label "culture".'

Culture and nature

The main distinction to be drawn in the culture versus nature debate concerns the historical concepts of race, gender and instinct. Throughout the colonial period it became fashionable to refer to the colonized people as a 'race' that was thought to be distinct from the colonizing group. These 'races' were often defined by attributing qualities to them, and we thus have the lazy African race or the happy-go-lucky Malay race (Peacock 1986). Within the British Isles we often hear of the dour Scot, the talkative Irish, the hot-headed Welsh and the stiff upper lipped English. Attribution of these cultural variations to genetic determinants formed the basis of nineteenth-century racism (2:11), and although scientific knowledge has revealed no such genetic basis, racism continues today. As Peacock (1986: 25) observes, 'racism is rife throughout the world, whether among American whites describing blacks; Australians, the Aborigines; Chinese, the Malay; or Hindu Brahmins, the "untouchables" '.

In terms of gender (2:5) we note the many differences that were supposedly genetically determined, such as men being dominant and assertive and women submissive and delicate. Until the current generation in the UK a woman's place was deemed to be in the home, while men went out to work. In this type of thinking, where these differences were considered genetically determined, education and learning to create change was considered a waste of time. Instinct was also a simplistic genetic explanation for behaviour, which could be attributed to racial differences. For example, kind or selfish, aggressive or passive, brave or cowardly, leader or follower are behaviours, which, it was argued, were given genetically at birth rather than being learnt through one's upbringing.

It is now accepted that all people on Earth probably originated from an African source and that any physical variations are adaptations in response to the extremes of environment in which people have lived over thousands of years. The way in which we live, i.e. different lifestyles, dress and foods etc., are what we know as cultural variations.

Culture and personality

We have dealt with personality in more depth in 3:3 and in this current context we refer to personality simply as a set of persistent characteristics of an individual, which can be inferred from a sample of a person's behaviour (Bock 1980). Psychological anthropologists have studied culture and personality for many years and suggest that the behavioural characteristics that determine a personality can be viewed in three ways: as traits (distinctive behavioural patterns), as character (interpersonal dispositions) or as modes of organization (the integration of behaviour and experience). To map the relationship between culture and personality, Bock (1980) highlighted three ways in which to express this.

- A culture is *like* a personality; that is, a culture needs to be explored on many different levels in order to understand it. As in our usage of the word 'personality', in which many behavioural regularities are assessed before we conclude on a person's personality, a culture requires the analysis of many behavioural systems.

- The patterns of a culture are connected by symbolic and logical linkages. To analyse these a person must be alert and sensitive to the linkages and they must get behind the explicit meaning of a word, a gesture, a belief etc., in order to explore the implicit level of linkage.

- Culture and personality are human systems that seek and create meaning. Anthropologists, as well as psychologists, study human behaviour at an individual level. That is, they observe the individual as a cultural microcosm.

In the study of cultures one is attempting to analyse the form or pattern of human behaviour, above and beyond the individual action. This is similar to 'knowing' a piece of music, not by the individual notes, but by the overall melody. This is achieved by appreciating *the relationship between* the notes, just as one would know the melody even if it were transposed into a different key, as long as the relationship between each note was maintained. The meaning is maintained in the pattern.

The relationship between culture and personality reveals itself when we observe cultural human behaviour in relation to child rearing. This was particularly important for Freudian theory, in which childhood experiences determined adult personality. Three examples should suffice. The first is the Russian behaviour of swaddling infants tightly, which is said to be undertaken to encourage an adult character who is prone to extremes of emotion (Gorer and Rickman 1949). The second concerns Balinese mothers' habit of sexually stimulating their child to arouse them and then undercutting their aroused desire to encourage a withdrawn personality in later adult life (Bateson and Mead 1942). Finally, it is said that in American families, rearing children to be independent and self-reliant serves to encourage self-blame, whereas rearing them in group activities and environments encourages them to blame others (Whiting and Child 1953). Although these detailed studies are reduced to single simple sentences here, the basis on which they are offered in full is complex.

Further reading

Bock, P. K. (1980) *Rethinking Psychological Anthropology: Continuity and Change in the Study of Human Action*. New York: W. H. Freeman and Co.
Elias, N. (1970) *What Is Sociology?* London: Hutchinson.
Macbeth, H. and Shetty, P. (2000) *Health and Ethnicity*. London: Routledge.

4.6 Tradition

In the previous section (4:5) we saw how cultures perpetuated themselves through shared learning and we follow this, in this section, by focusing on the specific concept of tradition. Tradition is that body of knowledge and practice that comes from the past, and it usually refers to information and action that are handed down from generation to generation. Tradition can be seen in a positive light as opinions, beliefs and behaviour that are held in high regard and link us to our ancestors. However, tradition can also be viewed as negative, with the links to the past needing to be severed, as in a revolution. If they are viewed as positive they will tend to reinforce behaviour, and if seen negatively they will tend to change behaviour. An important aspect of tradition concerns the way in which cultures are reproduced from generation to generation. They carry the weight of authority in the present in relation to the perceived high regard in which they were held in the past. This authority is the very point on which traditions are challenged by those who seek to overthrow them. Tradition can be seen as subtle and flexible deployments of reason in some spheres, but can also be viewed as indefensibly irrational strategies to maintain a particular status quo. We now deal with these issues in a little more detail.

Cultural reproduction

Tradition is an educational strategy that is taught both formally and informally. Children spend the majority of their time, especially in early childhood, either in school or at home, and it is in these two institutions that the importance, or not, of tradition is taught. Illich (1973) argues that in schools children are indoctrinated with what he termed *passive consumption* based on the organization, discipline and regimentation that the schools involve. This passive consumption, Illich argues, leads to an uncritical acceptance of the existing social order. The information that is taught in this scenario is not the formal curriculum but the hidden one, which is implicit in the school's procedures. Illich suggests that obligatory schools teach children 'to know their place and to sit still in it' (Illich 1973: 42). The learning of values, attitudes, beliefs and ideologies is fundamental to the notion of tradition and schools make reputations for themselves in relation to what they believe to be the rights and wrongs of life.

Cultural reproduction (Bourdieu and Passeron 1977; Bourdieu 1986, 1988) refers to the way in which schools and other social institutions maintain social and economic inequalities from generation to generation. The school is the disciplinary authority, with the teachers seen as those who are in charge, and children get an early glimpse of what the future world of work will be like for them. Those children from lower-class backgrounds experience a greater cultural clash when they first go to school and develop ways of talking and behaving that are different from those from higher-class environments (Bernstein 1975). In the latter group higher academic standing would generally prevail to a larger extent than it would in the lower-class group. An example should serve to reinforce this point.

Paul Willis studied a school in Birmingham in an attempt to explain how cultural reproduction works. He set himself the question: 'how do working-class kids get working-class jobs?' As a fieldworker Willis spent a long time at the school getting to know the pupils, and he spent a considerable amount of time with one gang of boys known as 'the lads'. Willis found that this gang had an excellent understanding of the school's authority system and used this knowledge to fight it. They enjoyed the conflict with the school and constantly battled against the teachers' weak points. They knew just how far to push and also knew when they themselves were vulnerable. Willis describes this thus: ' "the lads" specialise in a caged resentment which always stops just short of outright confrontation. Settled in class, as near a group as they can manage, there is a continuous scraping of chairs, a bad-tempered "tut-tutting" at the simplest request, and a continuous fidgeting about which explores every permutation of sitting or lying on a chair' (Willis 1977: 12). 'The lads' saw their future work in the same light, as a constant conflict with authority. However, it should be noted that they were actually looking forward to it and would only recognize in later life that they were trapped in a working-class job. Willis showed that the cultural tradition of lower-class kids getting lower-class jobs was based on the values that 'the lads' held while in school.

Tradition and authority

As we have briefly mentioned above, tradition carries some element of authority that is based on power and status. Weber (1922) identified three types of authority.

- *Traditional authority*. This is based on the unquestioning acceptance of the distribution of power in any given society. A type of legitimacy is given to the power, through the person who holds a particular position, because it has 'always been that way'.

- *Character authority*. In this scenario the person holding a particular position is considered to have very special qualities and there is commitment and loyalty towards them. The word of the charismatic person is considered all important.

- *Rational-legal authority*. This type of authority is based on a legal framework in which the distribution of power among individuals and groups in society is maintained by regulation. The organization itself, rather than the individuals in it, is seen as supreme, and there is an emphasis on rules and procedures that must be obeyed.

Tradition and health

Traditional beliefs about medicine and health are briefly mentioned above (2:13), but here we outline two anthropological studies that have reported on what are considered traditional beliefs. The first example is a study of Navaho Indians, who believe that health is a relationship between man and his environment. This environment includes the supernatural world as well as the world around him. A healthy state is closely associated with good, blessing and beauty, which are all viewed as positive values in life. On the other hand, illness is related to evidence that the person has fallen out of this balance. It is usually associated with the breaking of a taboo or contact with the spirits of the dead. It can also be related to another member of the tribe who has resorted to witchcraft. Thus, religion and medicine are seen as aspects of the same thing, unlike in our system where they are seen as separate entities. Western medicine has failed to understand this, and some contemporary Navaho Indians who have interfaced with modern medicine have been antagonized by this ignorance (Adair *et al.* 1957).

Our second example is from an Indian village in Hyderabad state, where an anthropologist reports that most of the common illnesses are associated with a fault in the physical system, which includes a strict adherence to the ritual cycle of festivals. Certain conditions, such as common colds, headaches, stomach ache, scabies, gonorrhoea and syphilis, are considered to be natural ailments and attempts to cure them are via medicines. However, other conditions, such as persistent headaches, intermittent fevers, continual stomach disorders, wasting diseases among children, menstrual disorders and repeated miscarriages, are associated with supernatural forces. In these conditions medicines and appeals to these forces are attempted together. Other conditions, such as blindness, smallpox, cholera and plague, are seen as the result of the wrath of a number of goddesses and no medicines are given, as worship is seen as the cure (Dube 1955).

No matter how much some might dismiss traditional beliefs about medicine and health, they maintain their cultural legitimacy through the weight of ancestral authority. They are a source of social stability and are seen as a communal inheritance.

Further reading

Hayek, F. A. (1988) *The Fatal Conceit*. London: Routledge.

PART TWO: APPLICATION TO PRACTICE

4.7 Nursing cultures

We saw above (4:5) that culture can be defined in an all-encompassing way to include the knowledge, belief, art, laws, customs and so on of a particular group, but we also noted that although accurate definitions of culture are difficult we tended to know it when we saw it. In terms of nursing cultures we can say that they are based on the traditional values that give the profession its identity and evolve in relation to the changing environments and supportive frameworks that surround practice. However, as we will see, there is nothing in this to ensure that nursing cultures naturally become positive entities. In the quest to become accepted as a profession in its own right nursing has attempted to throw off its long established image of being a handmaiden to the doctor. Stacy (1988) suggested that the nursing profession emerged out of the religious orders that used to care for the sick during the eighteenth and nineteenth centuries. The early nursing role largely being domestic work. Throughout the twentieth century the main nursing role mainly involved intimate contact with the patient's body surface and their various bodily waste products (Helman 2000), whereas the 'doctor' rarely had contact with bodily wastes and developed a specialized knowledge of the inner biological workings of the body. Contemporary nursing is keen to shed this traditional role and develop specialized knowledge and skills in equipment, technology and procedures. In this the culture of nursing, and the development of nursing cultures, will now be discussed.

Nursing cultural formations

Social anthropologists have studied nursing cultures for some considerable time, but these have largely focused on psychiatric ward cultures (Richman 1989). The published work on general nursing cultures is sparse, but what we can glean from this source is that the human dynamic is complex. For example, Littlewood (2000) suggested that nursing cultures form in relation to the patient group being cared for. She argued that in a search for a more hermeneutic method of nursing children, in a culturally sensitive way, nurses themselves develop their own 'children's nurses' culture. This is interesting, as it leads us to ponder whether all specific patient populations can have an effect on how we develop our own nursing cultures. In another study, Olson

(1993) examined three nursing cultures in three separate hospitals in Oregon. This author used multiple research methods, including a quantitative 15-item questionnaire and a qualitative cultural assessment inventory. The findings indicated that while two of the hospitals' nursing cultures operated in harmony with other professions, one of the hospitals' nursing culture had considerable elements of disharmony. The findings were used by managers to devise organizational strategies, to facilitate change and to educate nursing staff.

In a descriptive study of two nursing units in Pennsylvania, Wilson (1989) analysed nursing cultures in relation to their organizational structure. Certain elements emerged from this work that give us some indication as to how nursing cultures are formed and maintained. This author suggested that the nurses' view on their power status was a major factor in shaping the nursing culture. Autonomous working and influence in decision-making enabled nurses to work more effectively, it was suggested. Other factors included the relationship between the head nurse and junior staff, leadership accountabilities, group decision-making and the nursing curriculum under which they were taught. Thus, we can see that the nursing culture is finely tuned in response to a wide array of factors, including the values of traditional nursing, the patient population, the environment in which practice is performed and the organizational structure, which would include rules, regulations and sanctions. In another study, Mason (1993) investigated the formation and maintenance of a nursing culture and identified certain strategies by which nurses attempted to resist challenges to their culture. Humour was employed as derision towards anyone, or any strategy, that attempted to create positive change. This derision was self-reinforcing, as more and more of the peer group joined in the laughter. A second strategy was the use of the concept of 'dangerousness', which was employed to create fear of any change by suggesting that it was dangerous. Although we need much more work in this area of nursing cultures, we can begin to see that it is a highly complex area and this was neatly outlined by Burnard (1995), who analysed the nursing conference and suggested that it functions as a microcosm of the overall nursing profession. Although only a short, and tongue-in-cheek, paper, it gives some interesting glimpses into the nursing cultural world.

Explicit and implicit nursing cultural forms

If, as we note above (4:5), cultures are concerned with forms or patterns of human behaviour that are linked to traditions, values, morals and so on, then we need to explore the development of nursing cultures in relation to the images representing these behaviours. For example, the long-standing explicit image of nurses as 'angels' is clearly seen in relation to the dedication that is socially expected in the care of the sick. However, as we note above, the implicit reference point is that nursing is a 'vocation' based on the management of bodily wastes (Helman 2000), and does not need to carry secular rewards, as the later divine reward will be greater. Thus, sacrifice is an intrinsic element of many nursing cultures. But what of the representation of nurses in pornographic material? Many pornographic pictures display women in nurses' uniform producing the image of overt sexual desire, sauciness and availability (Orr 1988; Mercer and McKeown 1997). The dichotomy between 'angel' and 'tart' was neatly displayed in the *Carry On Doctor* film of the 1960s, with Hattie Jacques as the matronly figure of dedication and Barbara Windsor as the ebullient sexual being. From the heavenly to the earthly; yet there is another dimension that needs a mention before we proceed, and that is the nursing cultures that go beyond these boundaries. These are represented by the many inquiry reports into allegations of abuse undertaken by nurses and the numerous nurses who are struck off the professional register each year. These are predominantly, but not exclusively, nurses working with the mentally ill, mentally handicapped, elderly or children, in short, nurses caring for vulnerable groups. As an example, in this short space we focus on psychiatric nursing cultures.

Psychiatric nursing cultures

The research on psychiatric nursing cultures has a reasonably long lineage, although more commonly used terms for culture are 'milieu', 'atmosphere', 'climate' and 'organization' (Richman 1989). As early as 1954 Stanton and Schwartz were indicating the naming of a ward, the behaviour of nurses and the organizational philosophy as contributing factors in the development of nursing cultures. For example, wards labelled as 'disturbed', 'chronic', 'rehabilitation' and so on carried expectations as to what nursing behaviour was required. These descriptors are also known by patients, who employ their own evaluations of the nursing cultures that emerge (Richman 1989). Throughout the 1960s and 1970s scales were developed that claimed to measure cultural activities, such as interactions between staff and patients and structured programmes on the wards, the most influential of these being the Ward Atmosphere (Climate) Scale (Moos and Houts 1968). Probably the best known research into psychiatric cultures is Goffman's (1961) *Asylums*. In this ethnographic work Goffman undertook a series of studies at a mental hospital and described how such organizations can become total institutions. That is, they supply all elements of life for patients, including food, shelter, finances (meagre), shops and recreation, thus making the person become dependent and institutionalized.

We finish this section with a study of non-professional nursing care in a psychiatric setting, which was titled 'The tradition of toughness'. Eileen Morrison (1990) studied the relationship between organizational factors and violence, and reported an incisive taxonomy of cultural behaviour. She identified two staff norms: (a) the need for physical restraint; and (b) it's not you we don't trust. In the former new nurses are socialized into behaving in a controlling manner by emphasis on the need for control. The latter is concerned with socializing patients into the hospital system through explication of a set of rules and regulations. Morrison goes on to outline the primary role for unqualified (non-professional) staff as being 'enforcing', this having three components:

- *Policing*. This refers to the process of ensuring that the rules of the hospital or ward are adhered to. This is undertaken to maintain control of patients' behaviour.
- *Supermanning*. This involves a leader emerging from among the 'enforcers'. This is usually the toughest person and the one who sanctions physical behaviours that are deemed necessary to maintain control. Another aspect of the 'superman' role is to protect the other staff, which brings high status.
- *Putting on a show*. This involves the nursing staff giving textbook answers about therapeutic approaches to any official visitor to the ward, but behind the scenes being rough and abusive to patients.

Although we cannot generalize to all psychiatric settings, nor would we wish to, we feel that these strategies identified by Morrison are common enough to warrant attention in many psychiatric nursing cultural settings. We would argue that many nursing cultures, including general nursing areas, have nurses who like to enforce rules (i.e. strict visiting procedures), who like to be known as 'supernurses' (i.e. able to handle the most difficult of 'cases') or who like to 'put on a show' of therapeutic knowledge but engage in chicanery (guessing the patient's temperature etc.). In any event, there is sufficient anecdotal evidence to suggest that there are many aspects of nursing culture yet to be explored, and anthropological methods offers us one approach to engage in this.

Further reading

Beattie, J. (1989) *Other Cultures: Aims, Methods and Achievements in Social Anthropology*. London: Routledge.
Goffman, E. (1961) *Asylums: Essays on the Social Situation of Mental Patients and Other Inmates*. New York: Anchor Books.
Holden, P. and Littlewood, J. (1991) *Anthropology and Nursing*. London: Routledge.

▌4.8 Exploding nursing myths and taboos

Myths and taboos have complex meaning above and beyond the often simplistic story that accompanies them (4:2, 4:4). Myths are communicative strategies to inform and teach about long-standing beliefs, values and ideologies, and taboos communicate messages about right and wrong, good and bad, and ways of behaving in our cultural setting. Nursing myths and taboos are no different, but we should remember that nursing itself is a part of the wider society and has developed alongside the other professional groups. Therefore, myths and taboos within the nursing profession often mirror those in other disciplines, as well as those in general society. Myths and taboos are communicated through stories, and the philosophy of the 'story' is a complex matter indeed. Before writing materials emerged the word of mouth was the only means of passing down histories and information regarding ancestors. Yet since the invention of the written word we still enjoy a good story being told, often repeatedly. We know that stories differ according to the teller and that they are often embellished as to the details. However, the fundamental message, often implicit, will remain the same. Humour is frequently employed and is itself a complex concept, alongside the serious nature of the message being conveyed. Witty remarks, jokes and comedy, although hidden from 'official' view, are often utilized in the most serious of situations to alleviate stress. There can be few readers of this text who have not told such a story or enjoyed listening to one. On the propriety of such story-telling we would not comment, but on its role and function in creating and maintaining nursing myths and taboos we will.

Rational and irrational configurations

Robert Graves, in his role as the editor of the *New Larousse Encyclopedia of Mythology* (1986), claims that myths have two main functions. The first concerns answering the awkward questions that children pose, such as 'who made the world?', 'when will it end?' and 'where do souls go when bodies die?' The ability to provide an answer to these questions gives the teller enormous power and profundity. The second function of myths, according to Graves, is to provide a justification for an existing social system and meaning for traditional rites, customs and practices. If Graves is correct, and we do not have any reason to doubt him, myths and taboos employ both a rational and an irrational component, or put another way they have both a credible and an incredible element. This would link into the serious nature of the message and the use of humour, mentioned above, as juxtaposed concepts. Myths and taboos will differ according to context; for example, in cold climates the first humans were created through the licking of a frozen stone, and the afterworld is described as cold and featureless. Myths from warmer climes claim that humans were created by kneading mud on a flowery river bank, and see the afterworld as warm, celestial meadhalls (Graves 1986). What these myths share in common is the underlying 'explanation' for life and death.

We will outline a traditional myth to emphasize the rational and irrational components. Most people would have heard of Pegasus, the winged horse. However, few of us would be able to recall that Pegasus is supposed to have sprung from the blood of Medusa, a gorgon who had her head severed by Perseus. Pegasus is said to have carried numerous gods away from danger or towards a destiny, and is also said to have created the spring of the Muses (goddesses of poetry, art, literature etc.) on Mount Helicon by a blow of his hoof. Eventually Pegasus flew off and was transformed into a constellation. In contemporary astronomy Pegasus is the large constellation of stars in the northern hemisphere and is the seventh largest in the sky. In the myth of Pegasus the irrational elements are clear, in that a flying horse springing from someone's severed neck is rather incredible. The need for speed in avoiding danger or travelling to an assignation is clearly logical and the creation of an animal based on the strength of a horse and the speed of a bird is obvious. Some nursing myths and taboos will now be outlined in relation to these properties.

Some nursing myths and taboos

The starting point, for us, in dealing with the types of nursing myths and taboos involves 'tall tales'. Hewison (1999) called these the 'tales of the expected' and claimed that they were a feature of all organizations. In terms of the NHS he argued that many of these stories were apocryphal tales, including such themes as 'Heard about the nurses who lost a body on the way to the mortuary, or the student who cleaned patients' dentures in a washing-up bowl?' (Hewison 1999: 32). In describing these apocryphal tales, otherwise known as urban myths, Hewison gives us the example of a new student nurse caring for a patient with myocardial infarction who was confined to bed. As the patient needed to have his bowels opened the student sought advice from the staff nurse. The advice was to help the patient on to a commode. A few minutes later the staff nurse noticed the patient's head peeping above the curtain drawn around the bed for privacy. The student had stuck to her instructions by helping the patient on to the commode on top of the bed! This type of nursing myth is concerned with the limitations of following instructions to the letter.

Of course, not all nursing myths and taboos can be taken in a light-hearted manner. In dealing with the nursing taboo of euthanasia, Louis (1992) highlighted a clear tension: 'allowing a patient to die means nurses are torn between their responsibility to preserve life and judging when that approach can no longer be sensibly applied' (Louis 1992: 37). Passive euthanasia is the point where it is accepted that the patient cannot be cured and that palliative treatment should begin. However, this is increasingly difficult to ascertain given the advancements in medical technology. Whatever nurses are taught in terms of the legal and professional position relating to decisions on the subject of withdrawing treatment and allowing someone to die is one thing, but there is evidence, or at least a hint of it, that they do make such decisions (Goldberg 1987; Anonymous 1988; Thom 1989). Stories of these taboos abound in nursing and highlight a tension between practice and law, morality and theory.

Another area of nursing, as well as other parts of life, in which myths and taboos thrive concerns sexual matters, or more accurately issues related to sexuality. For example, there is often a reluctance to raise psychosexual issues with patients, particularly those with disabilities. Glass (1995: 251) suggested that 'a major reason for this failure centres around the cultural and social taboos concerning discussion of sexuality and the common misconception that the sexual needs of those with disabilities are lower'. He went on to argue for the adoption of supportive practices within rehabilitation units to address psychosexual dysfunction in neurological disorders, and outlined a strategy for this. There are a wide range of neurotraumas in which this strategy could help, including spinal injury, multiple sclerosis, spina bifida and lower motor neurone difficulties. It is not only for those with physical problems that myths and taboos can hinder patient care, but also for some with mental health problems. McCann (2000: 132) argues that 'while mental health professionals should recognize that people suffering from schizophrenia have sexual and relationship requirements, there appears to be a failure to address adequately the subject of human sexuality, particularly in the area of psychosocial rehabilitation'. The apparent reluctance on the part of the mental health professional to address this issue is based on the myth that schizophrenic patients have a reduced capacity, and desire, for sexual intimacy and personal relationships, which provides the justification to prevent involvement. Finally, on the sexual issue, O'Dowd (2000) reports on a pioneering initiative in Glasgow: a one-stop shop for sexual health. This programme aims directly at removing sexual taboos and under one roof its range of services includes family planning, sexual health advisory service, a centre for women's health and one for men's health, a young person's clinic, vasectomies and a drop-in clinic for prostitutes.

In the early 1990s a scoring system for assessing the severity of illness in young babies under 6 months of age was developed, known as Baby Check. It comprised of 19 observations, one of which was the taking of rectal temperature. It was based on four years of scientific research but at its launch in 1991 it was 'hi-jacked by an unexpected fierce attack from the Royal College of Midwives' (Handysides 1993: 673). The Royal College of Midwives argued that rectal thermometry in such young babies would cause an increase in parental anxiety, rectal damage and allegations of sexual abuse. Handysides (1993) claimed that this was clearly a battle between science and social taboos. There are many other areas of nursing that we could outline in relation to myths and taboos that the discerning student may wish to pursue; for example, depression in the elderly (Anonymous 1997), female circumcision (Jackson 1991) and food beliefs (Abdussalam and Kaferstein 1996). Unfortunately space does not allow us to develop these here.

Further reading

Healey, P. and Glanville, R. (1994) *Urban Myths Unplugged*. London: Virgin.
Williams, S. J., Gabe, J. and Calnan, M. (2000) *Health, Medicine and Society: Key Theories, Future Agendas*. London: Routledge.

4.9 Rites of passage

Rites of passage (*rites de passage*) concerns the rituals that are associated with the social transition from one status to another in society. They are said to exist in all societies, in one form or another, and involve rituals of pregnancy, childbirth, puberty, menarche, weddings, funerals and severe ill-health (Helman 2000). These rituals help to prepare the person to act in a new role, say in the move from 'adolescent' to 'adult', or from 'wife' to 'mother'. Although some transitional roles are not clearly delineated – for example, between pre- and post-pubertal states – others are; for example, when a couple are pronounced 'man and wife'. None the less, the rituals that are performed at these times are underscored by the values that represent the expected behaviours attached to those roles. Van Gennep (1960), a leading expert in this area, identified three stages in the rites of passage: (a) separation; (b) transition; and (c) incorporation. The stage of separation involves isolating the person from the normal social sphere, the second stage is concerned with the actual change in status, or new role, and the third involves a return to normal social functioning but in the changed circumstances.

Nursing rites of passage

Initiation rites are often painful. For example, the passage rites for a young Native American brave achieving a warrior status involve the setting of numerous challenges that the young male must overcome. Similarly, in many of our industrialized organizations workers set a number of informal 'initiation ceremonies' in which newcomers are subjected to performing a particular task. The task is, of course, a 'sting' and the newcomer displays ignorance and naivety. The new student nurse may be sent to the next ward for a bucket of Fallopian tubes or taught to test for glucose in urine by tasting the sweetness of it. Although the propriety of these actions is questionable the important point is that the operation of these rites serves a function. They contribute to the in-group solidarity for those employing the deception and they also reinforce the idea of the superior wisdom of those 'in the know'. The targeted person is expected to display embarrassment but is also expected to take it in good spirits, in order for them to be incorporated into the group. Unfortunately, they also carry some negative connotations, as they can lead to isolating the person and maintaining them as a member of an out-group. These initiation rites may leave the person ostracized and socially excluded, particularly if the target person does not react in the expected way or if these rites are undertaken malevolently.

Hospital rites of passage

When a person becomes seriously ill they may be taken away from their community and admitted to hospital (separation). The role of the health care worker is to help the patient to make the change from being an ill person to a healthy one (transition). Once this is achieved the now healthy person is reinstated into their society (incorporation). Seen in relation to van Gennep's (1960) stages we can now note a number of rituals that may be undertaken in the three stages of the patient's hospitalization: admission, treatment and discharge.

When someone is admitted into hospital they cross a threshold from their normal lives into a hospitalized existence, which is characterized by a lack of control for them. The admission procedure is an administrative process that removes the main aspects of their social identity. Their outdoor clothes may be removed and their prized possessions locked away. Night-wear is usually the order of both day and night and is a dispossessor of power and control. Choice is greatly reduced and patients await orders of what they must do, and when. They are given an identity band that must not be removed and allocated a bed and locker that defines their space. During the transition stage the patient becomes a 'case' to receive all manner of investigations. They receive a diagnostic label and a treatment programme, which they are expected to comply with. They should accept advice from all health care workers and move through the treatment programme at the expected pace towards recovery. Incorporation is achieved through the ritual of discharge once the patient is considered healthy enough to be reintegrated back into their society. The patients must await permission for discharge and be the recipient of the process. Travel arrangements must be arranged for them and they must await medications 'to take away' (known as TTAs). The ritual of goodbye is undertaken with expressions of gratitude, and often a token gift (flowers, chocolates), from the patient. In some hospitals mothers are not allowed to carry their own newborn baby out of the hospital but must allow a nurse to carry it (ostensibly for insurance purposes), to be ritually handed over to the mother at the threshold of the door. Thus, we can see that rites of passage have an important part to play in being hospitalized.

Health care issues and rites of passage

The first issues to be dealt with are pregnancy and childbirth in relation to the rites of passage, as in most societies they are as much social events as they are biological ones. They involve the social transition, particularly in the case of the first newborn, from 'woman' to 'mother'. During the transitional period of her pregnancy she is considered vulnerable to dangers and in some cases a danger to others. In many cultures taboos of diet, dress and behaviour are in evidence at this stage. In modern Western obstetrics the ritual symbols used are those involving medical science and technology, but they can clearly be seen as part of the ritualism associated with a rite of passage (Davis-Floyd 1987). Davis-Floyd shows how the philosophical basis of contemporary childbirth was rooted in the seventeenth-century mechanistic idea of the body, which involved the separation of the mind and the body into two distinct entities, and thus allowed the removal of the soul to the realms of religion and the body to the 'men of science'. This, it is argued, allowed male domination over midwifery. The technological focus on separating the baby from the mother in childbirth ignores the birth of the new social status of the mother. Pregnancy and childbirth, then, can be viewed as a social birth but in some cases, particularly young teenage pregnancies, they are also considered a 'social death' (Whitehead 2001).

Death is another area that carries rituals associated with the rites of passage. It is now recognized that in most societies we have two 'deaths', the first biological and the second social. The latter comes weeks, months or even years after the former. This is the transitional period in many belief systems, in which the soul is in a state of limbo, continuing to have some social rights. Many rituals and taboos exist, including the prohibition of marriage until a sufficient length of time has passed to allow for a social death to take place. In Western cultures too these social prohibitions occur but like childbirth itself death in our society has become an increasingly medical affair. Death is now considered a medical condition pronounced by medics alone. As stated above, Kubler-Ross (1970) outlined five stages in the rite of passage to death: denial and isolation, anger, bargaining, depression and acceptance (3:15) When someone is moving towards death, she argued, they can be greatly comforted by sharing emotions and coming to terms with their fate. This was alluded to, more recently, by Money (2000), who focused on shamanism as a complementary therapy in illness and healing, and death and dying. Working in a hospice, Froggatt (1997) explored how the nature and function of rituals could assist in relation to palliative care. Froggatt argued that using a rite of passage framework within a hospice can facilitate change for individuals, and is also helpful in allowing them to explore issues relating to the transition from life to death.

Another example of a health care issue and rites of passage comes from the work of Gutman (1999a, b) with males with traumatic brain injury (TBI) in relation to gender role strain. Young men (and women) with TBI may experience difficulty moving through adolescence into adulthood via the usual rites of this passage, e.g. dating/courtship experiences, independent community travel and shared apartment living in the community (Gutman 1999a). Through the development and evaluation of an occupational therapy programme aimed to assist this specific problem, Gutman (1999b: 101) reported that the intervention enabled them to achieve the following.

- Enhance their gender role satisfaction through newly rebuilt roles and activities.
- Attain certain long-held personal goals.
- Feel more like members of society.
- Perceive a greater congruency between their internal self-image and external post-injury roles.
- Learn more about their personal skills and values as men.
- Feel more comfortable using help-seeking behaviour.
- Feel a sense of shared experience and affinity.
- Feel more understood and accepted.
- Contribute to others through community member roles.

The excellent work of Gutman is a timely reminder of the overlay of anthropological theory and clinical health care practice.

Finally, two other related areas of health care can be briefly mentioned, and these are nurse education and organizational structure. People come in to nurse training, become student nurses, qualify as staff nurses and develop their careers. This is a socialization process that requires many rites of passage through many stages of this career development. The move from one status, in which one may feel comfortable and knowledgeable, to another status, in which worry and fear of the unknown feature large, can create stress and tension (Tradewell 1996). Many nurses will recall tales of the rite of passage known as the 'first day on the ward'.

Not only individuals but health care organizations as well may need to go through rites of passage. Moore (1991) provides an interesting account of corporate culture in which organizations strive for excellence in the delivery of patient care through improved productivity, recruitment and retention of staff, and financial returns. He argued that one way in which an organization can be helped towards such excellence is through rites and rituals that serve to strengthen group interactions. Some examples are given, which include every Friday being 'casual day', where no ties or suits are worn, positive myths and legends of previous great corporate leaders, and a spirit of freedom and learning from a reasonable number of mistakes. We may be able to recall some hospitals or departments that function in this manner, but we think it is fair to say that they are not in the majority. We can see that while rites of passage may be positive or negative, it is unlikely that we will ever be able to avoid them.

Further reading

Helman, C. G. (2000) *Culture, Health and Illness.* Oxford: Butterworth Heinemann.
Katz, P. (1981) Ritual in the operating room, *Ethnology*, 20: 335–50.
Walsh, M. and Ford, P. (1989) *Nursing Rituals, Research and Rational Actions.* Oxford: Heinemann.

4.10 Hierarchies and castes in nursing

Few walks of life do not have some form of hierarchical structuring, from religious groups to the armed forces, from schools to business cartels and from governments to families. The health care profession is no different, and all professions within this service structure their discipline according to such hierarchies. We have seen above (4:5) that caste systems are structured according to hierarchy, and although there may be a hierarchical structure within a particular group, that group itself may be part of a wider hierarchical framework. To take an example, say that all the heads of state of all the countries in the world were to form a group. Within that group a hierarchy of the most dominant, most powerful, most influential etc. may develop, with one head of state emerging as *the* 'top' person. Of course, in our example, heads of state are only one such powerful group, and if we were to do a similar hierarchical structuring with, say, religious leaders around the world it might be that a 'top' religious leader would emerge. Now, these political and religious hierarchies, with all their gradations from 'top' to 'bottom', could be butted against each other to see who would really come out on 'top', and where each subsequent grade within each hierarchy could be located in their counterpart hierarchy. This, of course, is hypothetical and would be highly complex to undertake in reality, as there are so many different factors and variables to deal with. The point we are trying to make is that we can, for the sake of example, replace these two hierarchies with the hierarchies of medicine and nursing, juxtapose them and consider who would be above the other at the differing levels, i.e. medical director–matron, or senior registrar, house officer, junior medical student–ward sister. Of course, again, this is hypothetical and would be difficult to achieve in reality, as, again, there are so many variables to consider. None the less, it helps us to begin to understand that hierarchies and castes are not only complex entities within themselves but also dynamically different when we attempt to view one group in relation to another.

Types of hierarchies and castes in health care

We have briefly mentioned the two obvious hierarchies in health care, those of medicine and nursing. However, many more exist; in fact, as many as there are disciplines and groups in the health care process. These include the professional groups of psychology, social work, radiography, pharmacology, physiotherapy, optometry, phlebotomy and paramedics, as well as the many technical services. Non-clinical professional groups include the support facilities, such as the hotel services (catering, laundry, domestics, portering). They also include the numerous hierarchies and castes within the business element of health care delivery, such as managerial, finance and personnel. Each of these groups will have its own hierarchical structure and taken together we can see that the whole can be viewed as a caste system. However, when we bring in that other group so central to the notion of health care delivery, the patients, the scenario becomes even more complex. Patients have been variously described as 'at the bottom of the pile', 'at the top of the pyramid' and 'at the hub of the wheel'. In fact, all are correct at one level or another.

In an emergency triage situation this hierarchical structure suggests that those most in need, from a life-threatening point of view, come first. However, in terms of the more mundane care delivery it is often the value system of the health care professional that determines who gets what and when (Stockwell 1972; Hartman 1992). Patients are sometimes treated not unsympathetically, but judgementally according to the perceived accountability that they are perceived to have for their illness or injury. For example, in terms of domestic violence on women they may sometimes be criticized for returning to the home to be further abused, and some health care staff may have difficulty in bracketing out their personal views on this (Warshaw 1993). Patients themselves can place their conditions in a 'pseudo-hierarchy' relating to how they perceive they have behaved in relation to their conditions (Lowy and Ross 1994). Finally, Mastro *et al.* (1996: 197) reported on a study of the attitudes of elite athletes with impairments towards each other in relation to a hierarchy of preference. They reported that 'the participants' responses toward other impairment groups, ordered from most to least favorable attitudes, were amputations, les autres, para/quadriplegia, visual impairment, and cerebral palsy' (Mastro *et al.* 1996: 197). It would seem that hierarchies and castes form a large part of health care delivery, as well as being ubiquitous in everyday life.

Aspects of professional and organizational health care hierarchies and castes

Professions are said to have certain characteristics, such as the use of skills grounded in theory, training and education regarding these skills, competence measured by examination, a code of conduct, providing a service for the public good and a professional body to which it is accountable (Millerson 1964). These characteristics set the scene in formulating the structural components below. Organizations are also said to have certain characteristics in terms of the ideal type of bureaucracy. These include: a distinct hierarchy of authority; rules and regulations to govern the conduct of members; members being employed and receiving a salary; separation of work within and life outside the organization; and non-ownership of the materials of the organization (Weber 1904). Drawing these two sets of characteristics together, we can outline a number of aspects of professional and organizational health care hierarchical structures.

- *Ability*. Within each role, at any level, it is expected that the person holding that position has the ability, skills and competencies to do so.
- *Knowledge*. It is anticipated that the functioning of the skills pertaining to the role is underpinned by knowledge based on scientific evidence or accepted practice.
- *Decision-making*. Each hierarchical grade carries some element of decision-making capacity that varies according to the level of responsibility.
- *Responsibility*. The higher up the role within the hierarchy, the greater is the degree of responsibility.
- *Status*. Each grade carries a degree of status commensurate with the scale of the hierarchy.
- *Power*. Accompanying the foregoing aspect, power, influence and authority are determined by the level achieved in the hierarchy.
- *Accountability*. The higher up the pyramid one goes, the more one is given, but the accompanying downside is that it is accompanied by expectations, and thus the greater the accountability.

Of course, we can see that it is difficult to locate where some of these aspects originate from, except to state that they fundamentally emanate from the society in which they operate. For example, in terms of status and power, who can give such power for the professions to wield over others, other than members of society, to which professions, organizations and governments are ultimately accountable in a democratic society? It is in the relationship between the individual in a hierarchy, the hierarchy and the profession, the profession and the organization and the organization and the society that the issue of accountability is located. Furthermore, when issues of abuse of hierarchical power are raised, as they often are, again it is probably within this accountability framework that the source of the problem is rooted.

It is when these aspects of the hierarchical structuring begin to have a negative impact on patient care that great concern is expressed. Akinleye (1991) studied differences between nurses and doctors in two hospitals in relation to their position in the organizational hierarchy and their decision-making capacity regarding selection and acquisition of medical equipment. The main relevant finding for us here is that there was a minor significant difference between levels within the hierarchy and decision-making, but no difference whether one was a nurse or a doctor. Thus, we can conclude from this that the profession itself made no negative impact on care delivery but that the hierarchical positioning did. One can assume that the higher up the hierarchy one goes, away from the clinical interface, the greater the role of diffusion and responsibilities regarding patient care.

Some specific nursing hierarchies and castes

Nursing hierarchies and castes cannot be fully appreciated without dealing with the relationship between nursing and gender. This arises in other sections of this book (2:5, 6:14) and we restrict ourselves here to the specifics of nursing hierarchies and gender. It has already been stated that nursing is predominantly a female occupation and that medicine is predominantly a male one (2:5), and this cannot be ignored in relation to the traditional father figure as head of the family and the role of the traditional mother. This is not to say that this dominant–submissive relationship has not been riddled with conflict, challenge and power struggles. Certainly, the medical and nursing professions are frequently engaged in such conflict (Chase 1995; West *et al.* 1999), although both professions aim to increase patient care. Furthermore, although we cannot cover these topics here we must not forget the fact that women in medicine may have conflict with the notions of their gender and femininity within a masculinized medicine, and that male nurses may have a tension between their gender and masculinity within a feminized nursing profession (Brown *et al.* 2000).

Two examples should suffice to show this complexity. Somjee (1991) outlined an excellent example of the complexities within the relationship between hierarchies and castes, and nursing and gender. Focusing on the social changes occurring in the nursing profession in India, she showed that in this culture the touching of the human body and its excretions were seen as highly polluting. Nursing was, accordingly, hierarchically divided into caste functions, the lower castes undertaking the menial jobs and the untouchables the 'dirty ones'. This downgraded nursing as a profession in India. Furthermore, females could not be nursed by males. Nursing carried a low-caste status. However, doctors were considered Brahman, as they fitted neatly into the categories of teaching and healing. Although lower castes did not have access to them on the grounds that they were 'untouchable', doctors could practise non-tactile, distance medicine. However, 'as physicians practising western medicine, the tactile requirement came back for them, but as physicians they were also considered socially high enough to have some kind of a non-stick, non-polluting armour round them' (Somjee 1991: 38). This 'armour' did not extend to nurses. However, things changed in the post-colonial period, but not because of it. For a number of reasons higher-caste women began joining the nursing profession, 'with encouragement from their parents, so that they might be able to get a doctor for a husband, either at home or abroad, preferably in the US' (Somjee 1991: 39). These changes in the nursing profession in India reflected the changes in their society at large at that time.

Our second brief example is the role of nursing within the armed forces. Gaskins's (1994) study related to the functioning of female nurses in the US military during the Second World War. The army hierarchy needed the female nurses for the wounded but within the male-dominated forces they tried every conceivable way to subjugate the army nurses. The army nurses used professionalization in an attempt to combat the army's gender discrimination, and although small successes were gained, the issue of gender remained the main focus from the army's perspective. When male nurses sought to join the Army Nursing Corp the issue of gender collided with professionalization, and 'in that collision military nurses demonstrated that professionalization alone would not free nurses from their subordinate status' (Gaskins 1994: 245). Thus, we can see the conflict here between the hierarchies of the army (male-dominated), nursing (female-dominated) and males becoming nurses within the army.

Further reading

Gunz, H. (1989) *Careers and Corporate Cultures*. Oxford: Basil Blackwell.
Holden, P. and Littlewood, J. (1991) *Anthropology and Nursing*. London: Routledge.
Leininger, M. (1967) The culture concept and its relevance to nursing, *Journal of Nursing Education*, 6(2): 27–37.

4.11 Breaking traditions

All that is traditional is not necessarily bad, or necessarily good. It would appear that the important point is having the ability to distinguish between the two. We have already noted that traditions are those aspects of human behaviour that are held in high regard, and have been passed on through generations, which gives them a feeling of being sacred (4:6). Nursing traditions are of a similar ilk and represent long-standing values conveying messages for those within the profession, as well as creating an image for society at large. Whatever the tradition is, it operates to evoke and maintain a certain authority that is above and beyond the influence of those who are currently engaged in it. It is as if the longer the tradition, the greater the power it has to perpetuate itself. Thus, its power is often a mantle that is passed on to the next generation and this responsibility can be taken on board as a serious matter, with those responsible not wishing to be the ones to break the tradition or to be seen to challenge it. Although, as we note, many nursing traditions can be seen as positive aspects of contemporary nursing, others can be viewed as negative and as contributing little to modern health care delivery. Before we proceed we must point out that it is not our place to begin to list certain traditional nursing practices as negative for the reader to agree with or not as the case may be. On the contrary, we would suggest that it behoves the reader to analyse their own nursing area of practice, decide whether these traditions are negative or positive and take the appropriate action should they wish to do so. This section is concerned with challenging these traditions and being aware of some of the pitfalls of doing so.

Another aspect of traditional authority concerns the notion of conformity. Most people conform because of one or both of the following mechanisms (Marsh *et al.* 1996).

- *Informal mechanisms of control.* These are part of the socialization process, where at a very early age in our childhood we learn the rights and wrongs of social behaviour.

- *Formal mechanisms of control.* These involve the legal and formally established sanctions of society, including the law, the police and the series of punishments that can be applied.

There is some overlap between these, as many law-abiding citizens would feel that the shame of the punishment would be greater than the punishment itself. Conformity is thus a more natural state of human action than non-conformity. Challenging traditional beliefs and behaviours can be a threatening undertaking, and those with a vested interest in maintaining the tradition, whether divine or secular, will wish to defend it. Much of this defence may be geared towards 'attacking' those who are seen to be threatening it, and one should understand that this is part of human nature. We now deal with some strategies for preparing those who wish to challenge negative nursing traditions to ensure that they operate in the highest professional manner.

Identifying traditional nursing actions

The main discrepancy in traditional nursing is the lack of scientific rigour that is applied to it. This distinction between nursing tradition and nursing science has been analysed by Sarvimaki (1994: 137), who argued that 'nursing knowledge is characterized as involving values, sets of beliefs, and procedural knowledge. Practical nursing knowledge is viewed as an integration of values, beliefs and procedural knowledge into action, whereas theoretical knowledge is viewed as a conception of nursing. Nursing tradition is described as the main organizer of practical nursing knowledge at the collective level, and nursing science as the main organizer of collective theoretical knowledge.' What this author is apparently suggesting is that the practice of nursing is predominantly traditional, while the science of nursing is predominantly conceptual. This would indicate that there is little to contemporary nursing practice that is science based. This is highly likely to be the case in the UK, as well as in Europe, where patients are demanding explanations of both medical practice and nursing traditions (Andersen 1994). This questioning is important for those who wish to break traditions, as it is founded on a challenge to the root of the action, which may receive one of the following responses.

- They don't know why they are doing it. It is often the case that no adequate explanation can be given for some traditional practices.

- It has always been done that way. In this scenario the evocation of history is seen as sufficient justification for the action.

- The illogical explanation. In this case the explanation that is given is implausible but imaginative, and taken with a 'pinch of salt' by most.

In the first stage of challenging negative nursing traditions this questioning is crucial to ascertaining the explanatory framework for this cultural action. The tradition may be viewed as mythological but, as we have seen, this gives some credence to it, and a challenge to it may be considered taboo.

Some examples of nursing traditions

Marilyn Williams (1995) considered a number of nursing traditions that needed to be challenged in contemporary health care practice. The first, she argued, was the traditional practice of the sister or charge nurse accompanying the consultant on the ward round, usually pushing the trolley full of case notes. This assumes that one nurse alone is responsible for all the patients on the ward and devalues the contribution made by others. The second tradition that Williams (1995) suggests might be challenged is the role of nurses in theatre, who function as targets for surgeons' 'tantrums', which resemble 'the spoilt child exerting his immature personality for the sake of it and trying to intimidate the assembled company in the process' (Williams 1995: 10). She mentions more, such as the fasting of patients from a set time irrespective of the time of the operation, the bed bath inflicted on patients without choice and task-centred nursing.

Nursing uniforms are a classic example of the embellishments of tradition. There has been a long-standing debate regarding nurses wearing a uniform. Those in favour argue that the public respects a uniform, that it creates an image of authority and confidence and that it enhances the professional image. Those against a uniform argue that it perpetuates the image of the doctor's handmaiden, that it is tight and restrictive and that it is a prop for nurses to lean on (Mahony 1999). Different colours of uniform may be used to designate rank, epaulettes and bands to highlight status and numerous types of headdress adornments to symbolize experience and rites of passage. Gelbart (1999: 26) goes as far as to say that nursing uniforms 'demonstrate commitment and dedication and, for many nurses, uniforms impart a sense of professionalism and status'. However, he also points out that contemporary nursing uniforms are a remnant of the militaristic past, with 'this host of meticulous restrictions [being] more concerned with social control than nurses' image' (Gelbart 1999: 26). Whatever the arguments for and against nurses' uniforms, there are a number of strategies for those attempting to break this, or any other, tradition.

Strategies for breaking traditions

When one is confronted with a traditional practice that ought to be challenged, a number of approaches can be recommended.

- *Ask others*. Talk to others not directly involved in the practice and ascertain their point of view. Question them about possible explanations or interpretations and try to understand the historical context.
- *Evidence*. Find the evidence relating to this practice. Search the literature and see if there is any published material for or against it. Enquire in different areas; for example, professional bodies, other disciplines, books and reports.
- *Careful management of material*. Once you have some information take care how it is used. Do not reveal it insensitively. Beware of people's egos.
- *Research*. If feasible, undertake a research project. Discuss the production of evidence-based practice.
- *Be prepared*. You might be isolated, ostracized, considered a troublemaker, a rebel, a maverick and definitely not one of 'us'!

To move nursing forward requires a deep understanding of the complexities of human action set within human cultures. Anthropological appreciation of customs, traditions, myths, taboos and so on will offer rich insights for the discerning nurse who wishes to explore the nursing enterprise.

Further reading

Gates, E. (1997) Handling problems, *Health and Safety at Work*, 19(6): 9–12.
Seymour, W. (1998) *Remaking the Body: Rehabilitation and Change*. London: Routledge.

4.12 Conclusions

By way of conclusion we offer a cultural group called the Nacirema, described by Miner (1956), and in particular their body rituals. We ask the student to read Miner's account, attempt to identify where the group come from and try to understand their ritualistic practices.

The fundamental belief underlying the whole system appears to be that the human body is ugly and that its natural tendency is to debility and disease. Incarcerated in such a body, man's only hope is to avert these characteristics through the use of the powerful influences of ritual and ceremony. Every household has one or more shrines devoted to this purpose . . . The focal point of the shrine is a box or chest which is built into the wall. In this chest are kept the many charms and magical potions without which no native believes he could live. These preparations are secured from a variety of specialized practitioners. The most powerful of these are the medicine men, whose assistance must be rewarded with substantial gifts. However, the medicine men do not provide the curative potions for their clients, but decide what the ingredients should be and then write them down in an ancient and secret language. This writing is understood only by the medicine men and by the herbalists who, for another gift, provide the required charm . . .

The Nacirema have an almost pathological horror of and fascination with the mouth, the condition of which is believed to have a supernatural influence on all social relationships. Were it not for the rituals of the mouth, they believe that their teeth would fall out, their gums bleed, their jaws shrink, their friends desert them, and their lovers reject them. They also believe that a strong relationship exists between oral and moral characteristics. For example, there is a ritual ablution of the mouth for children, which is supposed to improve their moral fibre.

The daily body ritual performed by everyone includes a mouth-rite. Despite the fact that these people are so punctilious about care of the mouth, this rite involves a practice which strikes the uninitiated stranger as revolting. It was reported to me that the ritual consists of inserting a small bundle of hog hairs into the mouth, along with certain magical powders, and then moving the bundle in a highly formalized series of gestures.

(Miner 1956: 503–4; reproduced by kind permission)

The Nacirema are, of course, the American (backwards), and the above ritual refers to cleaning the teeth at the bathroom sink (shrine) with the medicine cabinet on the wall. This natural behaviour, to us, can seem strange if taken out of context. The important point is that any behaviour can seem strange and unfathomable when viewed from an ethnocentric position. We hope that this chapter on thinking anthropology will launch the nurse into viewing many health care practices from a different perspective.

5 | Thinking public health

5.1 Introduction

There are a number of significant approaches within medicine that when brought together can be globally identified as 'public health'. To understand the basic principles of public health, we must explore both the theory and application of a number of discrete disciplines that fall under the overall umbrella of public health, and Figure 5.1 highlights a number of these disciplines.

At the beginning of the twenty-first century, public health finds itself in an exciting position, where the 'old soldier' of medicine has been called upon once again to investigate new diseases and re-examine the emergence of infections, such as tuberculosis, which were thought to have largely disappeared. The philosophy of public health continues to be characterized by the traditional forensic approach of discovering the nature and spread of disease. It also embraces the societal ideas and approaches of the 'new

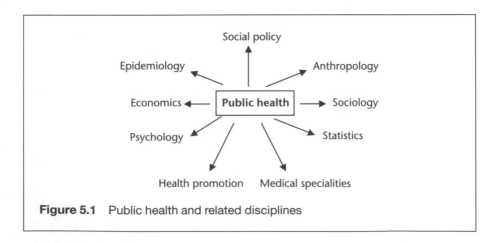

Figure 5.1 Public health and related disciplines

public health', which we discuss throughout the chapter. Nurses' experience of public health today is as much about health promotion, personal empowerment and lay knowledge as it is about understanding the incidence and prevalence of disease. Contemporary public health embraces the lifestyles, environmental influences and social change that are part of a dynamic process, which all communities experience to varying degrees. These factors have profound implications determining what we mean by the term public health and how the public health agenda should have a positive impact on everyday life. There are many factors that affect public health, and some of these are indicated in Figure 5.2.

In this paragraph, we introduce some ideas to help the reader to think about the factors that affect public health. As a society, we are increasingly composed of many cultures living within the broader culture of what we generally understand as 'British society'. Cheaper travel has allowed us to be more mobile and we travel both throughout our own country and to many different countries around the world, which has affected the nation's health. For example, we now have diseases, such as the most severe form of malaria (falciparum malaria), that are on the increase in the UK (Donaldson and Donaldson 1998). We are also involved in greater risk-taking behaviour, and public health follows certain social trends carefully, and therefore must be able to identify areas, and groups of people, who are engaged in certain behaviours, such as smoking, taking illicit drugs and abusing alcohol, and also those who are at risk of contracting sexually transmitted diseases, or unwanted pregnancies. Some of the antibiotics that were so potent in the latter half of the last century have now largely lost some of their efficacy due to overuse and misadministration by patients, and we are once again faced with inadequate treatments for some common infections. Public health strives to pick up the pieces of climate change, nuclear fallout and both civil

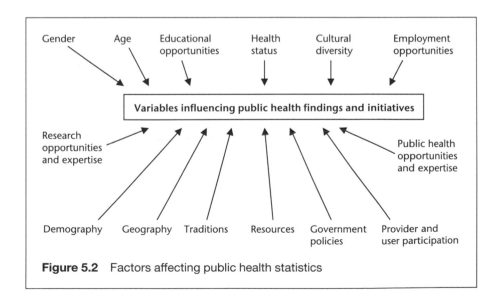

Figure 5.2 Factors affecting public health statistics

and global wars. This century has also begun with the health challenges of 1848, the year of the first Public Health Act, as so much of the world still does not have drinkable water and so many children die of diarrhoea. Whether in Mozambique or any of the socially deprived areas of Britain, the ravages of poverty continue to blight individual lives and damage communities, and therefore remain fundamental to the public health agendas in all countries, however well the agendas may be developed.

PART ONE: THEORY

5.2 Historical perspective

The history of public health is inextricably linked to the development of both the nursing and medical professions. Public health is the supreme example of how, when new knowledge is applied to practice, the results can be dramatic, and this is demonstrated later in this section by the story of John Snow, who identified and halted the cholera outbreak in London in 1884. For most nurses, our first introduction into the profession was probably learning about Florence Nightingale in a school history lesson, and unbeknown to us, it was when we also had our first taste of public health. Florence Nightingale incorporated the existing knowledge of public health into her nursing practices and policies, and this is clearly articulated in *Notes on Nursing: What It Is and What It Is Not*. This classic text (one of two books) is as much about public health as it is about nursing. In Chapter 2, Florence Nightingale informs her readers that there are five essential points in securing the health of houses:

- Pure air.
- Pure water.
- Efficient drainage.
- Cleanliness.
- Light.

She argues that without these 'no house can be healthy and it will be unhealthy just in proportion as they are deficient' (Nightingale 1980:16).

However, it is Hippocrates, the 'father of medicine', to whom we owe our first gratitude. Hippocrates was born on the Greek island of Cos around 460 BC. He based his teaching upon the science of medicine and the importance of clinical observation. Some readers will have heard of Hippocrates in relation to his famous four humours: blood, black bile, yellow bile and phlegm. Good health is dependent upon the humours working together in harmony and poor health occurs when there is a dysfunction of the four humours. The application of science to medicine was the thinking that underpinned the development of the understanding of health and disease in the Greek and Roman Empires. In public health, we look to the Roman

Empire, which introduced sanitation and clean water, and throughout history we have seen that these are the essential prerequisites to a society free of disease and promoting good health. The absence of sanitation and clean water in the Dark and Middle Ages of a poverty-ridden Europe was seen in the millions of deaths from every type of infectious disease, including smallpox, cholera and tuberculosis. As we discuss in section 5:13, we see that in areas of famine and war, where sanitation and clean water are unavailable, some of these diseases reappear and mortality rates rise.

Frazer (1950) has written extensively about public health during the eventful public health period between 1834 and 1939, and before we discuss some of his findings, we refer the reader to the time line illustrating the government's public health activity (Box 5.1). We begin our time line in the period of Elizabeth I and record the significant policies of the past 400 years that have pushed forward public health reforms.

Frazer argues that prior to the Industrial Revolution, England was fundamentally a rural country, where action by the state was unnecessary. Furthermore, he observes that in Lancashire and Yorkshire, where the first effects of the Industrial Revolution were felt, there grew up within 50 years a score of new industrial towns. The great rush to build accommodation for the rural incomers and their families, who were to work in the mills, resulted in the back-to-back houses that were once an important feature of the English urban landscape. The speed at which these houses were built, together with the economic prerequisite of providing only the most basic accommodation, resulted in housing stock without any regard for the sanitation needs of a fast growing and densely packed population. The lack of clean water and woeful sanitation conditions quickly gave rise to widespread disease and mortality, and public health became a national concern from every perspective. The Industrial Revolution was dependent upon a workforce whose existence was now seriously threatened by poverty, disease and death. The government knew it had to take drastic action, and the result was a series of legislative measures that resulted in a shift from local parishes being responsible for the poor, sick and old to the government taking more direct control. The time line in Box 5.1 shows the passage of the Poor Law Acts, which aimed to address the changing perceptions of how those in most need should receive their public funding and assistance.

Edwin Chadwick is the name most readily associated with the development of public health in Britain. Chadwick was said to be the most hated man in England and his personality was both his success and his undoing. Chadwick was a barrister without any medical training, who was inspired by the utilitarian philosophy of Jeremy Bentham (6:4). He was a member of the royal commission on poor law and in the first instance he is remembered for being the main architect of the Poor Law Amendment Act of 1834. Finer (1952) has argued that the purpose of this Act was to make public relief so unpleasant that most would refuse it. Chadwick focused his attentions on prevention of infectious diseases and linked this with a connection to poor sanitation and drainage. The journey from the Poor Law Amendment Act of 1834 to the Public Health Act of 1848 was complex and called upon

Box 5.1   Time line of public health activity and social policies influencing public health outcomes

1601   Elizabethan Poor Law. The 'impotent poor', including those who were old or sick, were to be cared for in almshouses and those paupers who could work were placed in houses of correction.

1751   The Gin Act placed a high tax on gin, which was held responsible for many social ills and a rising death rate.

1796   Manchester, one of the few cities to do so, establishes a board of health.

1832   The Reform Act.

1833   The Factory Act was the first Act to regulate hours at work (adult hours).

1834   Poor Law Amendment Act (The New Poor Law). Pauperism was replaced by workhouses. It was hoped that only those who were very poor would apply for relief in the harsh conditions of the workhouse, which had wards for those poor who were sick.

1840   Commission established to examine child labour in factories and mines.

1842   Edwin Chadwick (public health reformer) published Report on the Sanitary (5:1) Condition of the Labouring Population.

1843   Mines and Collieries Act prohibited the employment of women and boys under the age of 10 underground, created the mines inspectorate and set an age limit for tending machinery.

1844   The Royal Commission on the Health of Towns is established. The Health of Towns Association is founded.

1845   Final report from Royal Commission on Health of Towns is published. Public Health Act. John Snow identified the source of an outbreak of cholera to the Broad Street water pump in London and controlled the epidemic by removing the pump (5:1).

1848   First Public Health Act. Sanitary Act introduced.

1854   The second Reform Act.

1867   The Social Science Association (SSA) and the British Medical Association (BMA) influenced the establishment of the Royal Sanitary Commission, which led to the reorganization of public health.

1869   Local Government Board (later Ministry of Health) established.

1870   Education Act – beginning of board schools.

1871   Public Health Act made it compulsory for every district to have a medical officer.

1872   A significant shift in emphasis of the Public Health Act required rather than allowed local authorities to take public health measures.

1875   Under the Education Act, the provision of school dinners and the school medical service are introduced.

1880   Compulsory elementary education.

1890   Housing of the Working Classes Act.

1891   Free elementary education.

1897   Artisans Dwellings Act – promoted slum clearance.

1901   Ministry of Health (previously Local Government Board) established. Scotland – Infectious Diseases (Notification) Act.

1902   Education Act – beginnings of state secondary education.

1905   Unemployed Workmen Act.

1906   Public Health Act (Scotland). School meals for poor children.
1907   School medical inspection. Scholarships to secondary schools – 'free places'.
1908   Children Act – protection of children, juvenile courts, probation service.
1909   'The People's Budget' – graduated taxation. Trade Boards – for fixing wages in 'sweated industries'.
1911   Seebholm Rowntree published his findings on his fieldwork in York: Poverty: a study of town life. National Insurance Act – insurance against sickness and unemployment.
1918   Education Act – leaving age fixed at 14.
1919   Dawson Report recommended local authorities to set up health centres where doctors and health care staff could work together. Subsidized Housing Act – local authority 'council houses'.
1920   Registrar General in Britain used for the first time a hierarchical classification of social class based on occupation.
1926   Hadow Report – recommended state education for all.
1929   Local Government Act – abolished Poor Law Unions and Guardians of 1834.
1934   Milk Act.
1942   Beveridge Report on Social Insurance and Allied Services recommended a comprehensive social security system.
1943   Government announces its acceptance of the principle of a free national health service.
1944   The NHS White Paper, a consultative document, addressed issues of a free NHS, including the employment status of GPs, local authority control and health insurance.
1945   Education Act – secondary education for all.
1946   The Family Allowances Act provides cash allowances for the second and any subsequent child. The NHS Bill is published, under the determined leadership of the Minister of Health, Aneurin Bevan. The nationalization of hospitals, introduction of salaried GPs and establishment of health centres were among the reforms. NHS Act. New Towns Act.
1947   School leaving age raised to 15 years.
1948   5 July is the Appointed Day for the inauguration of the National Health Service. The Charter for the Family Doctor Service introduces a new payment system for GPs with incentives to work in areas where there is a shortage of doctors. The National Insurance Act establishes a contributory national insurance scheme.
1952   Town Development (expanding towns) Act.
1956   Clean Air Act.
1959   Mental Health Act – voluntary admission to a psychiatric hospital being one of the major developments.
1961   Graduated retirement pensions introduced.
1965   Circular 10/65 promoted comprehensive schools.
1966   National Insurance (Industrial Injuries) Act made provision for insurance against injuries from accidents and illness from a person's employment.
1967   The Abortion Act allows legal termination of pregnancy by a registered medical practitioner in an approved premises (e.g. hospital).

1970   The Local Authority Social Services Act requires all local authorities to set up social service departments.

1973   School leaving age rises to 16 years.

1974   Lalonde Report – A new perspective on the health of Canadians identifies the environment as fundamental to health. Control of Pollution Act. Health and Safety at Work Act.

1975   Earnings Related National Insurance scheme.

1977   Child Benefit scheme replaced family allowances.

1980   The Black Report identified the widening inequalities in health in Britain and argued for improved conditions for those living in poverty. It became a best selling book that was largely rejected by the then Conservative government. Inequalities in Health Report by Margaret Whitehead confirmed the findings of the Black Report and included new findings on poverty in Britain.

1983   Mental Health Act – nurses holding power is introduced and requirement of psychiatrists to plan care that would improve patients' mental health or prevent a deterioration in their condition.

1985   The WHO launches its Health for All programme.

1987   Public Health Alliance formed.

1988   Acheson Report created the post of Director of Public Health.

1989   Children Act fundamentally reformed child care law and practice. All those working with children were to be aware of the changes, particularly in relation to child protection. The NHS and Community Care Act developed a greater emphasis for developing polices of care within the community, across all ages.

1990   The AIDS (Control) Act gave new responsibilities on health authorities to report to the Department of Health on statistics, prevention measures and treatment undertaken. The Human Fertilisation and Embryology Act amends the 1967 Abortion Act. The pregnancy must not exceed the 24th week of gestation. Environmental Protection Act

1992   Control of Substances Hazardous to Health (COSHH). The Association of Public Health formed, with a remit for a wide range of disciplines to promote public health policy.

1995   Nurses, midwives and health visitors report to the government on their contribution to public health (Standing Nursing and Midwifery Advisory Committee).

1997   The first Minister of Public Health appointed. The WHO Jakarta Conference identified priorities for global health. Green Papers – 'Our Healthier Nation' health strategy for England.

1998   'Working together for a Healthier Scotland'.

1999   'Better Health, Better Wales'. 'Fit for the Future' (Northern Ireland). Health Action Zones (HAZs). The introduction of the Public Health Association (incorporating the Public Health Alliance and the Association for Public Health proposed).

2002   Draft Mental Health Bill – proposing 'approved clinician' rather than Responsible Medical Officer and introduction of dangerous severe personality disorder.

Chadwick's qualities of tenacity and determination, which finally resulted in the profound legislation of 1848. The Public Health Act focused on improving the nation's health through the improvement of sanitation and the delivery of clean water.

The famous Broad Street pump story demonstrates how even after the Public Health Act there continued to be public health problems of disease attributed to poor sanitation. John Snow is remembered for being the first doctor to use anaesthesia in childbirth, and gave chloroform to Queen Victoria during the birth of several of her children. In public health terms, Snow is noted for his success in tracing an outbreak of cholera in 1854. Snow meticulously plotted the incidences of cholera deaths and noted that many of them occurred near the Broad Street pump, which provided a communal water supply. However, Snow had to account for the 535 people who lived in a local workhouse, of whom only five died of cholera, and he identified that the workhouse had its own pump. He also found that the local brewery workers did not contract cholera and that they did not use the Broad Street pump. However, there was an isolated case of a woman who died in the same epidemic and lived some way from Broad Street. Snow found out that this woman liked the Broad Street pump water and sent her son to the pump for water every day. The story ends with John Snow providing evidence to the people who were in charge of the pump, the Guardians of St James' parish, the pump was subsequently removed and the cholera epidemic duly ended.

David Blane has identified the period 1870–1914 as being significant in the history of public health, as it was during this time that 'mortality rates fell more dramatically than in any other period since the introduction in 1837 of reliable recording of death' (Blane 1989: 20). The mortality rate fell from 9.6 per thousand in 1870 to 4.4 per thousand in 1914. Exceptional cases to this were the age groups of from birth to 5 years and those over 45 years. Despite this dramatic fall, Blane draws upon Oddy's work to remind us that at the beginning of the First World War 40 per cent of young men were unfit for military service (Oddy 1970).

In this brief history section, we have seen how public health has developed and continues to develop, and its progress is determined by increased knowledge, social and political change and the pressures and perceptions of individuals and groups. All these factors influence the public health agenda. The health education and health promotion section are fundamental to the recent history and present position of public health, but with the episodic and global outbreaks of tuberculosis, cholera and other infectious diseases, we are constantly reminded that the past is still with us.

Further reading

Frazer, W. M. (1950) *A History of Public Health: 1834–1939*. London: Bailliere, Tindall and Cox.

Nightingale, F. ([1860] 1980) *Notes on Nursing: What It Is and What It Is Not*. London: Churchill Livingstone.

Timmins, N. (1995) *The Five Giants: A Biography of the Welfare State*. London: HarperCollins.

5.3 Epidemiology

Epidemiology is fundamental to public health and we suggest that readers should study the discipline of epidemiology carefully before any relationship between epidemiological findings and public health policy can be understood. Our definition of epidemiology comes from the International Epidemiological Association: 'the study of the distribution and determinants of health-related states or events in specified populations, and the application of this study to control health problems' (Last 1995: 55). However, West reminds us how steeped in history epidemiology is: 'the Greek origin of the word simply means the study of people' (West, as cited in Craig and Lindsay 2000: 15). Donaldson and Donaldson (1998) have gone some way to enlarge upon the umbrella term 'epidemiology' and also discuss the term *descriptive epidemiology* (Donaldson and Donaldson 1998: 36). Descriptive epidemiology prompts us to ask questions about the data we have collected. For example, if we are examining a particular indicator for the incidence of teenage pregnancy or mortality under the age of 60 years from clinical depression, we will want to ask a number of questions involving comparisons between other populations and time periods, and it is from this information that we will be able to consider formulating a hypothesis. We must also take a stepwise approach with descriptive epidemiology in our interpretation of findings before we draw any conclusions (Donaldson and Donaldson 1998). Mulhall (1996) reminds us that epidemiologists are interested in all members of a group, be they 'healthy' or 'sick', and adds: 'another difference between epidemiology and medicine is that the former often wishes to know whether something has occurred, rather more than the mechanism through which it occurred' (Mulhall 1996: 1).

The gathering of data is fundamental to any epidemiological study. Yet the data made available to 'understand' the nation's health are sometimes supplied out of the context of epidemiological science. The result is that the public are led to believe that everyone is at risk of carcinoma of the lung or that the country is in the grip of an HIV epidemic. These public health scares often occur because of the manner in which they have been reported. It is therefore crucial that nurses are able to understand public health issues and relay accurate information to the general public (5:4).

Without epidemiology, our understanding of the patterns and nature of disease would be based upon hunches and opinions. Understandably, many people shy away from the statistics and language of epidemiology, but a basic comprehension of this population science is an essential requirement of public health. Throughout this chapter we include commonly used epidemiological terms, employed in reports, statistical information and health research papers. These provide the base line for your understanding of and thinking on public health.

In order to study the distribution and determinants of health and related states we need to have at our disposal extensive data that are both broad and detailed. The census is the most common and most well known method of collecting information. The census serves not only to count the number of people in Britain in one particular time frame, but also to provide a baseline of information about housing, family structure and the economic and educational status of everyone in Britain. A considerable amount of data can be gleaned from the census, the comparison over past years can ascertain social and cultural trends and the findings can also assist in providing data for future social and health policy. The 2001 census introduced a new question, which related to health, and respondents were asked to give their own opinions regarding their health status. People's perceptions of their own health are valued as a significant barometer of the real state of the overall nation's health. We can identify such factors as who, in what social class, in what geographical location and of which sex feel that they are the least or most healthy. The census, then, can be seen as the most widespread up-to-date epidemiological study – a snapshot of the nation's health.

There are other types of surveys that are used in epidemiology, such as cross-sectional screening and case finding surveys, and these are conducted in relation to the detection of populations at high risk of disease. These are representative samples of a given population where it is known that there is a high incidence of heart disease, for example. Using questionnaires and follow-up interviews, the prevalence, contributing factors and services can be assessed. Readers may recall reported surveys that are concerned with environmental factors, such as the epidemiology of people living near electricity pylons, and these are known as ecological studies.

The extended role of nurses means that they participate fully in all aspects of public health, including epidemiology, whether as research nurses, public health nurses or managers. This section provides some introductory concepts that are essential for understanding epidemiological terms, reports and analyses, and these are briefly mentioned under the following sub-headings and dealt with in more depth later in the chapter.

The incidence and prevalence of disease

In our consideration of measurement of the frequency of disease we need to take into account two fundamental epidemiological terms, *incidence* and *prevalence*. First, incidence, refers to 'the number of instances of illness commencing or of persons falling ill during a given period in a specified population. More generally the number of new events, e.g., new cases of a disease in a defined population, within a specified period of time' (Last 1995: 82). Second, prevalence can be defined as 'the number of events, e.g., instances of a given disease or other condition, in a given population at a designated time' (Last 1995: 82). The term incidence is used in outbreaks of acute disease to refer to the number of cases, i.e. the greater the number of cases the greater the incidence. Examples of this include outbreaks of food poisoning and the number of heart attacks per year. By contrast, prevalence is used to measure the burden of chronic disease, such as chronic anomalies and osteoarthritis (West, as cited in Craig and Lindsay 2000).

Morbidity and mortality statistics

Morbidity simply means to be diseased, and the morbidity rate refers to the number of cases of that disease. The latter is usually per unit of population (usually per 100,000) in a given period of time (usually one year). Mortality is related to death, and the mortality rate is expressed in the same manner as the morbidity rate of a particular disease, but usually for an age-specific group. Clearly, morbidity and mortality are related but, more importantly, it is the relationship between our understanding of their causes and the extent of the rates of them that give us an indication of what needs to be done to reduce them. Morbidity and mortality statistics are often the first epidemiological terms students become familiar with, and this is often in relation to national and international statistics. Many students will seek statistics for various projects and theoretical assessments, and they will find the Office for National Statistics (ONS) a valuable reference source.

Further reading

Beaver, M. (1997) Misuse of epidemiology, *Public Health*, 111: 63–6.
Chief Medical Officer (1998) *Report to Strengthen the Public Health Function in England*. London: Department of Health.
Unwin, N., Carr, S., Leeson, J. and Pless-Moli, T. (1998) *An Introductory Study Guide to Public Health and Epidemiology*. Buckingham: Open University Press.

5.4 Health education and health promotion

In this section we introduce the terms *health promotion* and *health education*. In our experience, the terms have been, and continue to be, used interchangeably by many factions of the health caring professions. However, we begin by asking if this custom is justified or if there is a tangible difference between health promotion and health education. Health education is often regarded as the forerunner to health promotion and this reflects the sea change in how public health has been, and continues to be, both perceived and practised. Health education is concerned with teaching the public on matters relating to health, particularly conveying health information and health choices of lifestyle. Many nurses and other health professionals are currently involved in health education programmes, whether they are at international, national or regional level, and their expertise has been utilized to implement government or locally led programmes. Many of these government initiatives require health professionals to dispel ungrounded fears and public health scares that have no foundation other than misinformation. This misinformation then becomes entangled with specific health education advice, leading to a confused population who are unsure as to how to respond. The disadvantage that health education has is that it is delivered through a very hierarchical route of communication. Tones and Telford (1994) have summed up the process of health education succinctly in relation to disseminating information from the 'expert to the ignorant'. By contrast, the experience of health promotion is altogether more recent than health education, with its changing expectations of a society where good health is dependent upon personal decisions and a more holistic lifestyle. Our contemporary thinking on health promotion has its roots in the following five principles.

- Health promotion actively involves the population in the setting of everyday life rather than focusing on people who are at risk of specific conditions and in contact with medical services.

- Health promotion is directed towards action on the causes of ill-health.

- Health promotion uses many different approaches, which combine to improve health. These include education and information, community development and organization, health advocacy and legislation.

- Health promotion depends particularly on public participation.

- Health professionals – especially those in primary health care – have an important part to play in nurturing health promotion and enabling it to take place (Ashton and Seymour 1988: 25).

The World Health Organization's Declaration of Alma-Ata (WHO 1977) and *The New Public Health* (Ashton and Seymour 1988) are major public health milestones, with health promotion focusing more upon the individual and how that person can work towards reaching their own health potential. Health education is rooted in educating sections of the population about particular health issues, and this is contrasted with health promotion, which is concerned with empowering people to reach their own health needs. In section 6:4 we discuss empowerment in detail and provide readers with further explanation that will help us to consider health promotion in greater depth.

For many nurses, their first connection with public health is through the experience of health education and health promotion. It is often in students' first meeting with a health visitor, health promotion officer or practice nurse that they begin to see what public health means in both a theoretical and a practical sense. For example, at the time of writing we are observing two major health concerns in the north-west of England: the rise in the number of people with tuberculosis and the increasing numbers of children who are suffering from obesity. Both these public health alarms are relevant to all nurses and Figures 5.1 and 5.2 explain the breadth of disciplines and influences concerned when we consider the reasons why there is a rise in these very different social diseases. Clearly, nurses are a crucial resource in work to reduce tuberculosis and obesity and to do this they must have the skills to understand the public health picture.

At this point we ask readers to think about the notion of empowerment, which is a significant aspect of health promotion. We begin by giving a baseline definition of empowerment for our discussion, and refer to the work of Rappaport: 'the mechanism by which people, organisations and communities gain mastery over their lives' (Rappaport 1984: 1). We suggest that readers refer to sections 6:13 and 6:14 on empowerment and ethics respectively to support this section. If we take the issue of obesity in children, as discussed above, and how we would implement health promotion, we are immediately faced with issues of empowerment. For example, we need to ask how young people and their families choose their lifestyles, make decisions and receive information on health and diet. The move towards nurses considering health choices *with* their clients/patients rather than *for* them is one of the most significant steps in the 'new public health movement'. Indeed, Ashton and Seymour (1988: 21) have argued strongly that 'the New Public Health goes beyond an understanding of human biology and recognizes the importance of those social aspects of health problems which are caused by life-styles. In this way it seeks to avoid the trap of blaming the victim. Many contemporary health problems are therefore seen as being social rather than solely individual problems.'

In our consideration of childhood obesity, it is clear that nurses thinking about appropriate health promotion strategies must address potentially sensitive issues, such as parental income and resources, cultural practices and parents' knowledge and experience of food and diet, including its purchase and preparation. We are all aware of the problems that arise when health promotion strategies are considered insensitive to both the target populations and the individuals themselves. Those that a programme intends to help may feel more excluded and victimized than before the programme began. At this point we ask students to think how they might put together a health promotion nutritional package for children in a sensitive way. It should become clear that communication skills (3:5) are crucial when sensitive issues such as obesity are the public health focus. As well as wide-ranging programmes providing clear information about how the general population might reduce obesity, in terms of diet and exercise, we also need to be able to discuss the health needs of individual people and work with them as to how these needs may be met. The 1986 WHO conference on health promotion held in Ottawa published a Charter of Health Promotion, which included a strategy with five dimensions that demonstrated the extensive reach of health promotion that extends beyond a traditional medical view and stretches into personal choice and community participation. This Charter (WHO 1986a) has remained a template for many health promotion strategies, and the dimensions are:

- healthy public policy;
- supportive environments;

- personal skills;
- community action;
- reorientated.

If we deconstruct the above strategies laid down by the WHO we can see the breadth of involvement and participation that is required to put health promotion into action.

First, *healthy public policies* are concerned with working towards making policy and implementing legislation. For readers new to health promotion some policies concerning particular Acts (for example, the Children Act 1989) may seem somewhat removed from their ideas of what health promotion is. On the contrary, health promotion is a central strand of the Children Act 1989 and this is illustrated by the Act's position on children with special needs. These children occupy a unique and special position in society, and they must receive support from a wide range of services to enable each child to fulfil their potential. This is echoed by Donaldson and Donaldson, who assert that 'every effort should be made to work collaboratively in multi-agency structures so that an effective network of services is available for children in need' (Donaldson and Donaldson 1998: 259).

Second, *supportive environments* also demonstrate the full extent of health promotion and direct us to consider the environmental effects on health. In this context health promotion is about improving the quality of life for people who live in an urban environment that is challenged by pollution, heavy traffic, dangerous roads and inadequate housing, and also the changing face of the planet as seen in, for example, deforestation, increased ozone in the lower atmosphere and growing populations, all of which have profound effects upon global health (7:10, 8:11). This point demonstrates how important it is for countries to work collaboratively towards creating environments that are safe and pleasurable to live in.

Third, *personal skills* are vital to any health programme and we have already discussed how important it is for those involved in delivering health promotion strategies to be able to engage with individual people in deciding for themselves their own health choices. Helping people to cope with the many health challenges whether they be illness, injury, psychological, environmental or social, is a fundamental action required of all those who are involved in health promotion.

Fourth, *community action* is needed to ensure that the programme is valued and reinforced throughout the society that it is aimed at. Empowered individuals and communities are a key indicator of the efficacy of health promotion projects at all levels. The experience of the participation of people to take control of their own lives through activities and initiatives as a result of the work of those in health promotion is rewarding and satisfying for everyone involved.

Finally, *reorientated* refers to that which is concerned with all those who have an interest, and desire to work, in health promotion, from whatever their background, and are able to work together in the pursuit of good health for all. If those who are involved in promoting the health programme are not enthused and motivated by it then this will transfer itself to others and the programme will not be as effective.

This section has shown the differences and similarities between health education and health promotion. Readers will be struck by the vast expanse of health promotion and its application from the wide range of issues that we have discussed, such as childhood obesity and deforestation. As deliverers and receivers of health promotion we all have a crucial role to play from the conception to the delivery of each project.

Further reading

Ashton, J. and Seymour, H. (1988) *The New Public Health*. Milton Keynes: Open University Press.

Ewes, L. and Signet, I. (1999) *Promoting Health: A Practical Guide*, 4th edn. London: Balliere Tindall.

Naidoo, J. and Wills, J. (1995) *Health Promotion Foundations for Practice*. London: Bailliere Tindall.

5.5 Nature of disease

Many people's perception of public health is rooted in the notion of disease; that is, its causes, effects and outcomes. Indeed, health care staff may often think about disease in a rather general way rather than considering the particular breadth and depth of a specific public health issue. In its broadest sense, disease can be divided into two main groups; first, infectious or communicable diseases; second, non-communicable diseases (see below for definitions). However, before we deal with these we briefly outline two main theories of disease.

Two theories of disease

We like to think that the theory of disease is both scientific and well understood. However, in different periods of our history our belief in how diseases operate differs considerably. The first historical theory to be considered is the miasma theory, which has its origins in the work of Hippocrates. 'A "miasma", composed of malodorous and poisonous particles generated by decomposition of organic matter, was thought to be responsible for many diseases' (Beaglehole and Bonita 1997: 87). Beaglehole and Bonita argue that although this theory was supported by political and economic groups and achieved some important public health interventions, it was eventually discredited. The second theory, beginning in the eighteenth century, was the advent of contagious theory or 'germ theory'. However, the origins of this theory go back to 1683, when the microscope was first introduced and the discovery of microorganisms was made. Since these early beginnings, our understanding of the nature of disease has continued to develop and there have been some notable contributors who have worked tirelessly to enhance and develop our knowledge. A significant milestone was the appointment of Professor Ryle, the first Professor of Social Medicine, at Oxford University in 1943. Simultaneously, across the world the interest in the nature of disease continued to develop and various centres and laboratories were set up to pursue research into diseases, immunizations and the impact of disease on health. We have divided the remainder of this section into two subsections addressing communicable and non-communicable diseases.

Communicable diseases

We begin this section with a number of definitions that are used in association with communicable diseases. Readers need to have these most commonly used terms at hand, so that they can understand and interpret various public health reports and projects.

Definitions of issues of communicable diseases

- *Communicable diseases.* The term is employed interchangeably with 'infectious' or 'contagious' diseases. They are defined as an illness caused by a specific infectious living agent that is transmitted directly or indirectly either from person to person or from animal to human. Readers who work in developing countries will become familiar with many infectious diseases, such as measles and tuberculosis. Although infectious diseases are now responsible for only 1 per cent of deaths, this has not always been the case. In England and Wales during the middle of the nineteenth century infectious diseases were responsible for a third of all deaths (Logan 1950).

- *Epidemic.* No doubt many readers of this text have used the term 'epidemic' at some time during their clinical practice. The term 'epidemic' has many derivatives; for example, *epidemic curve* refers to a graphic plotting of the distribution of the cases from onset. At this point, however, we focus on defining 'epidemic', which comes from the Greek *epi* (upon) *demos* (people), and is used to describe an increase in disease in a given population, which is above its baseline for a specified period of time. Clearly, the baseline needs to be set for any specific disease and this reflects the importance of studying the health of all populations.

- *Endemic.* This refers to a disease that is constantly present in a specified area and may periodically increase to become an epidemic.

- *Pandemic.* This refers to an epidemic of worldwide proportions, crossing international boundaries and usually involving large numbers of people.

- *Sporadic.* This is a term that is used when an outbreak of an infectious disease is not associated with other outbreaks. The outbreak is considered to have occurred irregularly and haphazardly.

- *Exotic disease.* With the increase of foreign travel for either work or holidays, we are now alerted to the possibility of contracting 'exotic diseases', which are those diseases found overseas but not in this country.

- *Incubation period.* Nurses, and particularly health visitors, are often asked by patients and parents what the incubation period for a particular disease is. Parents are particularly keen on asking about incubation periods and may say: 'My child was in contact with a child with chickenpox. When will they come out in blisters?' The incubation period refers to the time between the person becoming infected and the appearance of the first symptoms. Different diseases have different incubation periods depending upon the route of entry of the infection and the type of organism.

- *Primary or index case.* This is the first case of an outbreak of a disease.

- *Carriers.* This refers to a person, or an animal, that does not display any clinical signs or symptoms of a disease, but carries the infectious agent. They are often unaware that they are the carrier of the disease and may infect others without knowledge of this.

- *Reservoir of infection.* This is the natural habitat of the infection, where the animal, plant or microorganism lives and multiplies, reproducing itself and transmitting to a susceptible host.

- *Droplet infection.* This refers to where people are infected by small droplets from the nose or mouth, usually by coughing, sneezing or breathing. The range is usually limited to a few feet but can be greater if the organism is carried by wind. The common cold is carried in this manner.

- *Airborne infection.* This is the transmission of an infectious agent by particles, dust or droplet nuclei that are suspended in the air. Droplet nuclei are very small residues of dried evaporation droplets.

- *Nosomial infection.* This occurs in patients, or staff, and has its origins in the hospital or institution.

- *Iatrogenic disease.* This refers to an illness, or injury, that has been caused by the activity of a health professional. A nurse may inject a patient with a particular prescribed medication but the needle punctures the skin and causes an iatrogenic 'injury'.

- *Zoonosis.* This occurs when an animal transmits a communicable disease to man. (The plural is zoonoses.)

- *Hosts.* Humans and other animals who become an environment for other living agents.

The transmission of communicable diseases

For a specific organism to cause an infectious dose, it must enter the body via a particular route to begin the process of infection. There are six methods of transmission of communicable diseases, as follows.

- *Direct contact communication.* This refers to diseases that are transmitted from person to person by direct touch, including scabies and impetigo.

- *Airborne communication*. This is by droplet infection and includes diseases such as influenza, chickenpox and meningitis.
- *Congenital*. The term congenital means 'born with'. Some diseases can cross the placental barrier and these include rubella (German measles), HIV and hepatitis B.
- *Sexual communication*. This refers to infections that are transmitted through sexual activity, including HIV, genital herpes and gonorrhoea. Sexually transmitted diseases are on the increase.
- *Ingestion communication*. Diseases can be transmitted through swallowing infected material. Salmonella is one of the most common types of communicable diseases passed on in this manner. The types are food borne, water borne, zoonoses and person to person contact.
- *Injection communication*. In recent years the effects of using contaminated needles have caused considerable concern among public health workers. Many people will think of the contraction of HIV from infected needles used by illicit drug users as a principle source of infection. We must also be aware that injection communicable diseases include bites from animals (rabies) and insects (malaria from the mosquito bite).

Notification of communicable diseases

When a particular infectious disease is confirmed, whether it be in a hospital environment or in the community, a first question that those involved with the patient should ask is if the disease has to be notified. There are a number of infectious diseases that by law have to be notified to the Proper Officer (in England and Wales) of the local authority and the Chief Administrative Medical Officer (in Scotland and Northern Ireland) of the relevant health board. The Office of Population, Censuses and Surveys is subsequently informed, and issues and analyses the received data. This information is important for identifying diseases and their accompanying epidemiological data. It is at this point that we can see the significance of applied statistics to public health. Knowledge of disease trends, including their geographical location and the number of cases, is crucial in the planning of public health prevention programmes and attempts to control outbreaks. Box 5.2 outlines the notifiable communicable diseases in England and Wales.

Preventing communicable diseases

The task of preventing communicable diseases has been, and continues to be, one of the most significant issues on the public health agenda. We appreciate that, for many readers, the first time they begin to think about preventing communicable diseases is in relation to childhood diseases and the immunization programme. The terminology used within immunizations

Box 5.2   Communicable diseases notifiable in England and Wales

Acute poliomyelitis	Acute encephalitis
Anthrax	Cholera
Diphtheria	Dysentery
Food poisoning	Leprosy
Leptospirosis	Malaria
Measles	Meningitis
Meningococcal septicaemia	Mumps
Opthalmia neonatorum	Paratyphoid fever
Plague	Rabies
Relapsing fever	Rubella
Scarlet fever	Smallpox
Tetanus	Tuberculosis (all forms)
Typhoid fever	Typhus fever
Viral haemorrhagic fevers	Viral hepatitis
Whooping cough	Yellow fever

can be confusing and we therefore clarify some of the terms that we antici-pate readers will need to consider in relation to immunizations.

- *Immunization and vaccination.* The terms are actually synonymous. They refer to the protection of an individual from a communicable disease by administering a live modified agent (such as yellow fever), a suspension of killed organisms (such as whooping cough) or an inactive toxin (such as tetanus) (Last 1995).

- *Immunity.* This refers to a principle by virtue of which the bodies of certain humans and animals are protected from the invasion of certain diseases.

- *Natural immunity.* The patterns of natural immunity are of considerable interest to epidemiologists. It is well known that some animals have natural immunity to some diseases and poisons, while some humans have natural immunity to other diseases. For example, pigeons are only mildly affected by morphine and humans are not affected by swine fever.

- *Acquired immunity.* This term is used when an individual acquires immunity from previous exposure. A common occurrence is when a child has acquired immunity to measles because of prior infection with the measles virus.

- *Artificial immunity.* This is divided into two groups, active immunity and passive immunity. Active immunity is achieved by injecting a very small dose of a particular toxin or poison to stimulate the powers of resist-ance. Traditionally, the snake charmers of India inject themselves with increasingly higher doses of cobra poison, so they eventually build up a resistance. The most celebrated case of active immunity is the story of cowpox. Edward Jenner (1749–1823) was a doctor from Gloucestershire, who took some material from the sore of a milkmaid called Sarah Nelmes. Sarah, like many milkmaids, frequently contracted pustules on her fingers, which local people attributed to an infection from the cows. Jenner transferred this material from Sarah to a boy called James Phipps, who had cowpox, by scratching it on to his arm. James was later inoculated with smallpox. The experiment was repeated on other people. Neither James nor the others involved in the experiment developed smallpox. Passive immunity is that form of artificial immunity that is obtained by injecting into the body of one animal or human blood serum drawn from an animal already rendered immune by the active method. The diphtheria immunization is an example of passive immunity. Traditionally, children have been immunized from diphtheria by obtaining serum from horses that are already protected from diphtheria.

- *Herd immunity.* This term refers to the protection of the community as a whole.

Immunization programmes have two objectives: first, to protect the individual; second to protect the community. The nursing profession has a considerable role to play in this programme, both in health promotion programmes and in the administering of immunizations. Health visitors have traditionally filled these roles, but latterly nurse practitioners have also become increasingly involved in childhood immunizations. The immunization programmes vary from country to country. Box 5.3 outlines the immunization programme in the UK.

Non-communicable diseases

This term refers to diseases that are acquired by some means but are not infectious. These diseases may sometimes be called 'social diseases' and are frequently attributed to our lifestyle in contemporary society. An example of non-communicable diseases is hypertension. The reasons for high blood pressure include obesity, lack of exercise, smoking, stress and a high intake of cholesterol. These factors may exacerbate or cause hypertension and they are part of contemporary everyday life. When we reflect on the times when the Western world was not plagued by hypertension and its dangers (such as heart disease and stroke), we see that some of these contributing factors were not yet developed. For example, car ownership was uncommon and people took exercise through walking to work and school. Today, we have adopted a more sedentary lifestyle and the lack of regular exercise has led to a rise in obesity and subsequent cardiac disorders. Another contributing factor to contemporary problems with hypertension has been the huge changes in food preparation and consumption. Today we consume food that is frequently prepared with a high fat and salt content, much greater than home grown and cooked food of previous generations.

Box 5.3   Immunization programme

Age immunization is due	Name of immunization	Type of immunization
Two months	Polio	By mouth
	Hib	One injection
	Diphtheria	
	Tetanus	
	Whooping cough	
Three months	Polio	By mouth
	Hib	One injection
	Diphtheria	
	Tetanus	
	Whooping cough	
At four months	Polio	By mouth
	Hib	One injection
	Diphtheria	
	Tetanus	
	Whooping cough	
12 to 15 months	Measles	One injection
	Mumps	
	Rubella	
3 to 5 years (pre-school)	Measles	One injection
	Mumps	
	Rubella	
	Diphtheria	One injection
	Tetanus	
	Polio	By mouth
10 to 14 years (sometimes shortly after birth)	BCG (against tuberculosis)	Skin test followed by one injection if needed
School leavers, 13 to 18 years	Diphtheria Tetanus	One injection
	Polio	By mouth

Adapted from Health Education Authority and the Department of Health, March 2000.

Further reading

Davey, B., Gray, A. and Seale, C. (eds) (2001) *Health and Disease: A Reader*, 3rd edn. Buckingham: Open University Press.

Donaldson, R. J. and Donaldson, L. J. (1998) *Essential Public Health Medicine*. Plymouth: Petroc Press.

Unwin, N., Carr, S., Lesson, J. and Pless-Moli, T. (1998) *An Introductory Study Guide to Public Health and Epidemiology*. Buckingham: Open University Press.

5.6 Demography

Demography is a term used by many people to describe overall populations loosely. The considerable breadth of components within demography is illustrated by the following definition put forward by Last: 'the study of populations, especially with reference to size and density, fertility, mortality, growth, age distribution, migration, and vital statistics; the interaction of all these with social and economic conditions' (Last 1995: 45).

We can begin to see how significant demography is to public health when we consider the study of populations. Irrespective of the size of a given public health project, the significance of the issues of demography remains the same where information about growth and age distribution are crucial factors. There are two other demographic terms, which readers need to consider in this section. The first is *demographic transition*, where a specific country experiences a movement from high rates of fertility to low rates of fertility (and mortality). The reasons for this are not entirely clear, but it has been suggested that it may be due to technological change and industrialization or associated with the status of women and female literacy, but causes may also include war and conflict (Last 1995). The second term is the *demographic trap*. To understand this term we first need to grasp the meaning of *carrying capacity*, and this refers to estimating the number of people our planet or a specific country or region can sustain. The demographic trap is concerned with how the problems are faced by a population that has surpassed its carrying capacity. Populations that have exhausted their resources must turn to other communities and countries for food aid. These people may also become involved in conflict and become refugees.

This general sketch of demography has provided a baseline for us to consider the separate issues in more depth. The number of people, and their specific characteristics, in any given area when examined under the following headings will provide the baseline for understanding the particular health issue under scrutiny.

Population estimates

We have discussed the *population census* in section 5:3 and this of course provides us with a national statement of population size and specific characteristics. Unlike the census, which is carried out every ten years, *population estimates* take place annually. Population estimates are at their most reliable the nearer in time they are to the previous census, because the census is taken as the baseline and the estimates are achieved by adding births, subtracting deaths and taking into account the migration of people.

Population projections

Forecasts of the size and characteristics of populations are dealt with by population projections. Population projections can be reasonably accurate when forecasting population compositions in the near future but less so the further ahead we try to predict. For example, we can forecast the number of children who will be 16 years old in a given area because we have the birth records of those babies born. What will be less accurate will be our projection of the number of children those children will have in later life, and this is due to the uncertainty of their fertility. However, it is possible to give population projections based on different outcomes, so public health analysts can deliberate on the figures of low levels of fertility and intermediate and high levels of fertility.

Mortality

We have introduced mortality in section 5:3 and it is the statistic that not only nurses but also the general public are most concerned with. Indeed, many people will refer to the mortality rate as the *death rate*, and we can soon recall incidences, whether through the media or from hearsay, that the death rate from a particular disease is very high in a given area. The notification of deaths in the UK is rooted in public health history. Their recording began in 1532 and the registration of births and deaths began to be developed from 1538 (Mulhall 1996). The accurate gathering of mortality statistics is crucial to every aspect of public health and a legal requirement in the UK.

Migration

All countries, including the UK, experience migration at different times in their history. At the time of writing this chapter, here in the UK we are involved in the very thorny issue of accommodating asylum seekers. Migration has a significant effect on public health statistics. For example, a rise in the crude birth rate in a given area may be attributed to asylum seekers who have been given a temporary home. Migration is now an important public health factor, with much of the world's population on the move because of famine or conflict.

Morbidity

Most readers will have a general idea that morbidity is concerned with illness and disease. This is indeed true, but to focus on specific criteria, we offer the explanation put forward by the WHO Expert Committee on Health Statistics, who said that morbidity could be measured in three units: first, persons who were ill; second, the illnesses (spells of illness) that these persons experienced; third, the duration (days, weeks etc.) (WHO 1959). The relevance of morbidity becomes apparent when we apply morbidity statistics to our clinical work. Understanding morbidity rates and other statistics is our first introduction to planning and developing the health services of our area of practice.

Fertility and birth

We anticipate that readers who are also midwives or undergoing their mid-wifery training will probably find this section of public health the most relevant to their particular speciality. From their studies of the social and obstetric history of motherhood, midwives will be familiar with how maternal deaths, stillbirths and neo-natal deaths were, until the early part of the twentieth century, a not uncommon reality of everyday life. Understanding the reasons for the trends in fertility is one of the most important aspects of this public health issue.

Trends in fertility

Here the economic, cultural and social issues of the time can be analysed and predictions of future trends made. We begin with a historical account. The following extract from the historian Christopher Hibbert explains the situation from that period of time: 'contrary to popular belief families were not large, even though many women spent most of their adult lives pregnant. From the late sixteenth century until the early twentieth the average size of a household in England were less than five people' (Hibbert 1987: 386). The reasons for such small families are attributed to: first, a high infant mortality rate, where nearly a third of all children died before they were 15; second, birth control, which is thought to have been *coitus interruptus*, and the contraceptive effects of breast-feeding; and, third, a shorter period of fertility, from the mid-20s to the menopause, which was at about 40 years of age (Hibbert 1987). Hibbert also informs us of the notable exceptions, which included a Kentish woman called Ann Hackett, who having married at 18 gave birth 20 times in 23 years. An architect called James Smith had 18 children by his first wife, who died in 1699, and 14 by his second wife.

The fall in fertility in the UK during the 1930s occurred during the midst of a national economic depression, and it was feared that the population would not recover. However, the birth rate rose after the Second World War. Again the crude birth rate rose between the 1950s and the 1960s. The introduction and widespread use of the oral contraceptive pill contributed to the fall in the birth rate during the 1970s. Although the crude birth rate rose to 13.9 in 1990, we have never repeated the birth rate of 1960–2 of 17.6 (Office of Population Censuses and Surveys). The following subsections define these statistics and the reasons for the fertility trends are:

- cohabitation patterns;
- sexual practices;
- cultural beliefs;
- illness from sexually transmitted diseases;
- economic circumstances;
- lifestyle.

Recording and registering births

We have seen the significance of the population census to public health, and part of the census is the gathering of accurate data about births and deaths and still births, which are crucial for precise public health records. The first step in recording the baby's birth is carried out by the midwife or doctor who is in attendance at the birth. This is the Notification of Birth, which is completed within 36 hours of the birth and has the function of bringing into action the necessary services for mother and baby, such as the community midwife and health visitor services. The second step is the Registration of Birth by one of the parents or another informant to the local Registrar of Births, Deaths and Marriages, within 42 days of the baby's birth. This information provides statistical information for local and national surveys. A stillbirth is defined as 'a child, which has issued forth from its mother after the 24th week of pregnancy and which did not show at anytime after having been completely expelled from its mother, breathe or show any other signs of life' (Stillbirth Act 1992). A neonatal death is a baby who is born alive but who died within the first four weeks of birth (Donaldson and Donaldson 1998: 267).

Understanding the many types of fertility rates is essential in order to be able to grasp their application to public health information. These include crude birth rate, general fertility rate, age-specific rate and total fertility rate, and these are explained below.

Crude birth rate

Most readers will have come across this statistic, as it is very widely used in public health reports. However, we ask readers to be aware of its 'crudeness' because this statistic includes males, children and post-menopausal women. The annual crude death rate is the number of births per 1000 total population per annum.

General fertility rate

This statistic is a more reliable indicator of the fertility rate, because it focuses upon women of child-bearing years and excludes males, children and post-menopausal women. The general fertility rate refers to the number of live births per 1000 women in the population of child-bearing years (the age range is taken as 15–44 years or 15–49 years, the former being the more common).

Age-specific fertility rates

This is a very exact statistic and readers will see the importance of it when the public health issue under scrutiny involves obstetrics and gynaecological issues. For example, understanding teenage sexual activity and teenage pregnancy is one of the significant remits on the public heath agenda, where the age-specific fertility rates are crucial. The age-specific fertility rate is achieved by calculating the number of births from a specific age group per 1000 women of that age group. For example, the fertility rate of women aged 16 to 19 years is calculated by taking the number of live births occurring to mothers aged 16 to 19 years and expressing them per 1000 women aged 16 to 19 years in the population.

Total period fertility rates

This statistic summarizes age-specific fertility rates. The total period rate is used when comparisons are required over a period of time and between countries; for example, to understand the effects of nuclear fall-out in Russia during the post Chernobyl era, where it was anticipated that fertility rates would be affected. Unlike the other statistics we have thus far discussed this rate is not measured per 1000, but as the number of live births per woman of a single age. The total period fertility rate 'measures the average number of live-born children per woman which would occur if the current age-specific fertility rates applied over the entire thirty years of the reproductive span' (Donaldson and Donaldson 1998: 268). These authors go on to explain that the replacement of the British population requires a total period rate of 2.1, rather than 2.0, to allow for the deaths that occur prior to the beginning of their reproductive years (Donaldson and Donaldson 1998).

Cohort measures of fertility

Before we begin explaining cohort measures of fertility, we discuss the meaning of the term *cohort*. This commonly used term within public health statistics refers to what is sometimes known as a *prospective study*. In this instance an identified group of people are followed over a period of time to observe particular characteristics; for example, causes of death. In this statistic the cohort is the population of women who were born or married in a specific year; the study will then document the timing of births in their reproductive lifetime. Unfortunately, because it is a prospective study, the findings are not available until the cohort of women has passed their child-bearing years. This allows us to observe fertility over a period of time and also to predict future fertility trends.

Fecundity

Fecundity refers to the ability to produce offspring. 'If a woman produces a live birth, it is known that she and her consort were fecund during some time in the past' (Last 1995: 63).

Maternal mortality

Again readers who have an interest in midwifery will understand the enormous devastation that maternal deaths inflict on the hearts and minds of all those involved. This is demonstrated by Margaret Myles in her classic text-book for midwives: 'a maternal death is a tragedy. The childbearing woman is probably the most important person in the community, for the baby, hus-band and family all depend for their health and happiness on the mother's care. A maternal death also does harm indirectly by creating fear of child-birth in the minds of relatives and neighbours. Midwives must therefore do all in their power to prevent maternal death' (Myles 1981: 683). The role of midwives in preventing a maternal death involves their considerable skill in observation and detecting the abnormal. This is particularly relevant, as the two biggest causes of maternal mortality today are hypertension and pul-monary embolism.

Infant mortality

It is not only midwives, but also many other specialities, that have a particu-lar interest in mortality in the first year of life. As these statistics are one of the most fundamental indicators of health worldwide, it is important that readers fully understand how they are expressed. We suggest that readers familiarize themselves with, first, the classifications as expressed in various time periods and, second, the different mortality rates of infancy.

Classifications of infancy as expressed in time periods

The *perinatal period* refers to the time around the birth and is taken from the 24th week of gestation to the end of the first week of life, and the *neonatal period* is the first 28 days of a baby's life. This latter period is subdivided to include the *early neonatal period*, which is defined as the first week of life following birth, and the *late neonatal period*, which is defined as the end of the first week following birth to the 28th day of life. The *post-neonatal period* is defined as from the end of the 28th day of life to the end of the infant's first year. With these classifications in mind, readers should find that the specific rates of infant mortality will become clearer.

Classifications of mortality rates of infancy

The term stillbirth conjures up, for many people, visions of a Dickensian England of poverty and disease. Yet the term stillbirth is still used today and refers to a child who is delivered from its mother after the 24th week of pregnancy and does not breathe or show any signs of life. The stillbirth rate is the number of stillbirths per 1000 total births per annum. The mortality rates of the neonatal period are outlined as follows. The neo-natal mortality rate refers to the number of deaths in the first 28 days of life per 1000 live births per annum. Early neonatal mortality is the number of deaths in the first week of life per 1000 live births. The late neonatal mortal-ity rate refers to the number of deaths between the 7th and 28th days of life per 1000 live births, and those deaths that occur after the 28th day of life but before the end of the baby's first year of life per 1000 live births per year make up the post-neonatal mortality rate.

Childhood mortality

Statistically, childhood is divided into subsections from 1 year to 15 years. These are 1 to 4 years, 5 to 9 years and 10 to 15 years.

Trends of illness and disease in infancy and childhood

Whatever the period in history, for some it is childhood that will be the time where a significant amount of illness will be experienced. As the centuries have passed, living conditions have improved and poverty, although still present in our society, is not at the desperate levels that it once was. These factors together with immunization uptake and a more affluent society have contributed to the fall in infections and diseases among infants and children. Today our public health agenda for children is less about tackling the problems of childhood malnutrition and more about childhood obesity. Yet there are reminders of past illnesses from time to time when there are sudden outbreaks of diseases thought to be under control.

Further reading

Meredith-Davies, B. (1995) *Public Health, Preventative Medicine and Social Services*, 6th edn. London: Edward Arnold.
Unwin, N., Carr, S., Leeson, J. and Pless-Moli, T. (1998) *An Introductory Study Guide to Public Health and Epidemiology*. Buckingham: Open University Press.

▌5.7 Social exclusion

Any debate that is concerned with poverty and deprivation has the notion of social exclusion as a central tenet. Yet the term 'social exclusion' is a relatively new one, and is wide enough to embrace many varying perspectives creating social anxiety. Indeed, the phrase social exclusion is now so widely used that for many people it has become a convenient hook to hang social deprivation of any description upon. In this section we discuss the origins and theories behind the common usage of social exclusion and its place within public health. Many people welcome the introduction of 'social exclusion' as a replacement for the pejorative term 'the underclass' (Byrne 1999). Social exclusion is a societal experience found at the interface of sociology and public health, and Chapter 2 provides the sociological perspectives, giving further understanding of the societal constructs that are influential in determining public health policies.

The theories of social exclusion are grounded in a number of disciplines, including sociology, criminology, economics, gender studies, theology and anthropology. There are now significant leaders of various groups who have become champions for their cause, including directors of various charities, such as those for the homeless and people with mental health problems. These groups represent vulnerable members of society who, because of poverty, mental illness or both, are at risk of becoming socially excluded. Social exclusion is, in reality, a multilayered and multidimensional experience (Walker and Walker 1997; Madanipour *et al.* 1998; Byrne 1999).

Historically, social commentators, political activists and writers of moral conscience have observed and commentated on the most poor in society. The diarists, storytellers, biographers and autobiographers capture our imagination as we read and listen to those in society who because of their social exclusion unsettle our consciousness, creating feelings of sadness, sympathy, hatred, disgust and morbid curiosity. This passage from the novel *Angela's Ashes*, which was later made into a film, is a fine example of, first, the experience of poverty in twentieth-century Ireland, and, second, our desire to know how the socially excluded live.

> There in the middle of the crowd in her dirty grey coat is my mother. This is my own mother, begging. This is worse than the dole, the St Vincent de Paul Society, the Dispensary. It's the worst kind of shame, almost as bad as begging on the streets where the tinkers hold up their scabby children. Give us a penny for the poor child, mister, the poor child is hungry, missus. My mother is a beggar now and if anyone from the lane or my school sees her the family will be disgraced entirely. My pals will make up new names and torment me in the schoolyard and I know what they'll say. Frank McCourt, beggar woman's boy scabby-eyed dancing blubber-gob Jap.
>
> (McCourt 1997: 288–9)

As nurses we carry the responsibility of working with all sectors of society who are socially excluded. Our clinical practice takes us to all walks of life. For example, consider the role of the nurse in the following scenario. The nurse in the accident and emergency department cares for a lone teenage pregnant woman who arrives in the late stages of labour. The father of the baby is being counselled by the psychiatric nurse, because he has attempted suicide, and the community nurse finds the pregnant teenager's grandmother in an inner-city flat; she is cold, hungry and living in poverty. This brief vignette illustrates that nurses at every level, and in every speciality, whether in hospital or primary care, may come into contact with people who are socially excluded. Socially excluded groups, or individuals, are found throughout society and as nurses we work with those who have very profound experiences of social exclusion; for example, people with mental health problems or physical needs, those who are homeless, have a physical disfigurement or chronic illness, especially those who may be associated with risk-taking behaviour such as alcohol and substance misuse.

Social exclusion is closely related to the concept of stigma. It appears that we cannot go far along the analytical road of either of these concepts without introducing the relationship between them. The result of being socially excluded is the profound and isolating experience of being stigmatized. It is only by spending some time thinking about the effects of stigmatization on individuals and groups that we see how people's lives can be damaged both socially and emotionally. Erving Goffman, in his classic work *Stigma: Notes on the Management of Spoiled Identity*, offers us the following explanation, from which we can build our understanding of human interactions in contemporary life:

> While the stranger is present before us, evidence can arise of his possessing an attribute that makes him different from others in the category of persons available for him to be, and of a less desirable kind – in the extreme a person who is quite thoroughly bad, or dangerous, or weak. He is thus reduced in our minds from a whole and usual person to a tainted discounted one. Such an attribute is a stigma.
>
> (Goffman 1990: 12)

Our understanding of stigma has developed considerably since Goffman's work, and as new stigmatizing conditions come to the fore, we need to explore new ways of overcoming prejudice and social exclusion. The contribution made by Scambler to stigma has deepened our thinking considerably. An example is his work on 'the force of a label' (Scambler 1997), where the power of stigma becomes so strong that stigmatized people are defined by their condition. In this following extract Scambler draws our attention to how such a label dominates the perceptions of others: 'an individual's deviant status becomes a "master status": whatever else she may be – for example, mother, teacher or school governor – she is regarded primarily as a diabetic, cancer victim, or whatever. In other words, her deviant status comes to push into the background her other statuses' (Scambler 1997: 173).

When we pause to consider stigma in contemporary society our minds may turn to HIV, AIDS and drug misuse. However, we continue to carry a legacy of the past differences of appearance and behaviour that Goffman also observed during the 1960s in the United States. For example, facial disfigurement caused by burns, the colour of a person's skin, the experience of a gay man or woman 'coming out', or a child in a wheelchair – these and many other forms of difference divide our society into the accepted and socially included and the stigmatized and socially excluded. The complexities of stigma are illustrated in an analysis of the feelings of social exclusion felt by breast-feeding mothers. Consider why the totally natural process of a mother feeding her baby should give rise to antagonism and alienation. Mary Smale's (2001) work on stigma and breast-feeding introduces ideas of cultural difference, while relating the social exclusion felt by many breast-feeding women to perceptions of concealing, appearance, disruptiveness, blame and the potential for blame, as identified by Jones *et al.* (1984).

As nurses, we are faced with three difficult issues of social exclusion and stigma. We are concerned with: first, the identification of social exclusion; second, understanding its complexities; and third, how we can play our part in helping those who experience it to overcome it.

Figure 5.3 puts forward a model for change, where nurses can play a direct role in the intervention of stigma and social exclusion. We ask readers to consider where they would place themselves in this model to change a particular area of difference that they feel most strongly about.

The formation of the Social Exclusion Unit (SEU) in 1998 was an acknowledgement by the government of the problems of social exclusion in

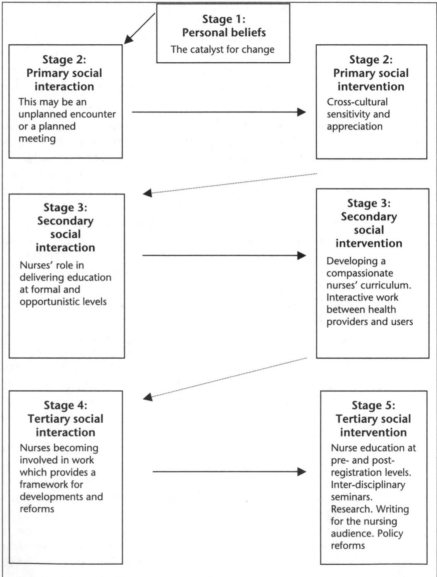

Figure 5.3 Stigma and social exclusion in health care practice: a model for change (adapted from Mason *et al.* 2000)

British society. The remit of the SEU has been to prioritize certain areas of social exclusion, including truancy, school exclusion, sleeping rough and the deprivation of housing estates. They attempt to achieve change by bringing together the work of various departments, local authorities and agencies to address the multifactorial issues that each area presents. The concern of various governments, and all political parties, is reflected in several significant reports, illustrated in *The Independent Inquiry into Inequalities in Health Report* (Acheson 1998), the *Black Report* (HMSO 1983) and *Our Healthier Nation* (HMSO 1998).

Further reading

Acheson, D. (1998) *Independent Inquiry into Inequalities in Health Report*. London: The Stationery Office.

Benzeval, M., Judge, K. and Whitehead, M. (1995) *Tackling Inequalities in Health: An Agenda for Action*. London: King's Fund.

Mason, T., Carlisle, C., Watkins, C. and Whitehead, E. (eds) (2001) *Stigma and Social Exclusion in Healthcare*. London: Routledge.

5.8 Public health and the sociology of health and illness

Students who choose to study public health in depth will quickly appreciate how the sociology of health and illness (traditionally known as medical sociology) has a significant impact on contemporary health issues. In this section we discuss public health within a framework of the sociology of health and illness and by doing so provide a qualitative perspective on the often stark statistics of public health. We argue that the public health of any community can only be understood in both its widest and deepest sense when we examine epidemiology and demography within a social context. Figure 5.4 demonstrates our approach to understanding the relationship between the two disciplines of public health and medical sociology.

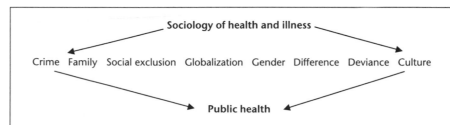

Figure 5.4   The influences of the sociology of health and illness on public health

Side one: the societal relationship to public health

In this subsection we consider how society both drives and responds to issues of public health. It is worth remembering that behind every public health statistic there is a story of individual or collective decision-making. To illustrate this we offer the example of a health visitor's caseload, which has been identified as having 16 per cent of babies who are not immunized. But when this statistic is broken down into individual cases, we can begin to understand the reasons why each child has not been immunized; for example, parental objection to immunizations or failing to keep clinic appointments. Choices are influenced by many factors, and social issues play a very large part in this. Chapter 2 provided an analytical discussion of the breadth and depth of influences that underpin contemporary British society, and here we assert that these influences, when applied to public health, help us to understand society and help with planning public health policy.

Side two: the health care receiving relationship to public health

In its early years, the hallmark of the NHS was paternalism, a status quo that was apparently accepted for many years by a grateful society, which uniquely could expect 'free health care' (7:6). However, over time we have witnessed considerable changes in the attitudes to and experiences of how we receive public health care (7:7). Since the beginnings of the NHS in 1948, our expectations have carried on rising and we demand more of the public health services that are provided for us. The reasons for this lie in our continually developing society, which is more affluent, educated and subsequently more greatly empowered than at any other time in history. As a result, the public health measures that were once set in stone and followed almost unquestioning by a grateful post-war public are not only rejected but seen as infringement upon personal liberty. For an example of this shift in attitude we return to the role of health visitors, who in the middle of the twentieth century gave a vast amount of 'paternalistic' advice about child-rearing practices and health care. In the post-war days prescriptive advice was the norm, where health visitor and client engaged in a very hierarchical relationship in which 'the professional knows best'! Today's mothers have rejected this unequal relationship and now question public health information and demand an equal stake in the decision-making process. The relationship of the deliverers and users of health care has become complex and we examine the effect this has on the providers of public health care.

Side three: the health care providing relationship to public health

When we consider the ways in which nurses deliver public health care, one method immediately springs to mind, and that is through giving health information. At this point we refer readers to section 5.6, where we see how changes in society led to reforms in the delivery of health education. We take the issue of informing the public about the importance of immunizations as an example to illustrate the health care providing relationship to public health. In the subsection above we discussed how our society has greater empowerment, and this influences the way that we deliver our public health. The MMR (measles, mumps and rubella) immunization has received considerable attention and been the focus of much debate. The MMR debate has brought home to health professionals how important it is for them to be fully informed in public health issues that they are involved in. In contemporary society, our patients and clients will no longer accept standard advice from nurses and other health workers. As the lay knowledge of the service user continues to grow, the relationship between service providers and users becomes more one of equality. The relationship between providers and receivers is now closer and more egalitarian than at any other time in our history. In the instance of MMR, most parents now feel more at ease discussing with health professionals their concerns and asking penetrating questions.

Thinking about public health within a framework of the sociology of health and illness allows us to begin to formulate ideas about the reasons behind many public health statistics. To help us in this process we will compare two different model of health. First, the medical model views ill-health and disease as being determined by the profession of medicine through the process of identification, classification, diagnosis, treatment and prognosis (2:13). Illness is seen as located within a framework of biological disorder and disease, and located within a nosological framework that gives the illusion of knowledge. It is paternalistic and autocratic, and informs the patient what they are suffering from, rather than the patient telling the doctor what is wrong with them. By contrast, the second model, the social model of health, is very much enmeshed within the sociology of health and illness, where one takes a wider perspective of society, seeking to understand cultures, people's behaviours and other factors within a social framework. Diseases and disorders, or at least a community response to them, can be socially constructed. Values are often attached to certain diseases; for example, AIDS carried the 'punishment from God' scenario in the early 1980s when it was viewed by some tabloid press editors to be a 'gay plague' (Giddens 1989a). The social model of health and illness allows us to understand differences within societies through the qualitative life narratives that surround many of the public health statistics. Finally, and to reinforce the foregoing points, we ask the reader to choose one particular public health statistic and consider the possible sociological factors that may contribute to its prevalence. Data from the *Independent Inquiry into Inequalities in Health Report* (Acheson 1998) can be used as a starting point:

> There is a higher prevalence of cigarette smoking in lower socio-economic groups. In 1996, 29 per cent of men and 28 per cent of women smoked but this ranged from 2 per cent of men (11 per cent of women) in professional occupations to 41 per cent of men (36 per cent of women) in unskilled manual occupations. Amongst smokers, men and

women in professional occupations smoke fewer cigarettes per week than those in unskilled manual occupations.

(Acheson 1998: 83)

Clearly, gender, socio-economic group and occupational status are important sociological considerations in analysing these statistics, demonstrating the significance of the discipline of the sociology of health and illness to public health.

Although the traditional domination of the general practitioner at the centre of primary care has been, and continues to be, difficult to shake, some degree of shift has taken place. The shift has been from a medical to a social model of provision of health care, alongside developments in community and primary care. The cracks of the medical model began to arise when the medical profession no longer found answers to problems presented to them by patients that were essentially of a social nature. We ask you to think of some examples and offer you the following vignette.

> Jane Davies is a lone parent with four young children. She lives in an inner-city area, which suffers high unemployment, bad housing and crime. Jane has come to see her GP and presents with symptoms of depression. Jane is also finding it difficult to cope with her children and cannot control their behaviour. Jane is trying to give up smoking, but says she is smoking more heavily than ever before.

What can the medical model offer Jane? It is a rigid and narrow perspective that involves the professional judgement of one person, namely the GP. The GP can offer anti-depressants but little else. Jane will not be invited to become involved in her own treatment and the decisions that her GP makes are likely be based on the inaccessible medical knowledge of a busy doctor. It is suggested that, in this instance, the medical model would indeed fail Jane and her family. By contrast, the social model looks more promising for Jane. As Jane confides her problems to her GP, he or she quickly appreciates that this is not a medical problem and therefore cannot have a medical answer. The problems and challenges faced by Jane and her family are social, by which we mean that Jane's depression is a reaction to many things, including living in the conditions in which she does. Her smoking and inability to cope with the children require help from a number of health professionals and organizations, of which her GP is only one. The successful outcome for Jane is dependent upon her being given the opportunity to make her own decisions about her life with the collaboration of others, with them sharing their knowledge, rather than using it as a source of power.

Further reading

Jones, H. (1994) *Health and Society in Twentieth Century Britain*. London: Longman.
Scambler, G. (ed.) (1997) *Sociology as Applied to Medicine*, 4th edn. London: W. B. Saunders.

Taylor, S. and Field, D. (1997) *Sociology of Health and Health Care*. Oxford: Blackwell Science.

PART TWO: APPLICATION TO PRACTICE

▌5.9 Community action: collaborations, partnerships and alliances

The successful outcome of the public health agenda, whether it is at local, national or international level, is dependent upon producing collaborations, partnerships and alliances with a range of relevant agencies. Our first task is to understand the process of creating an alliance. The five elements described by Funnel *et al.* (1995) are listed below and highlight their main suggested structure for a successful implementation of a public health policy initiative.

- *Commitment*. Those involved in the alliance demonstrate commitment by sharing their skills and resources.
- *Community involvement*. Participation from the community is essential in all alliance activities. Local people in the community must be represented, receive guidance where necessary and be treated equally.
- *Communication*. All those involved in the alliance must work in an open and honest manner.
- *Joint working*. Working together within a philosophy of equality is an essential feature.
- *Accountability*. The evaluation of the alliance is essential, so that the results are used positively to inform future policy.

Health alliances are most visibly seen in the community, where local participation is crucial in making the public health agenda work. The experience of community-led needs assessment involves examining the specific requirements of population groups identified by social class, age and geographical location. We now consider a national alliance called Sure Start. This national initiative involves a wide range of approaches and comprises over 200 programmes across the United Kingdom. It involves many local people, assesses local needs and responds to those needs through a series of programmes. Sure Start was established to address child poverty and social exclusion. It aims to improve the health and well-being of families and children, before and from birth, so that children are ready to thrive when they go to school. Sure Start is involved in two main activities: first, the setting up of Sure Start programmes for children under the age of 4 years; second, the dissemination of good practice from local programmes to everyone involved in providing services for young children. Sure Start is an example of how local people can become involved in the process of the planning of the provision and evaluation of services. Local families, local groups and professionals are involved in the planning and delivery of services that meet the needs of local people. There are four objectives and targets to the Sure Start programme and these are implemented in various ways depending upon the needs of the community.

- Objective 1. Improving social and emotional development.
- Objective 2. Improving health.
- Objective 3. Improving children's ability to learn.
- Objective 4. Strengthening families and communities.

We ask readers to consider the possible initiatives that they might introduce to fulfil these objectives in the communities where they live and the factors that they must take into account when they are planning services. For example, in objective 3, improving children's ability to learn, they must take into account the language(s) of the local population and how this can be incorporated into pre-school education. Having respect for a child's culture and language while ensuring that they are fluent in English requires mutual cooperation and the respect of all communities and educational authorities.

Further reading

Campling, J. (1995) *Health Policy and the NHS towards 2000*. London: Longman.
Lupton, D. (1995) *The Imperative of Health: Public Health and the Regulated Body*. London: Sage.
Naidoo, J. and Wills, J. (2000) *Health Promotion: Foundations for Practice*, 2nd edn. London: Bailliere Tindall.

5.10 Role of primary health care

The relationship, and the interface, between public health and primary care is an important one. Those who work in primary care, as opposed to those who work in public health, offer different definitions of what primary care means to them. This depends upon their specific roles and experiences as health care workers, whether they are nurses, doctors, clerical workers, midwives or ancillary staff such as physiotherapists. For example, a unique experience of general practitioners is that they act as the central referral system and that they are the gatekeepers to most of the health services provided to patients in the community. If we move away from the tasks people actually do within the primary care system to thinking about what the philosophy of primary care is, we can visualize its potential. Like so much of the current policies of the National Health Service, the delivery of services within the community is a legacy of its introduction in 1948. At this point in time, community services were still organized in an *ad hoc* manner and did not receive the attention that the new hospital system did. In the half-century since the beginning of the NHS, primary care has moved from a

Cinderella service of a family doctor, his indispensable district nurse/ midwife and a faithful caseload of patients (all of whom he knew from one generation to the next), to a vibrant and exciting system of health care involving the collaboration of a wide range of professional staff and local people. So we now take as our baseline for understanding what primary care is that defined in the Health for All strategy put forward by the WHO: 'essential healthcare based on practical, scientifically sound and socially acceptable methods and technology made universally available to individuals and families in the community through their full participation' (WHO 1985a).

When we think about public health in primary health care settings we see that at the heart of the most influential thinkers and policy-makers is the belief that participation and empowerment are the two most crucial ingredients. Note how the changes in traditional public health from pure disease prevention and control to community health alliances and public involvement, together with the shift in traditional primary care, from a service dominated by general practitioners and paternalism, to a community-led service empowering the local people, has brought the philosophies and aspirations of these disciplines closer together.

Kendall (1998) described research that demonstrated how public health could be implemented in primary care settings. The process by which this was achieved was through self-efficacy theory, which was described 'as having the potential to inform the work of health professionals in an enabling way' (Kendall 1998: 39). Giving professionals the knowledge and the power to exercise this knowledge in practice produces a higher outcome ratio of effective public health policies.

Public health practice in primary care

There are a number of well established public health initiatives within primary care, one of which is the screening programme, and we look at this in more depth, as most nurses will already be familiar with this from a user perspective.

Screening

One definition of screening is 'actively seeking to identify a disease or pre-disease condition in people who are presumed, and presume themselves, to be healthy' (Holland and Stewart 1990: 1). Five types of screening have been identified.

- *Protection of the public health*. This is particularly used for infectious diseases, such as mass chest radiography in TB (tuberculosis). An identified population might be immigrants settling in a country who have come from areas where TB is known to be a health hazard.
- *Prior to entering an organization*. Most people can recall a medical examination prior to entering an organization, and this is carried out to

protect the worker, work colleagues and, in the case of health care employment, patients. In social policy studies it is often claimed that many recruits for the Boer War, as well as the First World War, were unfit to fight, with large numbers of them plagued with bad teeth or anaemia, and some considered to be lame. Donaldson and Donaldson (1998) remind us that this army recruitment examination was the first pre-employment screening programme. There are a number of other professions where pre-employment screening is crucial to exclude particular health hazards; for example, myopia in airline pilots and salmonella in food handlers.

- *Protection of the workforce.* You might recall that there have been a number of industries that are potentially hazardous and continue to cause concern among the workforce, as well as those involved in public health; for example, workers in nuclear plants. Of course, there are also industries that traditionally have caused considerable health problems and these have been well documented in both public health and historical documents. The coal industry, which has all but disappeared in the UK, has left a legacy of pneumoconiosis and other respiratory conditions, which are experienced by ex-miners today.

- *For life insurance purposes.* Readers may also be familiar with this type of screening, which may only take the form of a simple questionnaire before insurance is issued or may be something much more complex, depending upon the type of insurance, the age of the applicant and existing medical conditions.

- *The early diagnosis of disease.* It is this type of screening that is possibly familiar to most. Examples are screening for cervical cancer, breast cancer or hypertension. These are among the conditions that do not present with symptoms, and hypertension, because it is pre-symptomatic, is often called the 'silent' killer.

We now ask you to consider the factors that you would take into account when deciding whether a particular medical condition should be screened for. We put forward a number of considerations that should be made before a particular screening programme is introduced.

- *Financial considerations.* There is only so much money in the pot and the decision to screen for one disease may put financial constraints on screening for another disease, or even in providing for a different service. Accurate budgeting is crucial in order to make accurate judgements about the delivery of all services.

- *Treating patients.* This is also a financial consideration in terms of treating those patients who have positive outcomes. One question that must be addressed is: are resources available to treat patients who are likely to have positive results, including professional time and expertise, clerical support, equipment, clinic space and monies available for the treatment package as a whole?

- *Ethical considerations.* The ethical considerations include the question of screening for a disease when there may be no treatment, when the treatment is ineffective and when it cannot be provided due to financial restraints. Donaldson and Donaldson argue: 'the reality is that only in a few diseases is there any convincing evidence that striving for early diagnosis on a total population basis, and hence early treatment, will truly benefit the person being screened' (Donaldson and Donaldson 1998: 123). It is therefore important to have a thorough knowledge of the disease in question, including the validity of the screening test and the benefit of the treatment available.

- *The significance of the disease in affecting a person's health.* The significance can be ascertained in two ways. First, the disease may affect many people in a general way. Second, the disease may affect only a small number of people, but its effects may be very profound in terms of seriousness to the individual and even society as a whole.

The following national programmes are widely used throughout the UK. First, pregnant women are screened to prevent death or disability to both the mother and the foetus. The tests are usually carried out by the midwife and doctor and include screening for hypertension, anaemia and diabetes in the mother and foetal abnormalities in the baby, such as neural tube defects (spina bifida) and Down's syndrome. Babies also undergo a screening programme in which the initial physical examination by the doctor, midwife and health visitor screens the baby for abnormalities of the heart, congenital dislocation of the hip, cerebral palsy, hearing and visual defects and metabolic diseases such as phenylketonuria. There are also other tests, such as screening for sickle cell anaemia and screening babies when there is concern over a particular genetic condition. Screening of babies is undertaken to prevent disability or treat disability through early detection, diagnosis and treatment. There are, of course, some conditions, typically phenlylketonuria, where early diagnosis is crucial in order to commence treatment and prevent disability. In middle and old age the screening of cervical and breast cancer, hypertension and osteoporosis aims to detect and treat disease early, not only to prolong life but also to work towards a good quality of remaining life.

We conclude this section by discussing one of the most well known national screening programmes in the UK: the cervical cancer screening programme. The health problem of cervical cancer is illustrated by the fact that it kills approximately 1400 women each year in the UK (Baggott 2000: 114). The programme has a long history of development commencing in the 1960s, and since that time it has had both successes and failures. The successes include a fall in the number of women with cervical cancer from 67.6 to 43 per million between 1990 and 1998 (Baggott 2000), but the failures include some high-profile cases where minor abnormalities and also some major ones have not been detected (Wells 1997). A large national programme, such as this has of course attracted much debate, argument and analysis. The questions raised are many and some of them include concerns over the cost-effectiveness of the programme, the recall system, the reliability of the diagnostic test and the expertise of those health professionals who both perform the smear and analyse the results.

In addition to the debates about the process of cervical screening there are also discussions regarding prevention of cervical cancer. It has been suggested that financial resources should be directed towards groups of women who are at high risk of acquiring cervical cancer. These groups include those women who smoke and those with a specific sexual lifestyle. As regards the latter, women who have their first experience of sexual intercourse at a younger age and women who have a higher number of sexual partners are acknowledged to be at significantly greater risk of developing cervical cancer. It is clear that, within primary care, practitioners of public health have a wide range of responsibilities and roles, including balancing the role of health promotion with the practice of clinical health screening. No doubt we can recall screening projects that have failed because some of the above issues have not been thought through.

Further reading

Baggott, R. (2000) *Public Health: Policy and Politics*. London: Macmillan.
Dixon, M. and Sweeney, K. (eds) (2001) *Primary Care Groups and Trusts*. Oxford: Radcliffe Medical Press.
Tudor Hart, J. (1988) *A New Kind of Doctor: The General Practitioner's Part in the Health of the Community*. London: Merlin.

5.11 Implementing health policy

We have seen throughout this chapter how the introduction of various polices has influenced the course of public health, from the appointment of the first medical officer of public health in 1848 to the appointment by the Blair government of the first Minister of Public Health almost 150 years later in 1997. The progress of the discipline of public health from Edwin Chadwick to present times has been a long journey, with times of great pace and times of apparent inaction. The change of pace has been dependent upon a variety of social changes, including war, politics and reform. Prior to the Second World War, the changes included legislation involving employment, education and pensions. If we spend a little time considering the state of public health since 1939, we can understand its present position in the UK and the subsequent strategies that have been developed. If this chapter had been written 20 years ago it would probably have been entitled 'Community medicine'. The reason for this is that Seebohm and Todd's Commission on Medical Education in 1968 promoted the 'new vision' of public health 'community medicine'. However, the progress of the new vision of community medicine was stifled by various reports and public health came into focus again, with an inquiry chaired by the then Chief

Medical Officer, Sir Donald Acheson, a public health epidemiologist. Those who have studied public health will probably see the Acheson Report (1998) as a very significant milestone giving public health a prominent role, which it continues to enjoy. This is the backdrop for public health legislation in the UK.

Students tend to have knowledge of a small number of well known reports, which they can draw upon for their various assignments and examinations. These documents frequently include *The Black Report* (1983), *The Health of the Nation* (1992) and *Our Healthier Nation* (1998). This section discusses the impetus and influences that drive public health policy and how this influences health care practice. We first introduce readers to the process of health policy-making structure and look at the landmarks of public health legislation, and we begin with a brief outline of how legislation is passed in the UK.

Legislation

Nurses of all levels of seniority are often perplexed and unsure about the process by which health policy is made. Here we clarify the uncertainties to provide a general understanding of how public health legislation is passed in the UK. We begin with some definitions. Common law is also known as case law because it occurs when a number of precedents have been derived from specific court cases; statute law is derived from Acts of Parliament and nearly all public health legislation is made through statute law. The stages of legislation are as follows.

- *Green Paper*. This is a consultative document that is issued by a government minister for discussion and comments within a set time frame.
- *White Paper*. This is the next stage on from the Green Paper. The recommendations of the Green Paper are incorporated into the White Paper.
- *Royal Commission*. Ministers can appoint a Committee or a Royal Commission if the issue is of sufficient importance. The purpose of the Royal Commission is to collect and synthesize evidence and interview witnesses. The Minister will incorporate the recommendations that he or she accepts into the White Paper.
- *Parliamentary Bill*. This includes the proposals from the White Paper for making positive steps to change the law. Each Member of Parliament is given a copy of this Bill.
- *First Reading*. This refers to the first reading of the Parliamentary Bill by Members of Parliament.
- *Second Reading*. This refers to the second reading of the Bill, where the main points of the Bill are discussed.
- *Committee of Members of Parliament*. If the second reading is approved, the Bill is referred to the Committee of Members of Parliament, who examine each clause of the Bill.

- *Report Stage*. The Committee of Members of Parliament return the Bill with any amendments for further discussion, and this is known as the Report Stage.

- *Third Reading*. The Bill receives a third reading before it passes to the House of Lords.

- *House of Lords*. The House of Lords then reads the Bill before it is submitted to the Monarch for Royal Assent.

- *Royal Assent*. Once this has been received the Bill becomes an Act. The previous 'clauses' become known as sections.

We would add to this process that an Act of Parliament consists of broad principles and it is the responsibility of the minister to ensure that the details are enacted. For a Private Member's Bill, an individual Member of Parliament, rather than the government, introduces the Bill.

Influencing public health policy

The description of legislation above clearly puts policy into a formal arena, which involves the procedures and the rules and regulations of Parliament. Ham and Hill (1984) define policy in terms of the decisions that allocate resources and how defined goals can be achieved. Many nurses may feel that they cannot influence policy because they do not have the power to make decisions or know the correct network of contacts, but we hope the following paragraphs will encourage nurses to think in a more ambitious way. Hennessy argued that 'many nurses are in positions to participate in the policy process, either by influencing policies as they are made or by getting involved with the implementation. Whatever the level of their involvement, nurses have to understand the policy processes so that correct actions can be taken at the appropriate time' (Hennessy 1997: 37).

Clearly, nurses, like all other health professionals, can only influence health policy if they are knowledgeable on the subject that they wish to influence. We cannot over-stress the importance of thoroughly knowing, and becoming an expert on, your specialist subject. By becoming known through your clinical expertise, research and publishing, you are more likely to be asked to join working parties and committees that are looking to reform existing, or to develop new, policies.

We have divided the formulation of policy into two sections: local policy and national policy. Contemporary nurses have never been in a stronger position to influence policy and the reasons for this are: (a) the study of nursing in higher education has brought a range of subjects not previously taught to nurses; (b) academic confidence from higher education is the route to becoming involved in research, and hence the development of new knowledge; and (c) the changes in the NHS have provided career opportunities and a higher status for nurses in the UK. This has facilitated nurses to take on new and more demanding high-profile roles, such as the new consultant nurse. All of these are empowering steps, giving many nurses a new belief in themselves and a confidence that they must be key players in deciding their own destiny, of which the formulation of policy is a significant part.

Local policy

Nurses, however experienced and qualified, may still feel excluded from making policy because they feel ill at ease in what is to them an unknown territory. Even at the local level, nurses have been known to say, 'I don't make the rules, I just work here!' The notion of being a key figure in policy-making can be daunting, but if nurses are introduced to the notion of being involved in making policy from an early stage then the prospect will be more readily received.

The successful development of public health policy is dependent upon the essential criterion that has been mentioned throughout this chapter, and that is the ability and willingness of all health care professionals (and interested parties) to work together for commonly agreed goals. In the past, the development of local policies has been frequently dominated by the presence of general practitioners, and their word was invariably the final decision. The reasons for this are historical and hierarchical, with nurses and other health care professionals taking on subordinate positions to the doctor, who used their higher professional status to capitalize on the situation.

There are very sound reasons why nurses should be involved in making decisions about local public health policy and the first of these is that nurses work in the area of the people that they care for. This gives them an opportunity to learn about the characteristics of the people and the environment with whom they work. Nurses (particularly nurses in primary care) understand the particular idiosyncrasies of the patients/clients they care for. These may include family networks and cultural differences that are known only to the local population. For example, in certain cultural groups the role of the grandparents is more paternal than in others. The implications for this are that doctors, midwives and health visitors must be mindful of the strong grandparental involvement in certain groups and when speaking to both generations they should take this into account. Historically, another example is found in rural areas, where traditionally women have taken on heavy farming duties to avoid employing farm labourers. The constant lifting involved in farm work results in farmers' wives sustaining chronic disabilities, particularly of the hips and spine. This 'local knowledge' is invaluable in the gathering of information to formulate new, or develop existing, public health policy. Second, nurses practising at a local level have a working insight into the particular issues that challenge their professional practice; for example, high levels of crime may threaten home visiting and the holding of evening clinics. Third, many nurses live in the area where they work and may be service users as well as providers, and this provides a further perspective for making policy. For example, a nurse in the role of user complained that the health needs of men were not fulfilled, and this eventually led to a range of services being introduced, including a well man clinic and a support group for lone fathers. Finally, nurses increasingly have a sound knowledge of theory within their area and this, together with the knowledge acquired within their nursing studies, gives them the confidence and ambition to become key players in the formulation of local public health policy. Some nurses will be encouraged to participate in local public health policy, and one such group of health professionals who have some history of being engaged in developing community practice are health visitors.

National policy

It is only with the increased professionalization of nursing that we will have a real stake in implementing national policy. Nurses must become proactive at all levels of professional development and attempt to become members of committees, working parties and other relevant groups. We certainly have a long way to go before we can be accused of having too much power and influence over policy. This criticism has been, and continues to be, targeted at the medical profession, who have been charged with dominating health policy (Illich 1990). They cannot be blamed for this, but it is up to nurses to challenge this position and put their views forward to influence developing policy.

Further reading

Berridge, V. (1999) *Health and Society in Britain since 1939*. Cambridge: Cambridge University Press.

Blackmore, K. (1998) *Social Policy: An Introduction*. Buckingham: Open University Press.

Dixon, M. and Sweeney, K. (eds) (2001) *Primary Care Groups and Trusts*. Oxford: Radcliffe Medical Press.

5.12 Government initiatives

We have seen (5:1) how public health strategies are influenced and driven by events that have exposed episodes of ill-health in a particular time and place. The timeline illustrates how legislation has both preceded public health issues and emanated from health concerns; for example, the introduction of health visitors in the first 20 years of the twentieth century. They were first known as lady sanitary inspectors and were employed to help to reduce the high rates of infant mortality. Their role of working with mothers was seen as an occupation for women and at the time this measure was criticized by the established male sanitary workers who were not allowed to carry out these duties. This famous piece of nursing history was one of the first initiatives that sought to address a major public health problem. The role of health visitors in implementing government initiatives has continued to expand throughout the decades irrespective of which political party is in government. Nurses, midwives and health visitors may also be involved in local initiatives that respond to the needs of the resident community, such as home safety campaigns where the incidents of childhood accidents in the home are high, or immunization programmes where the uptake is low.

Frequently, initiatives are the result of an 'unacceptable' statistic that makes a media headline, and readers may well be able to recall examples of reports of high rates of teenage pregnancy, high alcohol consumption among teenage boys or increased dependence on anti-depressants among middle-age women. We have already discussed the importance of understanding statistics before action is undertaken, but many of these headlines provoke a public reaction that finally results in a government initiative.

All initiatives require considerable thought and deliberation before they are introduced. The vast expenditure in many public health interventions may not be money well spent if the initiative was implemented on the hunch or whim of an impetuous practitioner who, say, had seen four male patients that day admitting to smoking 40 cigarettes a day and subsequently organized a range of anti-smoking initiatives involving clinics, poster campaigns and counselling. Consider the possible outcome for such an action, which may include cost, ethics and evidence; and what would be the outcome if, the following day, the practitioner had five female patients with chlamydia!

Further reading

Gray, J. A. M. (2001) *Evidence-based Healthcare*, 2nd edn. Edinburgh: Churchill Livingstone.

Klein, R. (1995) *The New Politics of the NHS*, 3rd edn. London: Longman.

Upton, T. and Brooks, B. (2000) *Managing Change in the NHS*. Buckingham: Open University Press.

5.13 Environmental and global health issues

When we begin to think about the effects of the environment on public health it is not long before we are prompted to consider these issues within a geographical framework that is much larger than our own country. For example, when we turn our minds to the effects of radiation on the UK we analyse not only the challenges of our own nuclear power stations but the global effects of nuclear power stations around the world. The most striking example of this has been the health consequences of the Chernobyl radiation accident of 1986. Some readers will remember how areas of the UK continued to monitor levels of radiation within the soil and vegetation, which were much higher than prior to the accident. Our time spent thinking about health and illness is, for most of us, largely concerned with health on a national or regional level. We may be concerned with the health needs of the population that we serve, such as patients on our ward, clients on our caseload, those who are close to us and our own selves.

When we consider world health our first task is to see the various categories that are used to classify the various countries. Readers may already have some experience of classifications such as 'developed' and 'developing' (or underdeveloped), 'First World' and 'Third World', 'North' and 'South', and 'rich' countries and 'poor' countries. All of these articulate the opposing economic statuses of the vastly different countries of the world. We have used the simpler and clearer status of 'rich' and 'poor' throughout this chapter, as do Beaglehole and Bonita (1997).

We begin our thinking about the environmental issues of public health by providing the reader with a broad definition of what the environment is. The explanation by Last embraces all that is external to the 'human host'. He includes such categories as social, cultural, biological and physical, and all of these can influence the health status of individuals and populations (Last 1995). Baggott has argued that such wide reaching definitions as these make it difficult for us to make the link between the environment and health (Baggott 2000). We appreciate this challenge and acknowledge that in modern day nursing curricula environmental issues are often given scant attention. Yet we also believe that this omission from nurse education leaves a fundamental gap in our understanding of health in general and public health in particular. Exactly what effects the environment has on health are difficult to measure and there remains considerable argument among world experts about the gravity of specific environmental problems.

Environmental issues have always been of huge significance to the discipline of public health. When we re-read the 'historical section' we can see how highly public health pioneers regarded pure water and clean air in promoting good health. Today, the environmental concerns of public health continue to have pure water and clean air high on the list of priorities. Despite all the achievements that have occurred worldwide, many people still do not have access to the basic requirements of pure water and fresh air.

The 'dirty dozen'

The writer and broadcaster Jonathon Porritt has worked for many years to understand and inform the public about the problems faced by the environment. He argues that there are 12 significant problems that threaten the future well-being of the Earth and has aptly called his list the 'dirty dozen'. These are ozone depletion, global warming, the energy crisis, air pollution, soil erosion and desertification, deforestation, water shortages, chemicals, toxic wastes, arms spending, international debt and population growth (Porritt 1990). When we look at Porritt's list we can see how environmental health issues must be seen in their widest context to be fully appreciated. As we try to make sense of this list we quickly become aware of how complex the issues are, due to a number of causes. However, economic factors play a very significant part and no one should underestimate what is probably the most fundamental challenge faced by all those concerned with global public health: poverty (7:10). Let us now consider each of these 12 issues individually.

Ozone depletion

This is associated mainly with the release of chlorofluorocarbons (CFCs). CFCs are the by-product of a number of industrial processes. The increasing ozone depletion in the high atmosphere is due to the release of CFCs in aerosol sprays and from refrigeration equipment. As the ozone layer continues to thin, particularly over the polar regions, we are exposed to a greater amount of ultraviolet light. The most well known side effect of this process has been an increased number of skin cancers. There are also other skin conditions, such as inflammation of the skin known as erythema. Less well known is the effect of ultraviolet B radiation on the immune system, with a rise in herpes simplex and also in cataracts. Some readers may have been involved in health promotion projects that warn people about the effects of over-exposure to direct sunlight. Health visitors, in particular, now have an established remit of talking with their clients about the dangers of babies and children being exposed to sunlight without wearing sunhats and protective clothing and using sun block creams. We must be aware that it is the rich countries that are most responsible for the ozone-destroying chemicals, yet the populations of poor countries undoubtedly suffer these effects to a greater extent.

Global warming

This is sometimes known as the 'greenhouse' effect and is caused by gases, including carbon dioxide, that trap heat radiation from the Earth's surface, leading to global warming. One of the most important health effects of global warming has been the rise of vector-borne diseases. Vector-borne infections are caused by the interaction between the human host and the vector. Their presence is affected by the variations of climates and seasons. There are six types of vector-borne infections: biological transmission, extrinsic incubation period, inapparent infection, mechanical transmission, overwintering and transovarial infection.

The energy crisis

For those people working in public health, persuading people to change their habits, so that there is less rather than more energy being consumed, has become one of the greatest challenges of modern times. As individuals, we frequently get locked into the idea that the actions of any one person are insufficient to make a difference. However, we must take responsibility for our consumption of energy, both as individuals and as collective members of the global community. We suggest that the significance of energy conservation is learnt in childhood, when it should be considered to be a vital commodity to be respected and used with care.

Air pollution

In section 5:2 we saw the significance that Florence Nightingale placed upon clean air. At the time of her writings, Victorian cities were overcrowded, as they recruited labour from the countryside to meet the manpower needed for the mills and factories of the Industrial Revolution. The urban air of Florence Nightingale's day was heavy with smoke pollution from the mills and the pungent odours of life in overcrowded conditions with little or no sanitation. Indeed, little was done to address the effects of air pollution until the Clean Air Act of 1956. The Control of Pollution Act of 1974 gave individuals greater legal power against those people (often companies) who polluted the environment. Legislation to combat air pollution has been slow, with much lobbying done by the Green Party and other environmental groups. The 1990 Environmental Protection Act introduced combined inspection and control and stipulated that those individuals or organizations found to be responsible for pollution must pay for the harm that they have caused.

Today, air pollution is recognized as a major health hazard. Although we no longer have the air pollution created by the Victorian factories, we have new threats to clean air, particularly exhaust fumes from motorcars. In poor countries the by-products of industrialization are not always regulated, and this continues to cause considerable harm to those who live near such factories and plants. Unfortunately, the owners of many of these sites are the sole employers, and local residents are forced to tolerate these conditions, as there is no other source of work. There are some particularly dangerous areas in the world, such as the countries of Central and Eastern Europe, where air pollution from large cities and industrial plants causes conditions such as chronic respiratory diseases, leading to a rise in mortality rates.

Soil erosion and desertification

The continuing change in the global landscape is usually only brought to our attention when we become aware of a 'natural' disaster. From our television screens we have all too often witnessed huge numbers of people standing in a land that used to be lush and green with enough crops to sustain its population, but that is now in the grip of a major famine. The United Nations is pessimistic about the challenges presented to us by the changing climate (United Nations Environment Programme 1999) and claims that the effects are greater than we first thought.

Deforestation

The reasons for deforestation are complex and very much related to soil erosion and desertification. Readers may be aware of only a proportion of the deforestation that has been, and continues to be, undertaken throughout the world. Much deforestation takes place in the poorer countries of South America, where there is a conflict of interest between those who seek to protect the forests and the indigenous populations who are dependent upon their forests for their livelihood. The methods of cutting down trees have changed drastically from traditional methods to a vast mechanical industry. Today, the destruction of forests is a massive business in which local people are merely pawns for huge companies that can deforest great areas of ancient trees in a very short period of time. The effects of deforestation are catastrophic, not only for the global climate, but also for habitats and species that become extinct. The lives of local people have in many cases been utterly destroyed, as they have been strangled by the greed and corruption of unethical organizations that obtain the precious wood at any cost.

Water shortages

It is estimated that 200 litres of water are used per day in each UK household. Our need for a constant supply of fresh water is insatiable. It has been estimated that 40 per cent of the world is already short of fresh water and by 2030 the shortage will rise to 60 per cent and in western Asia to 90 per cent (Donaldson and Donaldson 1998).

Trevelyan describes the state of living conditions experienced by the poorest citizens of Victorian cities and the ancient problem of obtaining clean water for everyone: 'these pioneers of progress saved space by crowding families into single rooms or thrusting them underground into cellars and saved money by the use of cheap and insufficient building material, and by providing no drains or, worse still, by providing drains that oozed into the water supply' (Trevelyan 1973: 127).

We have already seen how the purification of water has been, and continues to be, a fundamental public health issue and contaminated water remains a significant source of spreading disease (cholera, amoebic and bacillary dysenteries, enteric fevers, infective hepatitis and helminthic (worm) infections). Nurses who choose to work in poor countries may become heavily involved, not only in working towards providing water (for example, by drilling wells and sinking boreholes) but in ensuring that the water is pure (by filtrating and disinfecting water). There is some positive news. The 1980s was designated as the International Drinking Water Supply and Sanitation Decade, and the number of people receiving safe water and sanitation has increased (Beaglehole and Bonita 1997).

Chemicals

The release of chemicals through industrial processes continues to cause major concerns not only because of the direct effect on human health but also because of the devastating impact on the environment. The subsequent air pollution caused by chemicals being released from industrial activity, both on land and in water, includes dioxins and organochlorine compounds. The severity is dependent upon both the length of time individuals are exposed to chemicals (the longer the exposure, the greater the danger to health) and the resources available to countries to cope with chemical contamination. Poorer countries are particularly at risk of contamination from dangerous industrial plants and have few financial and human resources to deal with chemical accidents and prolonged exposures. Air pollution from industry and traffic may cause 'acid rain' and contains some of the most harmful chemical compounds, such as nitrous oxides, which cause both health and environmental problems, in particular the depletion of the ozone layer.

Toxic wastes

Like chemical contamination, the disposal of toxic wastes is a global issue of great concern. The British Medical Association's 1989 report on Hazardous Waste and Human Health raised anxieties over the relationship between a number of major health problems and toxic wastes. Despite the fears of birth defects, cancers and heart problems being linked to toxic wastes, such associations are difficult to prove (BMA 1989). At the time of writing the UK faces a new anxiety regarding toxic waste: the foot and mouth epidemic of 2001 cost the lives of over 1 million animals. These animals were burnt in pyres and their remains buried in large identified sites, causing concern regarding the seepage of toxins into the water supply. Landfill sites have always caused disquiet among the public. We have cited the Chernobyl incident of 1986 as an environmental disaster of massive proportions. Nuclear power continues to give rise to many fears among those working in the industry, interested professionals (such as health workers) and the general public. Baggott (2000) identifies the main health concerns as: first, the catastrophic consequences of a nuclear disaster; second, the effects of smaller emissions and leaks; third, problems arising from the transportation of radioactive materials and waste; and, finally, the issues associated with the storage and disposal of nuclear waste. In common with other environmental health factors, proving links with ill-health has sometimes been found to be difficult.

Arms spending

This is an extremely complex area, which can be summed up from two perspectives. The first concerns the fact that we spend a disproportionate amount of revenue on arms and defence in relation to health care in the UK. Second, the arms trade is such a lucrative market that we continue to sell weapons and weapon technology to many countries of the world, which we may well face on future battlefields. This irony is further compounded by the fact that should we engage in military action with these countries it is our health care system that will have to bear the brunt of treating our armed forces!

International debt

Many countries, in their attempts to provide food and resources for their own people, have been, and continue to be, strangled by the noose of international debt. The world's countries have recognized how the debts owed by poorer nations prevent them from gaining independence and some self-sufficiency. There have been a number of initiatives to reduce the international debts of the HIPC (heavily indebted poor countries) by the World Bank and the IMF (International Monetary Fund) (7:5).

Population growth

Understanding the growth of populations is a fundamental requirement of public health. We have seen in our discussion of the 'census' above the significance that is placed upon gathering baseline data to be able to make short-term and long-term (although less reliable) population projections. The growth in population throughout the world varies considerably, with the poorer countries having the most rapid increase. The population of the world in 1994 was 5.7 billion people. The highest projection given by the United Nations Population Fund is that by the year 2050, there will be 12.5 billion people in the world (Bonita and Beaglehole 2000). This is a startling statistic and we should pause to consider the effects of this on the world at large and the lives of individual people. It is clear that no one can afford to be complacent about how this will affect global environmental issues and world health. Both this and future generations of nurses have a crucial role to play in delivering relevant health care that will contribute to curbing the rise in populations. This may be through the use of contraception, the prevention of sexually transmitted diseases, increasing awareness of family health and involvement in changing women's status in society.

The Healthy Cities Project: a global environmental health alliance

In the latter part of this section we analyse the health of cities and look to the work of John Ashton and Howard Seymour, who in 1988 wrote a significant text that was, and remains, of great interest for all those people who study public health. Ashton and Seymour (1988) discuss the role of the WHO, the Alma Ata Declaration in 1977 and the recognition of a need to develop a new approach to public health that embraces and meets the needs of every citizen. From this there developed a Health for All Strategy. The Healthy Cities Project was a development of this initial work, and came out of the Beyond Health Care conference held in Toronto in 1984. The notion of 'healthy public policies' also began to be developed at this conference, where it was decided to move away from blaming people for their lifestyle behaviours. The Healthy Cities Project was borne out of this 'new public health'. A number of cities were brought together in a spirit of collaboration to enable the development of urban health promotion. There were 24 European cities involved, including Liverpool and the areas of Bloomsbury and

Camden in London, and these cities represented the UK. The significance of the impact of the environment became very significant in the definition of what a healthy city actually is. The individual qualities of cities were recognized as their culture, personality and spirit. However, it was suggested that all cities must have basic criteria that are necessary for each inhabitant, and these include:

- safe and adequate food;
- a safe water supply;
- shelter;
- sanitation;
- freedom from poverty and fear (Ashton 1992: 157).

These are very basic criteria and, indeed, Edwin Chadwick and Florence Nightingale had both found common aspirations a century before. Yet the objectives of the 'new public health', as translated in the Healthy Cities Project, take the above criteria not as all that is required by people who live in cities, but as a baseline for a range of ideas that can be expanded upon to build cultural, educational and social interests, where people are involved and participate in the decisions they make about their own lives. This became the 'New Urban Public Health', moving away from paternalism to partnership (Ashton and Seymour 1988). The cities project put forward five elements, which include implementing and formulating ideas that can be put into action, developing good practice, research, disseminating ideas and promoting collaboration and giving mutual support. The healthy cities project produced some wonderful examples of good practice and collaboration relating to environmental issues; for example, the creation of community gardens, allotments and small-scale animal husbandry projects.

We have discussed throughout this chapter the significance of collecting and analysing data to plan public health projects and initiatives. The following 11 points comprise the information that the WHO team use to measure what a healthy city is. The list includes traditional public health information, but readers will see some more creative ones.

- demography;
- quality of physical environment including pollution and the standard of housing and other buildings;
- the local economy, including unemployment levels;
- the quality of social support services, the type of social environment, the psychosocial stress and nature of local culture;
- personal safety;
- the appearance of the environment and the quality of life experienced by the inhabitants;
- educational services;
- the sense of community, including community participation and local government structures;

- health promotion indicators, such as physical exercise, diet, alcohol and tobacco intake;
- public health statistics, such as morbidity and mortality rates;
- equity (World Health Organization (1986b), adapted from *Healthy Cities Workshop*, Lisbon 1986).

The concern, of course, is that once a high-profile focus on a particular area is completed, everything will revert to its pre-state. Alas, this has happened in the past, but we believe that the key to preventing a return to the 'old ways' is in participation of the local community. Indeed, readers who have been involved in setting up support groups will realize the significance of both service providers and service users working together with mutual respect. In order for the support group to be maintained the service providers should gradually withdraw and allow the service users to take over the group themselves. The same principles of encouraging participation and giving empowerment to the local population apply to projects such as the Healthy Cities Project, where the local community maintains the support group that they have jointly established.

It is understandable that we focus our attention on the health of cities, but in doing so we are limiting our understanding of world health and fail to make comparisons with the health of people in all other countries. This is essential if we are fully to grasp global epidemiology, which is an essential component of global public health. The sociology chapter began with the old adage 'no man is an island' and we can equally apply this saying to public health, where no public health issue can be examined in isolation from the public health of the wider world. An example of this is where there is a case of tuberculosis and then we are prompted to examine the cases of tuberculosis occurring throughout the country. We may map the cases further afield and, in doing so, we can map the incidences, the locations, when the disease occurred and the progression of the disease, and take public health measures to halt it and where possible eradicate it altogether.

The World Health Organization is the body that brings together global concerns about health so that each country can contribute to world health strategies. One successful and memorable strategy has been the eradication of smallpox; this ten-year campaign led by the WHO resulted in the last naturally occurring case in Somalia in 1977 (Beaglehole and Bonita 1997). The Alma Ata Declaration of 1977 is symbolic of the collective sentiments of the WHO, and the declaration is remembered for the following ambitious statement, which did not become reality: the attainment by all the peoples of the world by the year 2000 of a level of health that will permit them to lead a socially and economically productive life (WHO 1977). There are other agencies that help shape the health status of countries. For example, the World Bank has an enormous influence on the problems of debt experienced by individual countries, particularly developing countries. The implications of world poverty for global health are enormous and, indeed, the WHO asserts that 'poverty is the greatest single killer' (WHO 1995).

Further reading

Ashton, J. and Seymour, H. (1988) *The New Public Health*. Milton Keynes: Open University Press.

Beaglehole, R. and Bonita, R. (1997) *Public Health at the Crossroads: Achievements and Prospects*. Cambridge: Cambridge University Press.

MacDonald, T. H. (1998) *Rethinking Health Promotion: A Global Approach*. London: Routledge.

5.14 Conclusions

As we draw the strands of this chapter to a close, the range of specialities that collectively come together to form the discipline of public health will surprise many readers. Public health is rooted in our social, medical and nursing history, but it is also a core discipline of contemporary health care practice. Public health can be likened to the wise family relative, who is always there, and in times of crisis will quietly work, often without thanks, offering support and compassion to those who need it. Finally, we ask readers to consider how often in their daily work they have seen or been involved in public health practices. For most of us the answer will be frequently. Public health is considered to be the eyes of health care practice, and it closes them at its peril.

Thinking philosophy

Glossary terms used in this chapter

Axiomatic · Consequentialism · Culpable · Deontology · Ensoulment · Epistemic · Hedonists · Metaphysics · Monistic · Normative · Pluralism · *Prima facie* · Rationality · Secular · Sentience · Volition

6.1 Introduction

Philosophy covers a wide topical area. In its simplest sense it is the study of knowledge, especially in relation to ultimate reality, general causes and principles of the state of being human in relation to the world. Furthermore, there are many branches of philosophy, including the philosophies of language, law, education, history, science, mind, psychology, religion, politics, space and time, to name but a few. To ask 'what is philosophy?' is to ask a philosophical question, and to attempt to answer this question is an undertaking in philosophy. We will see throughout this chapter that there are different levels of meaning and understanding, and in terms of establishing what philosophy is we can give two answers. First, we could say that everyone has a philosophy and knows what that is. Or, second, we could answer that philosophy is 'a matter of standing back a little from the ephemeral urgencies to take an aphoristic overview that usually embraces both value-commitments and beliefs about the general nature of things' (Flew 1979: vii). Both answers are probably correct but they require differing levels of interpretation.

Philosophy is important in nursing and other health care professions as the concepts that are often dealt with inform many ethical considerations that impact on practice. Given this central role in medical ethics it is, perhaps, surprising that it has not featured as prominently in professions allied to medicine as it ought to have. Certainly, during the course of a career in health care the majority of staff need the necessary philosophical knowledge to be able to give informed views. It is no longer acceptable to leave ethical decisions solely to 'men' of medicine; instead we need to offer intelligent responses from a multidisciplinary basis.

There are many philosophical concepts that could be drawn upon to give us some insights into how we should practise in health care settings, and this field is forever unfolding. However, we have identified a number of philosophical principles that have been addressed, not only by philosophers but also by many related disciplines, which are particularly relevant to medical and nursing practice, as they impact on other people's lives. They cannot be seen independently as they are often both inextricably entwined and often stand in opposition to each other. None the less, they must be dealt with despite their complexity, and they must receive serious attention given their consequences for all concerned.

PART ONE: THEORY

6.2 Autonomy

Autonomy is concerned with the principle of self-government or self-determination: the capacity to think, make decisions and to take action independently of others' let, hindrance or coercion. At face value this would seem a laudable position without serious challenge. However, as is usually the case with such concepts, once we begin to explore them we meet many difficulties, requiring qualifications to be made to the original position. For example, in this opening defining statement, what is the case for the growing child, or the bank robber, to act autonomously without hindrance when in the case of the child they may be endangered, or in the case of the thief they intend to harm others? Clearly in such instances autonomy must have some qualifications and we will deal with these in two sections: the differing types of autonomy and the conditions of autonomy.

Types of autonomy

The first thing to establish is that autonomy can be subdivided into three basic types. The first type refers to *autonomy of thought*, in which the person can engage in all aspects of thinking without interference from others. This will include having one's own beliefs, likes and dislikes, personal preferences and personal decisions. In short, it is 'thinking for oneself'. Yet even this requires some qualification, as it is difficult to imagine going through life without receiving some input from others via their attempts at persuasion. In fact, democratic societies are based on the very notion of persuading others to their point of view. However, as long as the end result is that the person is allowed to 'think for themselves' the principle holds true. Clearly, brainwashing and ideological indoctrination conflicts with autonomy at this level, but can be overcome, as we will shortly see (Chapter 8).

The second type is the *autonomy of will*, which refers to the idea that someone can make decisions based on their own deliberations. Although the concept of the 'will' is complex, it is generally regarded as the faculty of choice by which we decide what actions we will make (Kent 1996). Not without its critics, the notion of a 'will' (free will is dealt with in 6:5) in its pure sense is viewed with some scepticism. Notwithstanding this, we are reasonably safe in believing in a human 'will' that has a decision-making capacity, and that it is up to the individual as to how it is exercised. The freedom to decide is the autonomy of will (Dworkin 1988).

The third type is the *autonomy of action*, in which, as a corollary to the autonomies of thought and will, a person can take action independently. In this scenario we can see that a person may have autonomy of thought and autonomy of will but may be prevented from taking the action that he desires. Furthermore, we can also see that the prevention of action may be desired by others if the autonomy of thought refers to thinking about harming others (or self), the autonomy of will refers to deciding to take action against others (harming others/suicide) and the prevention is deemed justified. Here we can see where the principle of autonomy is difficult to reconcile in relation to paternalism (6:4). However, some degree of resolution is achieved when we employ the notion of rationality (Christman 1989).

The German philosopher Immanuel Kant (1724–1804) argued that rational beings had the power to act autonomously, while non-rational beings were acted upon. In this sense rational beings could be both rational and irrational, with the 'will' linking the two to enable people to reason. Thus, the rational has the stronger power to act upon the irrational (Gillon 1986). Therefore, autonomy of thought, will and action is reliant upon it being rational and/or *reason*-able. The child in danger, and the bank robber endangering others, are not considered rational or reasonable.

Conditions of autonomy

The philosophical concept of autonomy is linked to respect for someone else's autonomy, which is particularly relevant for those working in health care settings. Your autonomy is important for you and respect for others' autonomy flows from that. However, there are said to be 'three presuppositions that must be made by anyone who thinks that your autonomy should be respected in a present situation' (Glover 1988). These presuppositions are termed conditions and involve:

- the existence condition;
- the development condition;
- the possession condition.

The first, the *existence condition*, simply means that an autonomous person must exist. To have respect for autonomy one must consider the person to be alive. This would have a significant impact on, for example, how we view future generations or when we consider an embryo as a person. The second presupposition, the *development condition*, is concerned with the level of development that a person has achieved in order to have the wish or desire that would constitute his or her autonomy. For example, a growing child may one day want to win the Nobel prize for physics, but restricting her education today is not overriding her autonomy, as she does not yet have the wish or desire to become a physicist. It may well constitute bad parenting but does not constitute a disrespect for her/his autonomy. The third presupposition, the *possession condition*, follows on from the previous two conditions and refers to actually having the wish or desire that could be potentially overridden. It does not rely on a future time where you may be more knowledgeable or more intelligent, it is dependent on you actually having the desire whose satisfaction is in question. We can add a further rider to this possession condition, which would incorporate the person's disposition to that desire or wish. By adding this we can claim to respect a person's autonomy (his wishes or desires) when he is asleep, drugged, unconscious or hypnotized and is temporarily 'out of touch' with those desires (Glover 1988).

Further reading

Dworkin, G. (1988) *The Theory and Practice of Autonomy*. Cambridge: Cambridge University Press.

Christman, J. (ed) (1989) *The Inner Citadel: Essays on Individual Autonomy*. Oxford: Oxford University Press.

▎6.3 Paternalism

As we have seen in the previous section, full autonomy is conceptually difficult to accept, as some restrictions may be necessary in order to safeguard a person or to protect someone else. But this now raises questions regarding who is making these decisions and on what basis. Paternalism is a term that denotes the restrictions that are applied to a person's liberty of action when they are imposed for the good of that person. Of course, this again raises questions as to who is making these restrictions on liberty and how they have arrived at the measure of 'good'. Those in favour of paternalism argue that if one can prevent people from harming themselves then there is no reason not to do so. However, those in favour of libertarianism counter-argue that paternalism, even done with the best of intentions, does more harm than good in the long run. We will sketch out the main debate relating to paternalism under three headings: (a) the main arguments; (b) the risks and benefits; and (c) hard and soft approaches.

Three main arguments

In coming to understand the argument for paternalistic intervention we must make an early assumption. We must assume that we are dealing with an adult, who is rational, has the ability to weigh up the relevant information and can make clear choices. In this scenario what right have health care professionals to intervene in attempting to alter his or her choice of action? The paternalistic view would suggest that there are three main arguments for such intervention, but it should be remembered that the intervention must be considered as in the patient's best interests. As our example let us suggest that a person has made the choice to take a course of action that the majority of society would consider as a bad choice. In this scenario Glover (1988) uses the example of a person who has chosen to become a heroin addict, and in this case the argument for paternalistic prevention, he argues, is threefold.

The first paternalist argument is that the suffering that will be caused through the person's choice will be considerable, and paternalists would argue that they can be confident that those who have not made that choice would be better off than those who have. The second argument is that in making such a bad choice the suffering that is anticipated is almost certainly going to occur. That is, the probability of its occurrence is considerable. The third line of argument concerns the fact that reversing the choice, once embarked upon, is not easy and thus his future freedom of action will be greatly reduced. In choosing an example such as becoming a heroin addict, in which few would argue that attempting to persuade someone against such a course of action is wrong, it could be said that this is too 'black and white'. We would agree. However, it is a good starting point for the paternalist argument, from which position all manner of interventions are undertaken 'in the patient's best interests'. It has even been argued that 'if you agree that the physician's primary function is to make the patient feel better, a certain amount of authoritarianism, paternalism and domination are the essence of the physician's effectiveness' (Ingelfinger 1980: 1507).

Risks and benefits

The Hippocratic oath states: 'I will follow that system or regimen which, according to my ability and judgement, I consider for the benefit of my patients' (British Medical Association 1984: 69). As Gillon (1986) points out, the Hippocratic oath says nothing about doing what the patient requests, or not deceiving them, or asking them what it is that they would like, or informing them about choices or alternatives. However, this stark conflict, in reality, only rarely occurs, as the majority of doctors and other health care professionals do involve the patient, and take into consideration their wishes in the delivery of medical interventions. And in this there is a question of assessing the elements of risks and benefits in arriving at a paternalistic course of action.

In paternalistic decisions consideration must be given to the weight applied to risks and benefits for the person concerned. For our heroin addict above it is clear that, in his or her decision, the risks are great and the benefits are few. However, not all situations are as clear cut as this, as we have noted. Furthermore, as the benefits decrease and the risks increase, the case for trying to persuade the person against his or her decision also increases. In relation to the risks associated with not wearing a seatbelt and the reduced benefits of not doing so, the persuasion for actually wearing them takes the paternalistic form of legislation. Although most members of society do not welcome excessive state intervention, most would welcome the law on seatbelts or the wearing of crash helmets, as the consequences of not using these may draw heavily on health care resources that are in great demand from other less reckless situations. The final consideration is that the slight disadvantage of having to put on a seatbelt is very small in relation to the advantages gained in the event of a crash. In health care decisions the risks–benefits ratios are often highly complex, and frequently conflict with autonomous choices. Take a moment to think about the case of a smoker who continues to smoke, in which the risks are high, but so too are the 'benefits' for the smoker, and the disadvantages of having to give up are considerable for them. Furthermore, should smokers have the right to make those autonomous decisions when they are harming themselves, harming others through passive smoking and causing a drain on limited health care resources? Although we have legislation regarding smoking in public buildings we do not, as yet, have a law banning smoking completely. However, we certainly do have a powerful health promotion policy that paternalistically persuades people not to smoke or to cease if they do.

Hard and soft paternalism

A distinction is often drawn in paternalist arguments between what is called 'hard' and 'soft' paternalism. This distinction allows some advocates to be able to agree to a form of soft paternalism, while arguing against hard paternalistic approaches. Soft paternalism refers to the doctrine that paternalist interventions can only be justified when the person whose action is being restricted had not made a choice in a substantially voluntary way. Thus, if one considers that the person was not choosing voluntarily, paternalistic action might be advocated. Hard paternalism, on the other hand, refers to making decisions for someone else even if they had made their choice in a significantly voluntary way, but it was considered that their choice was the wrong one. This stance usually requires the paternalist to have some considerable power, either by legislation or by status, and some degree of control over the person. It is exercised in many walks of life, such as the police and fire services, armed forces, schools, families and even in some health care settings (for example, psychiatry).

Further reading

Buchanan, A. (1978) Medical paternalism, *Philosophy and Public Affairs*, 7: 370–90.

6.4 Utilitarianism

Probably the most widely, and popularly, known philosophical concept is utilitarianism, the roots of which can be traced back into ancient thought. Plato himself discussed the central tenet of utilitarianism in relation to the greatest balance of pleasure over pain. However, in more modern terms, utilitarianism grew out of the Enlightenment, with its three classical exponents being Jeremy Bentham (1748–1832), John Stuart Mill (1806–73), and Henry Sidgwick (1838–1900). Although now popularized, and simplified, under the common theme of 'the greatest good for the greatest number', it must be understood that in philosophical terms it is probably more accurate to refer to it as a cluster of concepts and ideas that have addressed the many and varied deconstructions of utilitarianism. For example, in relation to the central issue of pleasure over pain, Mill (1991) made a distinction between higher and lower pleasures in an attempt to answer the criticism of the Hedonists, who claimed that the concept was sensualist. Furthermore, many utilitarians argue for a further distinction between quality and quantity of pleasure, which shows how a basic idea can be constantly subdivided into ever more complex issues. However, the starting point for most utilitarians is in relation to the theory about the rightness of human actions according to which the only good result is welfare. Welfare is understood as well-being, or utility, which should, in their view, be maximized. We recognize today that there are two basic types of utilitarianism:

- act utilitarianism;
- rule utilitarianism.

Act utilitarianism

This is the simpler version of utilitarianism and is concerned with the view that each individual action that a person takes should be assessed on the results that it alone produces. In act utilitarianism an action can be assessed in relation to its rightness when its welfare or utility has been maximized. For example, if the action being assessed is donating to charity then it can be claimed to be right human action when the welfare of the greater number of people has been maximized over the detriment that the giver receives by his donation. At one level this appears as a straightforward analysis with a clear delineation between outcome of welfares. However, in reality, and in practical terms, problems arise with more complex frameworks of action. For example, in relation to taking action to save a person's life against his wishes, or to take a life in the form of an execution, both scenarios produce difficulties in the principle of maximizing welfare. This is due to the fact that in the former example the person does not wish to live, while in the latter he presumably does (6:11, 6:12). At this point some utilitarians have turned to the notion of a common-sense morality by which human action can be judged, but this leads them to look inwardly towards an intuitive state or an inherent set of principles of rightness. In short, this is referred to as rule utilitarianism.

Rule utilitarianism

Within this perspective the right action is that which is consistent with those rules that would maximize welfare or utility if all would accept them. Rule utilitarianism does not concern itself with the assessment of an individual's action but considers the utility of a rule for humans to act by. The fundamental idea is that everyone should do whatever is prescribed by the optimum set of rules even though on occasion less total happiness results. Whereas the act utilitarians would ask the question 'what would be the result of my action?', the rule utilitarians would ask 'what would be the result if everyone acted that way?' In our example of the charity donation above, the rule utilitarians could conclude that as a rule for human action donating to charity is right, as welfare is maximized within the principle. However, as in the case of the act utilitarians' more complex situations, such as the saving of the life and the execution, they continue to produce problems. For example, rules relating to abortion and capital punishment are notoriously complex and differ between ideological groups and across countries and creeds. This formation of rules to govern human action is very close to the concept of duty (6:7) (Brandt 1983).

Criticisms of utilitarianism

The major criticisms made against utilitarianism fall broadly into a number of groups for convenience, and these can be classed as (a) practical elements, (b) justice and (c) relativity.

Practical elements

In putting into practice utilitarian principles we immediately see some problems arising. The first concerns the notion of happiness. For example, what is it? What does it mean to be happy? How can it be measured? Do we need to be totally happy all of the time? Although Bentham equated happiness with mere pleasure, Mill later rejected this in favour of equating happiness with human flourishing. However, this simply raises more questions as to what flourishing actually means, and with the variability of human nature how does it take account of individuals' desire for autonomy? Modern utilitarians tend to overcome some of these problems by claiming the satisfaction of an individual's autonomous preferences 'as being the best way of maximising overall happiness' (Gillon 1986).

Justice

Maximizing the greatest good for the greatest number may well mean the sacrifice of an innocent party. To what extent can we accept that the state is more important than the individual? Is it morally correct to sacrifice one person in order to save one hundred? There seems to be an abundance of problems with the justice of utilitarianism in relation to the individual's right of autonomy, but there are also problems of a collective nature with the maintenance of unjust institutions in the quest for utilitarianism. For example, in maximizing the greatest welfare for the majority of a given society, who would consider the institution of the slave trade as just?

Relativity

The morality of human action is measured only in terms of outcomes, or results, and the issues of intent and motives are not dealt with. This makes it difficult to understand the relationship between happiness and suffering. For example, there are a group of people who prefer some legitimated suffering in the form of their religious doctrine, and although utilitarians would argue that their autonomous preference for suffering is being satisfied, thus maximizing their welfare, the problems of relative happiness and suffering remain (Smart and Williams 1973).

Although utilitarians have numerous counter-arguments to the many criticisms levelled against them, difficult philosophical problems do remain in this theory of moral action. It is probably safer, in philosophical terms, to conclude that the harder rigid versions of utilitarianism are less helpful in health care settings rather than the abridged versions that have developed over generations. It would appear to us that accepting that the individual has the right of autonomy, within the limitations set out above and below, is a fundamental construct in any theory of morality.

Further reading

 Scarre, G. (1996) *Utilitarianism*. London: Routledge.

6.5 Free will and determinism

Free will and determinism are apparently opposed philosophical concepts but are best dealt with together, as they are also inextricably linked. Both free will and determinism have long philosophical histories and most philosophical theories have addressed these ideas in the progress towards formulating conceptual frameworks. Certainly, they are as important today as they have always been and are central issues for those working in health care settings who wish to understand to what extent we may be held responsible for ill-health or to what extent we are culpable in law. By understanding free will and determinism we are in a position to make statements as to what we consider to be moral behaviour or moral action. Thus, morality features large in our philosophical understanding of free will and determinism and provides the framework for the many codes of practice by which we judge our professional behaviour.

Free will

We will attend to the notion of free will by making a distinction between the concept of 'free' and the concept of the 'will'. In the concept of free will we are mainly concerned with the extent to which we are able to choose a course of action freely, whereas the 'will' is popularly understood as an internal mental faculty that provides us with the basis for making choices. Of course, this is simply stated and in real terms has provided the foundation for complex philosophical debate for centuries. However, for the sake of our brief overview we are concerned with the notion of free will and determinism in terms of attempting to answer two fundamental questions: (a) to what extent are we truly free to make choices; and (b) to what extent are we morally responsible for our actions? (Strawson 1986). Before we tackle these questions it is worth pointing out that some philosophers have answered in the affirmative to both, some in the negative to both, and some have produced a range of permutations from 'possibly' to 'perhaps' (Kane 1996).

At an everyday level it is almost axiomatic that we have the freedom to exercise our own choice in either understanding an action or abstaining from one. Yet we must deal with questions relating to the extent to which we could argue that irrespective of our upbringing we are free to exercise our will according to our wishes at the time of making decisions. However, this appears to qualify the true notion of free will. In secular terms some argue that we are free agents, as most people are not intoxicated, imprisoned or forced to take a course of action, and thus we must be responsible for our behaviour. However, others have countered this by claiming that genetic inheritance and early upbringing have influenced the way that we are. The question really revolves around whether given our physical and psychological make-up we can still make free choices of action for which we are responsible. Given that mental illnesses, brain damage and altered states of mind can affect the exercise of volition, if these are absent can the exercise of choice be truly free? (Kent 1996).

Determinism

Determinism has been understood in different ways down the centuries, but basically holds that every event has a cause and that the future is predictable (Earman 1986). To understand determinism philosophers have looked to the physical sciences, such as Newton's physics, for explanatory logic. Determinists believe that all events, including human actions, are predetermined. If this is the case then it is difficult to see how we can be responsible for our actions, given that they have been predetermined and therefore are inevitable. However, to extricate themselves from this impasse the determinists argue the case for human action to be understood in terms of causal relationships that are formed from choices of action (Pink 1996). In both areas of argumentation involving free will and determinism, the question of one being true while the other being false is often posed the other way around. That is, why should one be true, or why should it be false? In a physical sense determinism may hold some truth for human action in terms of cause and effect, but what can it tell us of motivation, desires, artistic impression and so on? Furthermore, if we link determinism with the physics of the natural world, where does this fit with the indeterminism of the more recent quantum physics?

Compatabilists and incompatabilists

Some philosophers have argued that free will is compatible with determinism and suggest that free choice of action is essentially a question of merely not being constrained or obstructed in some way when arriving at a decision to act. In this scenario compatabilists would argue that under normal conditions or situations humans are free to choose one thing over another. They accept a degree of determinism, in that our genetic inheritance may govern our physical make-up and our upbringing may determine our socio-psychological frame of reference, but within these limitations we are free to choose what to do. Compatabilists tend to focus on understanding human action in terms of causality and make a claim that free will and determinism are often defined in ways that make one explicitly exclusive of the other. Thus, in terms of our two questions the compatabilists would answer in the affirmative to both; that is, to being free to make choices and to being responsible for our actions. On the other hand, the incompatabilists hold that free will is not compatible with determinism and point out that if human action was predetermined, even before we were born, then the idea of being morally responsible for those actions is nonsensical. However, incompatabilists fall into two types: (a) those philosophers who believe that we are free to make choices and therefore are clearly responsible for our actions; and (b) those philosophers who believe we are not genuinely free agents and therefore not totally responsible for our actions. Clearly these are opposite positions, but both argue that free will and determinism are incompatible. The former they argue that determinism is false but fail to say why the claim for falsity is any better than the claim for its truth. The latter group of incompatiblists argue that the falsity of determinism cannot actually help their case, and suggest that to be truly morally responsible one would need to be genuinely responsible for the way one is. In this case we would need to be responsible for the way in which we were brought up or responsible for our genetic inheritance, and clearly neither is the case.

This shows the complexity of the relationship between free will and determinism and the two central questions that are posed. It also shows the nature of philosophical enquiry and how in one sense there is a tension between such theoretical speculation and practical human action. For many human beings it is accepted that we can make free choices and are responsible for those actions irrespective of the philosophical argument to the contrary.

Further reading

Kane, R. (1996) *The Significance of Free Will*. New York: Oxford University Press.

6.6 Beneficence and non-maleficence

The extent to which we are driven to action is clearly a complex matter, and even our outline in the few short sections above would suggest either a force that 'pushes' us to action (propelled) or a force that 'pulls' us (ought). In health care settings we are very fond of making claims that we are there to 'act in the patients' best interests' or that 'the patients' interests always comes first'. However, we have already seen that we often act in a paternalistic fashion and act against the individual patient's autonomous state (6:2). Yet few would argue against the idea that the motivation for being involved in the health care professions is to do good for others, or at least not to do them any harm. But here again things are not as clear cut as they might at first seem and we must deal with the two issues of beneficence and non-maleficence.

Beneficence

Beneficence literally means to do good to someone, to show by actions a positive kindness and to behave in a way that produces a positive outcome for the person. We can see from this that beneficence must carry an element of action or behaviour that constitutes for the person an outcome that is considered good. In health care settings it does not involve the person merely wishing or desiring to do good, or feeling pity for the patient's plight, nor is it having sympathy, meddling in the patient's affairs or looking as though one may be doing something rather than nothing. It is worth emphasizing that beneficence means *doing good* (action) *for others* (not self). However, there must be some constraints to this, as what one person considers as good may not be viewed as such by another, particularly the recipient. Furthermore, we must be aware of the extent to which we might be contravening the patient's autonomy and acting outside of paternalistic boundaries. The three main constraints against launching ourselves, in beneficent mode, to do good for others are: (a) a respect for their autonomy (6:2); (b) a balance of costs (8:10); and (c) a question of justice (6:4) (Gillon 1986).

In dealing with the respect for a patient's autonomy (6:2), we only need to add here that the central issue revolves around understanding what the person actually subjectively desires, what he wishes to do or what he would like to be done to him. Although there might be cases in which the act of beneficence may override autonomous decisions, such as in the patient's desire to commit suicide, it is important to ascertain what their wishes actually are. There is often a conflict between their wants and needs (e.g. antibiotics for a viral infection), and we have already seen that the Hippocratic oath behoves the physician to act in accordance with what he or she considers is for the benefit of the patient (not necessarily what they desire). The second constraint refers to the notion of balancing the costs between acting beneficently and respecting the patient's autonomy. The weighing of bad effects in the quest to do good for the patient must be considered, and the balancing must involve the patient's wishes. Gillon (1986: 77) sums up this position: 'one person will choose laryngectomy and a 60 per cent three year survival rate for vocal cord cancer, whereas another will prefer radiation to spare his voice at the cost of a three year survival rate of only 30–40 per cent'. This balancing of costs is reliant upon good communication, which is grounded in honesty and integrity. The third constraint is a question of justice. In a system of health care, which has limited resources, decisions have to be made regarding how much is used to benefit one person at the expense of many others (6:4). With limited medical resources some form of just distribution must be achieved. This dilemma is faced on a daily basis by many health care professionals and, irrespective of the lines of argument relating to 'it's not my job to manage resources but to do my best for the patient', decisions are made within the system. These decisions are either managed or left to the adversarial approach in which everyone does one's best for their cause and winners and losers emerge (Kletz 1980).

Non-maleficence

Maleficence refers to the act of causing or doing harm to others. Therefore, the subheading of non-maleficence simply means doing no harm to others. We hope that the principle is clear here, in that if one cannot actually do good for others (beneficence) then at the least one ought not to do any harm (non-maleficence). On the face of it (*prima facie*) this seems a straightforward position where the avoidance of causing harm to others takes primacy over beneficence. We could possibly agree that we have a prime duty to avoid doing harm to others, whereas the duty to do good to others feels less of an imperative. However, it is not as clear as this, particularly in health care practice, as many procedures involve the risk of harm. We may balance those risks, and we would certainly involve the patients in those decisions. In fact, if doing no harm always took priority over doing good then many patients would be outraged at the ineptness of the health care professions. Thus, we can see that there may be circumstances in which non-maleficence does not take primacy over actually doing good (Owen 1984).

Often the moral objective that health care professionals are called upon to exercise involves both actions that do good and actions to prevent harm to others. The picture is further complicated by the fact that the quest to enact beneficence or non-maleficence may activate the opposite. For example, we may set out to do good to a patient and in fact cause harm, and alternatively we can prevent, or avoid, harm to someone which may be of benefit to them. We say 'may' because as we have pointed out above, avoiding harm may actually be non-beneficial to the patient. For example, refusing to operate on a brain tumour may lead to the death of the patient.

What is clear from the foregoing is that all human action is caught up in a balance of risks, assessing strengths and weighing pros and cons in relation to operating within moral codes. We may be clear as to what constitute the extremes of human action in terms of ethical boundaries, but the closer the poles converge the more complex the arguments become.

Further reading

Fried, C. (1978) *Right and Wrong*. Cambridge, MA: Harvard University Press.

6.7 Deontology

Deontology is the study of ethical frameworks that takes the notion of duty (Greek *deon*) as the basis of morality. We are all aware of the concept of doing one's duty, but on closer examination we need to understand that the duty being referred to is probably in relation to a specified code of practice. For example, a policeman or a soldier has a duty to carry out a task in relation to a specific operation, and that role is operationalized according to a set of rules that prescribe what is right or wrong action. However, in terms of understanding a moral code of practice by which all humans should act it is clearly fraught with philosophical pitfalls. The question of whether there is an absolute rule, or human law, that should govern all human action in all circumstances is a thorny issue indeed. This philosophical question is highly relevant for those in health care practice, as such stated universal laws pertain to the way in which others are treated. For example, can we make a claim that 'thou shalt not kill' is a universal law when clearly killing occurs through war, executions or euthanasia? Or, can we claim that 'causing no harm' should be a universal code when we have already seen that there are instances when some harm is undertaken to protect against a greater danger. In health care there are an abundance of codes of practice that insist on dutiful obeisance, such as the Hippocratic oath, the Declaration of Geneva and the World Medical Association's International Code of Medical Ethics. All of these call for a duty of care based on what are considered to be sound ethical laws, or laws of humanity (Fried 1978).

Appeals

The formulation of a duty is reliant upon establishing an appeal to a moral code. Most moral codes are structured around the idea of assessing the consequences of not abiding by certain rules. However, deontological theories are not consequentialist, as they justify their theories not according to consequences but typically because they are commanded to act in certain ways. For example, most religions insist on a code of human action by decree (e.g. the Ten Commandments of the Old Testament), and state that the universal laws of their faith require obedience. However, such deontological theories as these fall foul of certain philosophical objections, particularly in relation to the philosophical possibility of a religion commanding cruelty, killing or self-sacrifice. In these instances, suggesting that we are morally obliged to obey these commands would jar with most consciences. One way to overcome such difficulties is to agree that the moral code comes not from God but from nature. Setting human behaviour in natural laws makes the claim for a natural ethical code of human conduct and suggests a degree of objectivity. However, it is not clear what the term natural law actually means, and much of what occurs in nature is not necessarily desirable merely because it is considered 'natural'. This brings us in close proximity to the work of one central philosopher who wrote extensively in this area.

Immanuel Kant

Although a devout Christian, Immanuel Kant (1724–1804) constructed one of the most important non-religious deontological moral theories. The basis of his theory was that rational beings recognized that they were bound by a 'supreme moral law', which stemmed 'from the fact that rational agents (or persons) intrinsically possessed an absolute moral value (in contrast with inanimate objects and "beasts"), which rendered them members of what he called the kingdom of "ends in themselves"' (Gillon 1986; 16). Furthermore, Kant believed that rational beings not only recognized themselves as 'ends in themselves' but also recognized this value in others. The supreme moral law that forms the basis of Kant's belief could be formulated in three different ways. The first is that a person should 'act only on that maxim through which you can at the same time will that it should become a universal law' (Kant 1785: 67). This means that a person should act on the basis that his action should be the action that everyone else undertakes. This is very close to the Christian ethic of 'do unto others as you would have done unto you'. The second formulation is that everyone must be treated as an end in themselves and not only as a means to an end. This puts the human being on a high moral plane and means that no action should be done to a person in the quest to achieve another end, no matter how valuable that end is considered to be. Contrast this position with that of utilitarianism (6:4). The third formulation refers to human action that should be undertaken as if that person was creating a universal law of human action for everyone.

Criticisms of Kant's deontological moral theory can be summarized under four main points. First, some philosophers have argued that Kant's moral framework has no orientation for how humans should really behave in practice. In this line of argument it is suggested that there is a wide gap between the moral theory and actual behaviour. The second criticism is that the three formulations of a single principle as outlined by Kant were in fact three separate principles that required different action. Third, it has often been said that Kant's moral philosophy is far too austere and harsh, and it does not reflect the human capacity for such elements as, say, kindness. Finally, the theory does not allow for any exceptions to the supreme moral law.

Deontological pluralism

Of course, not all deontological moral theories adopt the universality principle. Some theorists accept that it is appropriate for a moral theory to contain more than one fundamental moral principle. For example, Ross (1930) argued that rational mature persons knew the moral obligations that they were under, and he distinguished between *prima facie* duties and absolute ones. Ross believed that rational human beings knew intuitively what these moral obligations were, and included in his list duties of promise, beneficence, non-maleficence, justice, reparation, gratitude and self-improvement. As long as these moral obligations do not conflict with an absolute principle, Ross argued, they ought to prevail.

Further reading

Fried, C. (1978) *Right and Wrong*. Cambridge, MA: Harvard University Press.

6.8 Idealism

Idealism incorporates a wide and varied philosophy that not only has a long history but also has undergone considerable changes from era to era. In dealing with this group of philosophical beliefs we first make a distinction between idealism and ideals. Ideals are, in short, models of excellence, and have their roots in Plato's notion of 'idea'. Plato considered the term ideal in relation to the Ideal State, which consisted of a number of qualities that when taken together produced a 'real' state. Thus, the term ideal in Plato's sense equates with something becoming real when it achieves a number of genuine qualities. However, idealism, as a philosophical group of theories, is concerned, at a fundamental level, with how the human mind creates the external world. Idealism does not quarrel with the simple view that external things actually exist but does take issue with the view that the material world is completely independent of the mind. We briefly outline this group of theories under four headings.

Berkeleian idealism

George Berkeley (1685–1753) was born in Ireland and eventually became the Bishop of Cloyne. In 1710 he published a book entitled *A Treatise Concerning the Principles of Human Knowledge*, in which he argued that there is no external material world and that items such as trees and stones are merely collections of ideas. Furthermore, he claimed that God produces these ideas in our minds. Although we may be tempted to dismiss Berkeley's views as outrageous, to do him justice we must see his metaphysics in relation to the time in which he lived. Science was on the march and many discoveries were being made that overturned traditional ways of thinking. Moreover, there was a popular move towards atheism that Berkeley foresaw, and he was concerned to develop a credible philosophy to counter this move. Whether he actually achieved this is open to debate, but his theory certainly merits serious attention. Berkeley argues that sight does not give us understanding of external objects but merely transmits appearances of objects, which produce sensations in our minds. Thus, in one sense, they are not 'real' but only sensations. He argued that 'all bodies which compose the mighty frame of the world, have not any substance without a mind, that their being is to be perceived or known; that consequently so long as they are not actually perceived by me, or do not exist in my mind or that of any other created spirit, they must either have no existence at all, or else subsist in the mind of some external spirit' (Berkeley 1948: 6). Throughout his life Berkeley opposed himself to inert senseless matter, to a world distinct from appearances and to a world that viewed science as equating with the reductionist explanation of all phenomena.

Transcendental idealism

Transcendental idealism, also known as critical idealism, is a term that was applied by Kant to his theory of the external world. Kant believed that objects of our experience do not exist in any sense other than as appearances in our own thoughts. This gives the person the power over such ideas, and this manner of thinking is often called subjective idealism. Transcendental idealism asserts that the dependence of the world of experience rests on the activities of reason alone. Transcendental arguments are based on answering questions related to establishing the preconditions that are said to exist in order to pose the question in the first instance. For example, Kant argued that the propositions of Euclidean geometry are true but that this is only possible if the human mind itself establishes spatial characteristics first. Transcendental idealism has been criticized, not surprisingly, along the lines that it is not always possible to establish all preconditions, in all cases, and critics point to the field of judgement as an example of this (Davidson 1984).

Objective idealism

Objective idealism, which is also called absolute idealism by some, is a philosophical position that was first developed by Georg Hegel (1770–1831). The former two types of idealism, Berkeleian idealism and transcendental idealism, are both pluralistic in that their theories accept the existence of multiple minds. However, objective idealism is a monistic theory which maintains that all that exists is a form of one mind, or one entity. To make sense of this in such a brief sketch is difficult, but what one needs to do is to tie this notion into the idea that single truths may exist independently of how many minds may think of that truth. For example, it might be accepted that a single truth is 'no one should harm another person', and this might be true no matter how many individuals might think of it. Objective idealism searches for single truths that form the idea of one existence (Dummett 1978).

German idealism

Finally, we mention German idealism, which refers to the dominant German philosophy extending from the late eighteenth century to the middle of the nineteenth century. It began as a project to develop Kant's revolutionary way of thinking that was to establish principles of knowledge from the independence of mind or spirit. However, philosophers of German idealism eventually expanded Kant's theory to such an extent that it could no longer be called Kantian, and their theories stood alone in relation to the wider body of philosophical knowledge (Solomon and Higgins 1993).

Conclusion

In conclusion, idealism is an important philosophical concept in health care, as it lies close to the notion of ethics. If one believes that general truths exist, or that single truths exist for all, then this will have an important bearing on ethical considerations in health care settings. However, as we have seen, not all believe this to be the case and each person's way of thinking will have an impact on the way that they practise.

As the reader progresses through the first section on theory above we hope that there is a sense of moving from relatively easy philosophical concepts through to more conceptually difficult ones. Furthermore, as these philosophical perspectives are deliberated upon it should become apparent that even the simpler versions have many more complex levels of interpretations. Finally, there should now be a sense that they intertwine with each other, producing a feeling of a dynamic cauldron of problems, contradictions and tensions. This reflects life in general, and certainly resonates in health care settings, and Part Two of this chapter is concerned with how this 'amorphous philosophical brew' impacts on practice.

Further reading

Kant, I. (1781) *Critique of Pure Reason*. London: Macmillan (1933 edn).

PART TWO: APPLICATION TO PRACTICE

6.9 Confidentiality

Confidentiality is, possibly, the single most revered principle in medical ethics, and forms the basis of the professional–patient relationship. In its simplest form confidentiality refers to respecting other people's secrets. However, the issues involved in this are complex. Confidentiality involves the element of trust, which is required from both parties in both giving honest information and maintaining its secrecy. However, its complexity becomes apparent when we begin to unravel some of the issues within the notion of a confidential relationship. For example, when is the information considered secret? If the patient tells the doctor something but does not consider it a secret, should the doctor keep the information in confidence? Furthermore, what is the case when this situation is reversed; that is, the patient gives information that they consider to be confidential but the doctor does not genuinely believe that it is? And again, suppose that the information was given in confidence, and understood to be so by the doctor, but the information contained a threat to a third party. Thus, we need to consider whether confidentiality is an absolute principle or whether there are occasions when it may be qualified and certain exemptions can be applied (Campbell and Rader 1999). However, before progressing to this we need to point out some of the underlying philosophical principles that drive the issues of confidentiality.

We can clearly see that respect for a person's autonomy must feature large within the debate on confidentiality, but also see that when it is qualified, and it is considered appropriate to break that confidence, the charge of medical paternalism may be levelled against it. Furthermore, the deontological duty of keeping a person's secret is broken when the doctor reveals that information to safeguard others on utilitarian grounds (6:4). In these situations the doctor may not be operating beneficently for the patient and may actually be causing the patient some degree of harm (maleficence) (6:6). Thus, the philosophical arguments become highly contentious, with no clear rights and wrongs.

Absolute principle

Confidentiality as an absolute principle would involve keeping the person's secret at all times, in all situations and for ever, even after the patient's death. Two codes of confidentiality that do involve this absolute principle are the Roman Catholic confessor–priest relationship and the doctor–patient relationship within the World Medical Association's International Code of Medical Ethics (British Medical Association 1984). However, most other codes accept some degree of qualification, as we will see below, or at least they allow an element of interpretive licence. However, before we move on to this let us deal with some of the philosophical issues that will guide us in the practice arena. Utilitarians and pluralist deontologists, by the nature of their incorporation of others, would argue strongly against an absolute confidentiality principle (6:4, 6:7). They would consider it appropriate to operate for the greater good and to override individual considerations, particularly when it involves harm to others. It would be a strange person who would remain quiet when informed by a confidant that they are going to murder someone. Even within the Kantian notion of the universal law there is some leeway against absolutism, as other rational beings must be taken into account in its application. As Gillon has argued, 'Kantians too would thus have no place for a maxim that demanded absolute medical confidentiality in all circumstances. Nor, incidentally, would there be any philosophical justification within these systems for the requirement of confidentiality to be absolute after a patient's death' (Gillon 1986: 109). It is apparent, then, that there may be some justification for arguing against absolute confidentiality and for some degree of qualification in certain medical codes of ethics (Thurston *et al.* 1999).

Qualifications

The Hippocratic oath refers to confidentiality: 'whatever, in connection with my professional practice, or not in connection with it, I see or hear, in the life of men, which ought not to be spoken of abroad, I will not divulge, as reckoning that all such should be kept secret' (British Medical Association 1984: 69–70). Although not unambiguous, it can be interpreted that within the phrase '*ought not to be spoken of abroad*' there is an apparent leeway that allows for breaking such confidence in extreme circumstances. Although we cannot be certain about this, there is some element of non-absolutism in the word '*ought*', which guides what we should do in usual circumstances. More modern day codes of ethics do give situations in which absolute confidentiality does not apply. For example, the General Medical Council in 1985 listed eight such exceptions: (a) when a patient or their legal representative under instruction gives consent; (b) when other health care professionals are involved in the patient's care; (c) when it is medically undesirable to ask the patient and it is believed by the doctor that a close relative should know about the patient's health; (d) when it is believed by the doctor that a third party should be informed and it is in the 'best interests of the patient', and when the patient has rejected 'every reasonable effort to persuade' them; (e) when statutory requirements dictate disclosure; (f) when a judge or equivalent legal authority instructs disclosure; (g) when it is in the public interest, such as in an 'investigation by the police of a grave or very serious crime'; and (h) when it is required for legitimate research that has been approved by a 'recognized ethical committee' (General Medical Council 1985: 19–21).

In making exceptions the governing body concerned is likely to be criticized on a number of counts. First, it may be accused of medical paternalism in overriding the patient's wishes and in deciding what the 'patient's best interests' are. Second, the charge of not respecting the autonomy of the individual in the face of divulging information to third parties may be levelled against the authors of such a code. Third, in breaking confidentiality for research purposes the doctor may be accused of utilitarianism, in which the views of the individual are subjugated to the greater good of the greatest number. Finally, while few would wish the medical profession to fall foul of the law, they can be charged with colluding with the police in operating as agents of social control. Of course, it is a relatively easy task to criticize a professional body that is attempting to formulate codes of practice that attempt to do the best for all concerned in the health care enterprise. Therefore, it seems unjust for Siegler (1982) to claim that confidentiality is a 'decrepit concept'. Certainly, absolute confidentiality may not be totally feasible, or acceptable, but to aim to achieve a state of confidentiality as close to this as possible seems to be at least desirable (Meier 1999). It is probably better to ensure that patients understand that it is not absolute and to inform them of the parameters in which information may be disclosed, either with their consent or without it.

Further reading

Brandt, A. M. and Rozina, P. (1997) *Morality and Health*. London: Routledge.
Gillon, R. (1986) *Philosophical Medical Ethics*. Chichester: John Wiley & Sons.

6.10 Consent

Like confidentiality, the notion of consent in modern health care delivery is central to our ethical code of practice, and at one level we would probably be outraged if an intervention was applied to us without our consent. However, we do not have to stretch our imagination too far to consider a number of situations in which consent is frequently overridden; for example, in cases of mental illness where the capacity for rational thought might be considered as impeded, in the case of a severely handicapped person with learning difficulties or where someone is intoxicated with drugs or is unconscious (Salladay 1998; Ardagh 1999). Thus, we can see that consent is underpinned by a number of concerns that must be taken into consideration when dealing with the issue. However, before we address these let us look at the definitional difficulties that are involved in this concept. First, we are drawn to the differences between positive and negative consent. The former involves a reliance on someone receiving information, deliberating on it and making an uncoerced decision to give consent to what is proposed. In the latter case of negative consent it is assumed that the consent is tacit, implied without direct expression and dependent upon the person actively withdrawing it. In many situations, and in many countries, this latter position is no longer acceptable, particularly in cases of medical interventions, but can be the case for such procedures as organ donations in the event of death (depending on country and religion). The second difficulty is that certain patients do not want a great deal of information, do not wish to know the intricacies of their 'problem' and merely want to say 'yes, now get on with it' as a type of uninformed 'consent'.

A third difficulty concerns the notion of 'informed consent' and what information actually constitutes 'informed'. How much can the patient understand? To what depth of knowledge does the professional attempt to explain? And how wide should that information be in relation to side effects, success rates, resources available etc.? Fourth, in those cases where we may be considered unable to give consent (e.g. mental illness, unconscious states) and others are going to make that decision for us, how do they arrive at that decision, through what body of knowledge, on what basis? To what extent are they deciding on what *we* may wish, or not, or on what *they* desire, or not? Finally, very serious difficulties arise when the person flatly refuses to give consent and the decision is made to override their refusal and apply interventions against their wishes.

We could spend considerable time attempting to apply definitions in all cases, which would be unwieldy and probably fruitless for all everyday applications in practice. Therefore, we will accept for the purposes of this project that consent in medical practice, whether these are investigations, treatments or research, is defined as 'a voluntary, uncoerced decision, made by a sufficiently competent or autonomous person on the basis of adequate information and deliberation, to accept rather than reject some proposed course of action that will affect him or her' (Gillon 1986: 113).

Acquiring consent

Asking someone's consent, whether it be in relation to them undertaking a medical operation or whether it concerns the donation of an organ in the event of their death, is a manifestation of a moral obligation to respect the person's autonomy (6:2). However, in the case of an operation it is also a legal obligation (Mason and McCall-Smith 1983). This respect for an individual's autonomy has a deep seated root in the ethical principles of our society, and it is interesting to note that, despite the Alder Hey Children's Hospital organ scandal in the UK, in which children's organs were systematically retained without parental consent for many years, most of the parents that were involved stated that they would have volunteered their children's organs if they had been asked. Of course, the practical question under this heading refers to whether we ought to give positive consent to our organ donation programme or whether consent should be automatic unless we actively withdraw our consent. It may be apathy that prevents most people from giving positive consent by carrying a donor card, but it is certainly showing more autonomy for the individual to seek that consent rather than assume it. Notwithstanding this, it is also accepted that recipients of the organs may have different opinions on this issue (Anonymous 1999a).

Informed consent

It is sometimes argued that the patient is unnecessarily alarmed by the number of side effects, probability of success/failure ratios, differential diagnoses, complications etc. Although this is certainly true for some, many others appreciate the expression of open information (Moskop 1999). The most practical way forward in delivering information, or not as the case may be, has been excellently summed up by Gillon (1986: 115): 'the doctor who really respected his patient's autonomy would discover in a sensitive way, which did not demand a particular answer, what and how much each patient really wanted to know and how much he wished to participate in the decision making'. This clearly links into respect for the patient's autonomy (6:2).

Consent on someone else's behalf

As we have noted, there are occasions when obtaining consent is not feasible and a third party must decide whether to give their consent, or not, on behalf of another person. Although there are clear cases in which the person (victim) can be said to have no autonomy, e.g. a baby, other cases become more difficult depending on the perceived degree of autonomous thought that they may have. For example, in the case of a person who has had severe brain damage since birth one is never truly certain as to the extent of mental capacity. Again, in the case of a brain damaged victim following a trauma in life, the consent-giver may have known the extent of the person's previous autonomy, and thus his or her wishes and desires etc. Finally, there may be the case of the mentally ill person who was perfectly rational before the onset of the illness, and whose condition now impairs rationality, but does not eradicate it altogether. The difficulties in these types of cases concern not only the degrees of autonomy of thought, of will and of action, but also the extent to which the third party decision-maker can take the victim's desires into account. This has to be coupled to the extent to which the decision-maker is basing their decision on what they would wish for themselves in that situation, but this is clearly not the victim's certain desire.

Overriding refusal to consent

There are some situations, but increasingly rare ones, where a person explicitly refuses consent to treatment but this is overridden by either the next of kin or medical professionals. Space does not allow us to dwell on these, but four examples are offered to highlight this difficult area. First, a child with a potentially fatal disease may not wish to have antibiotic injections, but this is likely to be overturned by parents. Second, a person with a mental illness who is going to kill themselves or someone else may refuse treatment, but this can be overridden by two psychiatrists under mental health legislation. Third, a child requiring a blood transfusion but not having parental consent on religious grounds is a more difficult scenario, and one that currently receives different legal and medical decisions in different cases. Finally, an adult with anorexia nervosa, and slowly starving to death, may refuse medical treatment, and this situation is ever more likely to be upheld in favour of the victim, even with psychiatric testimony. What these examples show are the ever shifting 'sands' of ethical decision-making in the area of consent (Moore 1997).

Further reading

Dunstan, G. R. and Seller, M. J. (1983) *Consent in Medicine*. London: King's Fund Publishing Office and Oxford University Press.

Lidz, C. W., Meisel, A., Zerubavel, E. *et al.* (1984) *Informed Consent*. New York: Guilford Press.

6.11 The right to life

In the following two sections we outline the major issues relating to both the right to life and the right to death debate, and these are closely related to the question of euthanasia. Obviously, this is a hugely complex area that rightly warrants the voluminous literature that concerns it in philosophical texts, medical and nursing publications and numerous legal adjudications. Clearly, we can offer only the briefest of overviews here, but we feel that even this is important, as it has such a large impact on everyday practice. We begin by establishing the principle of absolutism in relation to the right to life. As we have noted above in the theoretical section, the philosophical principle of absolutism would refer to all human beings having the right to life, in all circumstances, and human intervention that would contribute to ending life would be excluded (6:5, 6:8). For those who uphold this position this would include no killing in war, no executions and no killing in self-defence. Some individuals, as well as some religious groups, do adopt this absolute pacifist position and even extend it to include the animal (non-human) kingdom. However, for most believers in the right to life the absolute principle is tempered to a *prima facie* perspective that accepts that everyone has the right to life, *on the face of it*. This gives a strong hint that they view killing as wrong but certain circumstances may dictate its necessity, e.g. self-defence. But there are other problems with the absolute principle of right to life, and these concern such issues as when life actually begins, or when an embryo is a human being; and when life should end, or when we can cease resuscitation or life-support maintenance (Koehler *et al.* 1999). This brings into focus the issue of euthanasia. Euthanasia has two forms, passive and active. In passive euthanasia the person is allowed to die naturally (and painlessly) without modern equipment or techniques to maintain life. In active euthanasia there is an actual intervention that is applied to assist the person's death (Griffiths 1999). Although legal in certain countries, euthanasia is illegal in the UK. Euthanasia can also be voluntary, non-voluntary or involuntary. Voluntary euthanasia is said to be when a person requests their own death, non-voluntary where killing a person supposedly in their own interests occurs, but when they cannot express their views on the matter, and involuntary euthanasia is when the killing takes place in disregard of their wishes to stay alive. The latter case here can be ruled out of our discussions, as it falls foul of the law of autonomy and, as we are here concerned with the philosophical issues rather than the legal ones, it is clearly outside any moral position (Glover 1988).

Levels of life

In the debate on the right to life we must begin to deal with the issues revolving around what 'life' actually means and to whose 'life' we are actually referring. The first issue concerns the distinction between the lives of humans and the lives of other animals. While there are some who believe that all animals have as much right to life as humans most people accept the death of certain animals for food. However, Jeremey Bentham, writing on utilitarianism, believed that animals were equivalent to humans morally, and that the principles of utilitarianism applied as much to them as they do to us (6:4). The 'level' of Bentham's equivalence relates to the extent to which the animals are sentient. He asked not whether the animal could reason but whether it could feel pain. However, we must ask ourselves where the line is drawn on this, and to what extent it is counter-intuitive. For example, if we accept that higher primates can feel pleasure and pain, would we accept that lower forms of life such as slugs and snails also have the right to life on this basis? Taking the example further, can we claim that microbes, bacteria and viruses also have this right? While few would argue that this level of life can claim sentience, we do not actually 'know' and can only make assumptions regarding this. Therefore, the majority of human beings assume that human life is more morally important than animal life. However, even accepting this brings us to the thorny issues of when human life begins and when it ends.

At what point does a human being begin to be a member of the human species? This again depends on particular beliefs. For some (Roman Catholics and some other religions) this occurs when ensoulment or hominization occurs; that is, when the soul is infused. Precisely when this occurs is not explicitly extolled, but most believers of this doctrine behave as if it occurs at the moment of fertilization (Gillon 1986). There are varying stages at which others believe that membership of the human species begins, such as at the fertilized ovum stage prior to implantation, at the embryonic stage following implantation and at the later humanoid foetal stage. Still others argue that it may be at the stage when embryos are no longer able to divide into twins, when embryos are no longer able to coalesce or when mere cell division has ceased and cell differentiation has begun. Irrespective of one's own personal beliefs, what is important here is that there is extensive debate regarding this start of life, which impinges on such issues as types of contraception that may be acceptable, and approaches to aborting foetuses, up to the legal time in the UK, which is 24 weeks' gestation. However, this is not definitive, as 'in certain circumstances the Human Fertilisation and Embryology Act (1990) places no limit on legal abortion' (Donaldson and Donaldson 1998: 295).

Qualifications to the principle of absolutism

Thus far we have seen that although there are some who do believe in the absolute principle of the right to life, the majority of people qualify this in relation to certain circumstances and in relation to certain 'levels' of life. Now we will focus on qualifications that have been made on human beings and their right to life. The preliminary case concerns those who, both historically and today, have been killed because they are of another race, creed or culture and who are viewed as subhuman or simply different. Case examples include the Nazi holocaust, the Bosnian ethnic cleansing and the more recent Indonesian Dayak massacres. Although abhorrent, these fall outside of our general discussions on the right to life in health care settings.

However, having said that, let us not forget that the Nazi holocaust began with the killing of a mentally handicapped man by a paediatrician, supported by nursing staff, the killing taking place not in a concentration camp but in the Leipzig University Children's Hospital (Meyer 1988). Within the debate on the right to life we must not forget the role of health professionals in the many medical experiments and the many deaths during the Nazi regime, with the elimination of thousands of mentally ill and mentally handicapped people.

Let us now briefly look at a few contemporary examples in which a person's right to life is overridden by health care staff, with or without the patient's consent. We do not make any moral judgement on the complex examples stated here, but merely request that readers consider whether they believe that they do constitute overriding the right to life, consider the arguments for and against, and ponder what their own personal views may be on these issues. The first one has been briefly outlined above and concerns the aborting of a developing foetus. This, of course, is hotly contended in the prolife debate and we will not expand on this further here. The second example we ask you to consider is the case of vegetative states, in which modern technology is maintaining life and the decision is made to turn off the support (6:12). The third case concerns the current debate on writing 'do not resuscitate' in clinical notes. This decision may override the person's desire to live (6:2, 6:3, 6:4, 6:5). Finally, consider the separation of conjoined twins, one of whom will die due to the lack of organs. If left joined both may live a life, albeit qualitatively poor and short. Thus, we can see that the right to life is a complex area in which practical decisions are made on a day to day basis in health care settings. The situation is equally complex when someone considers that they have a right to die.

Further reading

Glover, J. (1988) *Causing Death and Saving Lives*. London: Penguin.
Lindemann, J. and Lindemann Nelson, H. (2000) *Meaning and Medicine: A Reader in the Philosophy of Health Care*. London: Routledge.

6.12 The right to death

In the previous section, on the right to life, the central issue appeared to be a respect for the person's autonomy, and if the argument is accepted that the person has a right to life, because it is their life and no one else's, then there appears to be a straightforward case for allowing them to do what they wish with their life. As long as they do not harm someone else then it appears relatively clear that they should be allowed to act autonomously. There are a number of general situations that fuse together in the right to die debate and these can be identified as:

- a situation in which a person commits suicide;
- a situation in which the person wishes to die based on what is considered an irrational decision;
- a situation in which a person wishes to die based on what is considered a rational decision;
- a situation in which a person wishes to commit suicide and requests assistance in doing so from others;
- a situation in which a person is dying from a terminal disease and wishes to terminate his or her life prematurely;
- situations differentiating between assisting the patient to die and allowing him or her to die by inaction.

Given that the decision to terminate one's own life can be made both irrationally through disordered thinking and rationally through a clear assessment of the circumstances, then denying people the right to die can be seen as a value judgement on the part of the person intervening (Goldberg 1987). Differences of opinion do exist between those who believe that they have a right to die and those who believe that they do not (Kissane *et al.* 1998). To intervene in order to terminate someone's life against their wishes is clearly wrong, but what is the difference in intervening to save someone's life against their wishes? In practical terms the answer may be that in the latter case they get another chance to fulfil their wishes, while in the former they do not. However, in terms of the moral argument there appears little difference (6:2, 6:3) (Wecht 1998).

Acts and omissions debate

We would like to emphasize again that we are concerned here with the moral debate and not the legal one. In this section we are dealing with the differences, if any, between actively assisting to terminate a life at their request and omitting to do anything while the patient does so himself or herself. A practical example may assist clarity here: say that a rational person with a terminal disease requests a bottle of tablets to take his life and you provide those tablets, place them in his mouth and help him to swallow them with a supply of water; or, in a similar scenario, you find the patient swallowing the tablets obtained from another source but you do nothing to prevent him from taking them. In these examples there seems little moral difference between the two (Gillon 1986) but, intuitively, despite the patient wishing to terminate his life, the actual assisting may appear as morally worse than omitting an action and allowing him to die (Robb 1997). Many people facing these moral dilemmas assess the situation in relation to 'harms' and 'benefits'. In assisting the patient to take the tablets the person is considered to be causing harm to the patient, despite the fact that they may argue it is for the benefit of the patient by bringing relief, and that they might cause harm if they did not assist the patient's death. Notwithstanding this line of argument, in the actual act they cause harm to the patient. However, in the latter case where the person does nothing and allows the patient to die, in the omission, they do no harm, although it could be argued that they do not benefit the patient and also allow the patient to harm himself. Despite this extremely fine distinction, this does appear to form the basis of an intuitive moral difference between acts and omissions (Galambos 1998).

The right to die and some consequences

Some religions do not differentiate between acts and omissions on the grounds that an omission is clearly a failure to do good. Thus, in their view, failing to prevent someone from terminating their life is as morally bad as actually assisting them to die. Therefore, in our practical examples above (bullet points), for some there is little moral difference while for others moral distinctions can be drawn. The consequences for health care staff making decisions on the right to die are complex beyond the basic moral positions outlined above. For example, legal action may be taken against the health care staff for intervening when a patient has exercised his right to die. This scenario was outlined by Donohue (1998) in a paper entitled ' "Wrongful living": recovery for a physician's infringement on an individual's right to die'. In this scenario a patient sues the physician for intervening to prevent the patient from dying. In terms of assisting the patient to terminate his own life, some courts adjudicate that those who do assist patients to die are in violation of the law, while other courts in the same jurisdiction are less certain (Candilis and Appelbaum 1997). What this shows is that, yet again, the situations that are often faced in health care settings are not always a question of black and white, and it is often a question of exploring the moral issues, with the aid of philosophical concepts, in relation to the legal concerns, and arriving at a reasoned decision to the best of one's ability.

Further reading

Glover, J. (1988) *Causing Death and Saving Lives*. London: Penguin.
Hardwig, J. (2000) *Is There a Right to Die? And Other Essays in Bioethics*. London: Routledge.

6.13 Empowerment

Empowerment is a popular concept in modern day health care delivery, and is closely related to the idea of patient advocacy. In an attempt to define empowerment we note that there is little agreement other than to pivot the issue on the notion of power. This was succinctly stated by Roberts (1999: 82), who argued that, 'whilst there is no consensus amongst analysts regarding how best to define patient empowerment, at the very least, this concept entails a re-distribution of power between patients and physicians'. Thus, we are immediately faced with the philosophical issue of power, which is anchored in the relationship between the patient and the institution of health care delivery. However, we must not forget that empowerment can also refer to staff working in health care settings and includes hierarchical relationships *within* disciplines as well as the power relationships *between* professions (Sabiston and Laschinger 1995). Empowerment has also been applied to a range of groups, such as the women's movement, the Black Power movement, gay and lesbian rights, AIDS victims and student groups. What these share in common is a perceived imbalance of power between the group to which they belong and a larger segment of society. However, in focusing on empowerment in health care settings we may wish to query what this power consists of, and question whether structures are in place to maintain the imbalance ratio.

Before undertaking this it is important to establish the links between empowerment in practice and the philosophical framework in which it is set. At a theoretical level empowerment is concerned with maintaining the autonomy of the individual (6:2). It is considered to be a strategy by which medical paternalism is, at least limited, if not kept at bay, and has some elements of beneficence as patients who are empowered, generally, respond better to treatments (6:3, 6:6) (Duncan 1996). The World Health Organization's Health for All policy (WHO 1985a) claimed that this was achievable by adding life to years, and by adding years to life. This was underpinned by five general principles, three of which are equity, empowerment and participation. These indicate the strength in balancing the relationship of power in health care delivery: equity refers to fairness and equal opportunities; empowerment means giving people the control over their own health decisions; and participation refers to the involvement of people in planning and running their health services.

Em-power-ment

This subheading depicts the central role that power plays in the decision-making process regarding health care issues, and it appears that the power is rooted in the vulnerability of illness and the perceived potency of medical knowledge in restoring health. Thus, those who are ill and ignorant of this knowledge feel powerless, and those who are healthy and have this knowledge are deemed to be powerful (Turner 1990b). Indeed, Turner (1990b) felt that this relationship, based on a power imbalance between doctor and patient, revolved around its temporary status. The point, Turner argued, 'is to show how the doctor and patient are committed to breaking their relationship' (Turner 1990b: 41). The temporary status is underpinned by the power of medicine to move the patient from the sick role to a state of health. This medical force is the fulcrum of power within the professional–patient dynamic. Historically, medical knowledge has been acquired by *men* who employed the knowledge to bolster the power that it brought (Krause 1977). In contemporary times it is considered that the imbalance of power is no longer acceptable and modern health care delivery is geared, or is being geared, towards a more equitable professional–patient status.

Of course, we must see the historical disempowerment of patients in relation to the socio-political context of the time, and similarly the contemporary move towards empowerment is set within the socio-political frameworks of today. The commodification of health care, the marketization of services, the bureaucratization of health management, the consumer driven society and the expansion of health care litigation are driving forces in the move to empower patients (Hogg 1999). Contemporary society comprises of people who are, generally, more knowledgeable about health care issues, more questioning, more interested and more desiring to be involved in the decisions regarding their health (Hagland 1996). Thus, the curriculum content of many health care courses includes issues of empowerment. Indeed, some courses are focused specifically on the delivery of care based on strategies of empowerment. In the design of course curricula in nursing studies Duncan (1996: 182) argued that 'these strategies provide a framework for teaching nursing students to promote the health of populations by shifting their focus of care to one that is compatible with principles of primary healthcare and health promotion within a context of healthcare reform'. This is why many influential professional bodies are making statements regarding the empowerment of patients, including the World Health Organization and the United Kingdom Central Council (McCormack 1993). In fact, in the quest to empower patients it has been deemed necessary to instigate structures aimed at facilitating this move, these being known as advocacy services.

Advocacy

Patient advocacy is concerned with providing active support for the patient in the health care enterprise. Advocacy will feature in the majority of textbooks on nursing, and most students will be taught that it is a central role of the function of the nurse: to act as a go-between, representing the patient when they cannot represent themselves, for the effective operation of the doctor–patient relationship. While few would argue against this, we need to take stock of the underlying forces that may be driving this scenario. Writing anonymously, a patient claimed that this sort of advocacy was little more than a subtle form of subterfuge in which health professionals exercise their power through a mechanism of persuasion (Anonymous 1999b). Health staff too have voiced a cautionary note on the advocacy role, with Alspach (1998) asking whether we have ascended to new heights or fallen to new depths. This question relates to the philosophical tension between doing good for the patient (6:6) and acting in a paternalistic manner (6:3). At one level advocacy relates to the concept of informed consent, in which health professionals provide as much information for the patient as he or she requires to make a decision (6:10). However, seen at another level it may appear as a sophisticated manipulative strategy that ensures that the patient complies with medical requests, and places the patient as an item in operationalizing the professional agenda (6:3). Furthermore, the concept of advocacy begins to look somewhat tenuous when it clashes with personal value-judgements (6:7). That is, how does one advocate for the drug addict who wants another 'fix', or a sectioned psychiatric patient who wishes to leave the hospital, without applying one's own professional value-judgement? One may respond with a call for negotiated care in these situations, and indeed negotiation may be an appropriate response, but negotiation is not advocacy. The application of another's value-judgement is a form of paternalism and the role of advocates in these situations requires careful philosophical reflection.

Further reading

Hunt, G. (1994) *Ethical Issues in Nursing*. London: Routledge.
Thomson, A. (1999) *Critical Reasoning in Ethics: A Practical Introduction*. London: Routledge.

6.14 Feminist ethics

For centuries traditional ethics have been devised by men, claiming to speak for all, and thus it is men who have decided on the questions that are asked, the manner by which they are analysed and their answers (Walker 1989). Feminist ethics, therefore, makes the claim that traditional ethics are biased against women. Couple to this the fact that Western medicine is a male-dominated institution and it can be fairly surmised that medical ethics are also male-orientated, and thus, it is argued, biased against women. This being the case, feminist ethics would be concerned with the role and status of women within the institution of medicine (Sherwin 1984). In a medical sense males have largely gained control of women's bodies and minds, and there is both a growing awareness of this and a growing urgency to address it. Feminist ethics is concerned to develop systems of thinking that place women at their centre, and adopts one of two approaches within a wider multi-approach perspective. It may:

• take traditional male-dominated medical ethics and employ a feminist analysis to draw different interpretations;

• or employ feminist thinking to develop a different focus, different questions and different answers.

We reiterate that there are many approaches within this basic subdivision of feminist ethics:

• feminine approaches, which place personal relationships and the role of care at the centre;

• maternal approaches, which focus upon the one relationship of mother and child as the fundamental moral paradigm;

• lesbian approaches, which focus on choice of action rather than traditional deontology;

- feminist approaches, which focus on changing, or overturning, the systems, structures and processes of male domination and female sub-ordination in all areas of life.

We should note the distinction between the feminine and the feminist approaches (first and fourth bullet points above) to ethics, which involves the difference between a feminine ethics of caring and a feminist ethics of power (Tong 1993). However, for the purposes of this chapter we employ the term feminist ethics, in the broader sense, to incorporate all the above perspectives.

Why do we need a feminist ethics?

For some, it is absolutely no surprise that in the male-dominated medical model the focus of attention is predominantly on cure, and that in the essentially female nursing model the focus is on care. Thus, caring lies at the heart of feminist ethics. As holders of this perspective see many subjugated and vulnerable groups within the health care system, such as the young, the old, the disabled and the sick, they feel that it is morally worthwhile to care for such groups. As there are many other oppressed and powerless groups in society, such as AIDS victims, gay and lesbian groups, as well as females generally, it is argued that feminist ethics are needed to help not only females, but all such oppressed groups. Holmes (1992: 3) summed up the position accordingly: 'as members of the globally oppressed majority, we must use what I call "epistemic empathy" toward oppression and offer other oppressed groups our help and insights – both theory and practice'. A second reason for needing a feminist ethics is that given the abusive nature of the male-dominated medical model and its relationship to the predomin-antly female care-givers it cannot help but work towards perpetuating the system. This system, in being viewed as corrupt and abusive, will also corrupt and victimize females within it. Thus, it is considered necessary to develop and apply a feminist ethics to prevent oppressed groups from being further subjugated and to overturn this abusive relationship. A third reason for requiring a feminist ethics concerns the role that caring plays in our society, and while we might have an 'epistemic privilege' in 'caring', we must ensure that it is based on a genuine set of feelings about others and not merely just because the caring role is stereotypically attributed to women. There is little doubt that this stereotyping is unhelpful in the power struggles against male-dominated systems but it cannot be dismissed, as it is central to helping people and changing the abusive institution of medicine (Holmes 1992).

What are feminist ethics and their impact on practice?

Traditional ethics are concerned with such principles as universality and generalizability; that is, establishing principles to guide human action that are fundamentally correct for all people. Feminist ethics, on the other hand, focus on the particular context in which that human action takes place. For example, whereas traditional ethics may be concerned with the rights and wrongs of abortion *per se*, feminist ethics would focus on the rights and wrongs of an abortion for the mother and foetus, in their given set of circumstances. Thus, in one sense, the principles of universality and generalizability are not incompatible with feminist ethics if the method of feminist ethics – that is, the application of an analysis of context – was applied to all. Thus, feminist ethics reshapes the questions that are asked, applies a different analysis and formulates alternative answers. Purdy (1992) suggested four central discussion paradigms for feminist ethics to address:

- To emphasize the importance of women and their interests – but this should avoid the rigidity that is resonant in traditional ethics. Purdy (1992) argues that we should avoid dismissing certain analyses as 'not really feminist', but critically appraise them and highlight how a feminist ethics analysis could be applied. This would help to incorporate feminist ethics into mainstream thinking rather than locating it as a 'specialism'.
- To focus on issues that are specifically relevant to, concerned with or affecting women. It is suggested that there is a need to adopt a broad brush approach that will incorporate many issues for feminist ethical analyses: AIDS and sexual rights, IVF and gestation issues, contract pregnancies, cloning and the production of life, and so on.
- To rethink basic assumptions. This will entail challenging fundamental principles and traditional methods in philosophical thought, and will ask such questions as: what is truth, and whose truth is it anyway?
- To employ feminist analyses from other disciplines. This will enrich all feminist approaches but is highly relevant in health care, as it naturally employs multidisciplines and multi-agencies.

In understanding this, feminist ethics will need to address both traditional areas and new issues as they arise from advances in technology and developments in theory. Warren (1992) has a mature outlook, suggesting that new feminist directions in medical ethics need not develop in one particular way, nor need there only be feminist interpretations. Warren cautions us in dealing with the issue of 'sexist ethics' and claims that sexism in male-dominated ethics, as well as the sexism in her own feminist ethics, is largely unintended. She makes the case for changing the way that ethical questions are framed and offers four new categories of ethical questions: (a) inequalities; (b) sexist occupational roles; (c) personal issues; and (d) relationship issues. What are needed are ethical questions that do not involve winners and losers in the struggle for power.

Further reading

Doyal, L. (1998) *Women and Health Services: An Agenda for Change*. Buckingham: Open University Press.

Held, V. (1993) *Feminist Morality: Transforming Culture, Society and Politics*. Chicago: University of Chicago Press.

Holmes, H. B. and Purdy, L. M. (1992) *Feminist Perspectives in Medical Ethics*. Bloomington: Indiana University Press.

6.15 Nursing ethics and morality

At first sight it may appear odd that in this section on applications to practice we begin to close the chapter with what seems to be a theoretical topic. However, this is arguably the single most important lesson that can be delivered in this chapter on 'thinking philosophy', and that is that ethics and morality are fundamentally important in governing human behaviour in action. Even Aristotle suggested that there appeared little point in studying ethics and morality unless they had an impact on how we lived our lives. Known as applied ethics, this approach to ethical and moral enquiry is of vital importance to us today as long as it influences how we treat patients in health care settings. This importance becomes striking when we consider the numerous life and death scenarios that are faced, as well as the complicated decisions regarding such issues as organ donations and embryo research. However, we must also remember that ethics and morals have a big influence, or ought to have, on the day to day interactions with patients, remembering, for example, the principles of autonomy, beneficence and non-maleficence mentioned above. Although we have used ethics and morality interchangeably, as most people do, we would like to point out a subtle difference between the two. John Skorupski (2000: 600) defined the difference as: 'morality is a distinct sphere within the domain of normative thinking about action and feeling; the whole domain, however, is the subject of ethics'. Thus, when the nurse directly interacts with patients he or she can do so with principles of morality in mind, and equally importantly, when they are in discussions contributing to decisions regarding patients they ought to remain aware of such concepts.

Practical reasoning

In the above definition we note that both ethics and morality, at whatever level, are concerned with 'normative thinking about action and feeling', and if this is accepted then we can see that it is a dynamic process rather than a fixed static system. Although we have observed in the theoretical section above that many philosophers have sought universal principles that remain in all cases and for all times, we can also appreciate that the changing nature of the human condition would suggest that 'normative thinking' evolves and changes over time. In health care new technological advances have demanded new considerations regarding how we feel about the practical impact of such developments for human beings. This practical reasoning takes place in many fields of ethics and morality, and law, education, environment, business, exploration, sport and many more all have their own specific branch of ethics. In the field of health care we often refer to our own branch of ethics as medical ethics or bioethics. However, bioethics as a part of the broader framework of applied ethics is really concerned with the moral, social and political issues arising from biology and the life sciences, which would incorporate the environment and animal ethics, as they impact on human well-being. Thus, in the wider framework of medical ethics more specific perspectives on nursing ethics have been developed (Hunt 1994); although, to be fair, Hunt (1994) pertains more to identifying difficulties and hurdles to good practice than focusing upon the construction of a theoretical framework of good practice. Notwithstanding, it highlights the close relationship between ethics and the practice arena, and is therefore worth a read.

Certainly, more work is required in the field of nursing ethics, although a few preliminary areas can be sketched to provide some direction. The first is concerned with the distinction that can be drawn between what nurses do in practice and what other professionals do. In this we would need to examine the ethical framework in relation to applied nursing as it impacts on the human condition. We would need to be perfectly clear about the difference *in* practice and not just the difference *of* practice; that is, the nursing 'normative thinking' about our action. The second, and closely related, area concerns the nursing perspectives on health care issues, and this entails locating an ethical framework of what it means to be a nurse attempting to influence those issues. This continues the applied ethics theme, as it would need to address the nursing perspectives on health care issues as they impact on human well-being. The third area concerns the nursing claim of a distinctive conceptual framework that revolves around the role of the nurse in relation to the application of care rather than the focus on cure. Again, this is a practical issue, as it centres on the relationship between 'carer' and 'cared for', with each interaction within that relationship being unique. It will be concerned with exploring the ethical and moral issues relating to ill-health, or disability, as a life crisis and the impact that it has for that individual within their social network (Hunt 1994).

Nursing ethics would also need to incorporate three other areas from general ethics, which could then be analysed in relation to nursing in practice. The first concerns the issues of praise and blame, which have at their philosophical centre justice, desert and free will (Klein 1990). These issues, although complex, lie at the heart of nursing, both from within the profession itself and from the wider societal view about nursing (nurses as being 'dedicated' or having a 'vocation' debate). The second is situation ethics, in which decisions regarding the right and wrong of a particular action are given a moral weight (Fletcher 1966). This entails a critical analysis of rules that prohibit a particular action. The third concerns the ethical duties of nurses, in which the intrinsic rightness or wrongness of nursing action can be explicated. This is closely related to the deontological position outlined above (6:7).

Practical ramifications

In this final section we outline three aspects of morality that seem important for developing a nursing ethical framework.

- morality and identity;
- morality and emotions;
- morality and the high ground.

Morality and identity have been linked in two ways by philosophers. The first concerns the extent to which a person remains the same over time, and has important consequences for making decisions as a rational being. As our views change so do our decisions regarding moral issues. The second relates to the way in which we understand the social contexts and personal attributes of individuals that produce meaningfulness in life. It is this attempt to understand the human element of life that links morality with identity, and we could extend this notion of identity from individual identity to professional identity. This would contribute to an overall nursing ethics. In the second area, morality and emotions are appropriately linked, as it has long been recognized that moral action is influenced by emotions such as anger, jealousy, envy and compassion. Emotions can affect judgements, beliefs and whole ideologies and can make people behave in ways that they otherwise would not (Solomon 1993). Finally, morality and the high ground are connected by posing a series of questions regarding to whom and to what we should apply moral standing. To all human beings equally or to some more than others? To all higher primates or to all creatures great and small? To institutional entities such as political states and cultural traditions? To professional groups equally? In deriving answers to these questions we will be forced to address the issues of claiming the moral high ground, which is a criticism often applied to many groups, including nurses.

Further reading

Edwards, S. (2001) *Philosophy of Nursing: An Introduction*. Basingstoke: Palgrave.
Hunt, G. (1994) *Ethical Issues in Nursing*. London: Routledge.

6.16 Conclusions

Until recently philosophy and nursing were not readily linked together, as philosophical concepts were probably seen as the domain of medics, with nursing seen as being fundamentally grounded in practice. However, through the ever increasing complexity of ethical decisions in health care settings and the move towards multidisciplinary involvement in decision-making, it is necessary that the modern day nurse is equipped with some of the general philosophical concepts. Furthermore, contemporary nurses also need to be aware of how philosophical concepts are closely related to practice, and they need to have not only the terminology available to them but also the conceptual grasp of the relevance of these terms. It hardly needs stating that this current chapter is merely a starting point for the philosophical exploration of nursing practice, and the discerning nurse is urged to read, and debate, further. Of necessity, we have had to omit many areas of philosophical areas that are also highly relevant to health care settings, and feel that in reading further the nurse will be well rewarded, with the emergence of new and exciting possibilities. Finally, we have stressed the strong relationship between philosophy and practice and would like to conclude with a further example of how philosophy can be used in an applied sense to shape developments in practice. Many nurses, as their careers develop, are engaged in the construction of policies and procedures, and it is beyond doubt that those who have wrestled with the philosophy of practice will be better equipped to contribute to the production of quality documents that are realistic, workable and influential.

7 Thinking economics

7.1 Introduction

Newcomers to modern day nursing will probably bring with them some preconceived knowledge of what nursing studies might consist of, and it is unlikely that economics would be part of that knowledge. All of us share a deep-rooted experience of nursing as being a caring profession that is concerned with looking after the sick without the burden of health economics, which is viewed as belonging to the domain of others. However, the contemporary nurse is forced to cast a wider net and embrace the realities of financing the delivery of health care, as economics will directly affect them on one level or another. The economics of health care covers a wide perspective, from the price of a bandage to the annual expenditure of the National Health Service, and from the building of a hospital to the salary of a nurse. Whichever aspect of care is under scrutiny the expenditure on health is of concern to all involved, including both users and providers. In recent times the nursing profession has developed new and extended roles requiring an understanding of economic principles and policies because of the close relationship between the practical aspect of care delivery and the availability of economic resources. Nurses soon discover that the issues underpinning the economy of health care provision are clouded by varying political agendas (Chapter 8). Whether it be in developed or developing countries, the health care systems are dependent upon the economics of financing them. The factors that influence the economy of health care delivery are wide and varied, and include public pressure, interest groups, politicians, high-status individuals in organizations and sections within the NHS, and all those who exert a powerful voice.

PART ONE: THEORY

7.2 Theoretical overview

An understanding of the economics of health care in Western societies must be underpinned by an appreciation of the political and social events that contributed to the development of the differing medical systems in the post-Second World War era. This is particularly interesting in European countries, as many of them were largely destroyed by the devastation of six years of war. In the UK these political and social factors were directly influential in the spirit of the National Health Service (NHS), which was based on the principle that there would be access to health care for all that would be free at the point of delivery. Theories of economics tend to emerge from the practicalities of everyday life, and the starker the physical conditions the more radical the theories tend to be. It can be said that economics affects all our lives and we understand this at the level of 'cutting our cloth accordingly' or our inability to satisfy all our physical needs, wants and desires without the resources to purchase them. A substantial lottery win may well alter our economic conditions! However, although economics does affect our everyday lives, economists, via politicians, attempt to influence our living and working conditions in positive rather than negative ways. Unfortunately, in most theories of economics there are usually winners and losers, and those who decide who these should be rely on politics, philosophy and the various ideologies that are contained within them. In this section we briefly outline microeconomics and macroeconomics and outline the dominant issues that have contributed to modern day economics.

Microeconomics

There is no clear boundary line between microeconomics and macroeconomics but for the sake of definition we can say that microeconomics is the study of economics at the level of individuals or groups of consumers, or individual firms (Bannock *et al.* 1987). Although microeconomics focuses on the small-scale, it none the less must deal with the major concerns that the world faces. As Sloman (2001: 21) puts it, 'despite being "small economics" – in other words, the economics of the individual parts of the economy, rather than the economy as a whole – it is still concerned with many of the big issues of today'. There are a number of approaches to structuring the constituent parts of microeconomics. For example, Sloman (2001) identifies the following:

- *Markets, demands and supply*. This deals with how different countries organize their economies to answer the three basic questions: 'what to produce', 'how to produce' and 'for whom to produce'. The answers to these questions will be restricted by many other factors, such as price determination and the free market economy, to name but two.

- *Markets in action*. This is concerned with the important concept of elasticity. Elasticity refers to the extent to which one variable in the economy will respond to a change in one of its determinants.

- *The supply decision*. Usually firms will make a decision to supply a product based on how much of the market they can command and how much profit will be made. However, it also involves other complex issues: short-term or long-term gains, pricing, availability of raw materials, labour and so on.

- *Market structures*. This involves the extent of competition, and the extent of monopoly, oligopoly and price discrimination. It also involves an assessment of the relationship between different types of market and the service to the consumer.

- *Wages and the distribution of income*. This focuses on employment factors, including the differences in wages between, for example, pop stars and hospital porters. It naturally involves issues of why some people are rich and others are poor.

- *Market failures and government policy*. This involves assessing why markets do fail and what remedial action governments may take in an attempt to correct them. It involves an analysis of policies of privatization, deregulation, cutting expenditure and taxation, for example. It also involves an examination of non-governmental action.

We can already see not only that, microeconomics is a complex field with many overlapping areas within the theory, but also that it has many closer relations with, or influences on, macroeconomics. Although there is a general agreement on certain factors that should be included within microeconomics there is also some leeway given by other authors on what might be included. For example, Lipsey and Harbury (1988) structured their approach by subdividing both microeconomics and macroeconomics into elementary and intermediate parts. This approach enables the student to have a good grasp of the basics before moving on to the more complex aspects. Within elementary microeconomics they deal with demand and its relationship to price, as well as income and other determinants that influence this relationship. They also deal with supply, elasticity and both market price determination and market equilibrium. Within intermediate microeconomics they include sophisticated concepts such as indifference curves, business decisions, international trade and principles and problems of microeconomic policies.

Dealing with the relationship between microeconomics and macroeconomics Harvey (1988) argues that, broadly speaking, economic systems comprise two parts: (a) 'firms – business units from the sole proprietor to the government deciding what to produce and employing the productive resources'; and (b) 'households – the consumers of the goods, the services produced and the suppliers of the productive resources' (Harvey 1988: 22). In simple terms, Harvey (1988) argues that microeconomics is concerned with the supply of a particular good or service, how this relates to the demand for it and how that demand for its production relates to its supply. Furthermore, 80 years ago this would have been the extent of the study of economics, but today we have macroeconomics due to the sophisticated developments of the world's markets, economies and the overall globalization process (2:8, 8:11).

Macroeconomics

The concept of macroeconomics, as noted above, is of more recent origin and from this perspective 'we examine the economy as a whole. We still examine demand and supply, but now it is the *total* level of spending in the economy and the total level of production. In other words, we examine *aggregate demand* and *aggregate supply*' (Sloman 2001: 243). Sloman (2001) argues that macroeconomics must deal with the determination of national income and the role of fiscal policy. However, a note of caution is observed, as there is no universal agreement as to how the economy functions at this level. Money and monetary policies are also involved in macroeconomics, including an analysis of the supply and demand for money as well as an examination of the equilibrium in the money markets at both national and international levels. Unemployment and inflation are also linked into macroeconomics, including a look at the relationship between the supply of money and the price of goods and services. Finally, within macroeconomic theory, Sloman (2001) deals with international trade, the balance of payments and exchange rates within the concept of free trade and fixing foreign currency exchange rates. He sets the study of macroeconomics firmly within the concept of globalization and produces a clear and comprehensive account of these issues.

Lipsey and Harbury (1988), as noted above, outline elementary macroeconomics, which involves circular flow, consumption and investments, and both equilibrium and changes in national income. They argue that there are six major issues to macroeconomics: (a) employment and unemployment; (b) inflation; (c) the trade cycle; (d) stagflation; (e) economic growth; and (f) the exchange rate in relation to the balance of payments. Finally, within intermediate macroeconomics they deal with banks, money, interest, inflation, exchange rates and so on. However these issues are examined and understood, they call upon a basic understanding of consumption and investments, and the relationship between income fluctuations and fiscal policy. Furthermore, there are numerous controversies within macroeconomics and differing views on how they should be addressed. These include the conflict between monetarist views and Keynesian views of the trade cycle, and these are dealt with below.

Feminist economics

There is very little written on the issue of feminist economics. However, there is a growing concern that more intellectual space needs to be given to this important area (Miller 1999). Historically, the workplace is a male-dominated environment, with women traditionally remaining at home, the latter not being considered a place in which work is carried out. Work brings income and whoever controls the money tends to hold the power. Again, this has historically been the domain of men. In terms of both microeconomics and macroeconomics, and the issues that we have outlined within them above, feminist interpretations have yet to make an impact. On a global scale the roles of men and women in many cultures remain within fixed demarcations. This can be seen even in the ravages of war, disasters and famines, when gender issues may override the necessity of survival (Porter *et al.* 1999). Iddi (1999) highlights this tension in Burkina Faso in an article entitled 'Mind the gap: how what we do differs from what we say'. In this intriguing work she argues that predominantly men, but some women also, in her culture will make positive comments regarding the need for flexibility in their gender roles, but appear unable to act this out in practice. However, from an economic perspective in Ethiopia, Tadele (1999) offers a glimmer of hope in a gender role reversal, with 'men in the kitchen, and women in the office'. This work was undertaken because 'despite their equal share with men in socio-economic life, Ethiopian women have little decision-making power and a smaller share of resources and benefits' (Tadele 1999: 31). This is a system that is reflected around the globe and feminists must make greater inroads into the field of economics if they are to make an impact on the future of women's lives. We may consider that the grand issues of freedom, equality, justice, fairness and so on are important on a global scale, and indeed they are; 'however, feminism typically goes further than this and advances views about how domestic relations should be ordered, about the image of women conveyed by the prevailing culture, and so on' (Miller 1999: 324).

Further reading

McCrone, P. (1998) *Understanding Health Economics: A Guide for Health Care Decision Makers.* Buckingham: Open University Press.
Sloman, J. (2001) *Essentials of Economics.* London: Prentice Hall.

7.3 Demand, supply and the market

Demand, supply and the market lie at the heart of economics and the study of these factors has been a focus of investigation for some considerable time. Of course, these factors are usually seen in relation to a specific material product, such as food, clothes or other goods of one description or another, but can also be the delivery of services. In the former, material terms, it is a relatively, and we must emphasize *relatively*, simple task to measure the demand, produce the supply and allow the market to govern the price. If we are dealing with the demand for computers, the supply will be produced and the market will dictate the price, given such factors as production costs, the availability of materials and so on. This extremely simplistic view is theoretically feasible with the production of goods, and may even be feasible with the production of services such as sports centres, restaurants and hotels. However, the question of whether such services as health care or welfare systems can be left to the vagaries of the market in terms of supply and demand, given the ability, or inability, to pay, is a thorny issue indeed. Before we deal with this, later in the chapter, we look at the concepts of demand, supply and the market in a little more detail.

Demand

Most of us will probably have had the experience of wishing to purchase an item along with many others who also wish to purchase the same product. For example, there may be a desire to buy a certain toy at Christmas and the manufacturers have not made a sufficient quantity available, or there may be a limited number of tickets available for a concert or football match. We can see that there is a relationship between the desire, or demand, for a particular item and its availability. In simple terms this relationship determines the price of it. The law of demand states that the quantity of a specific good that is demanded per period of time will fall as the price rises and will rise as the price falls, with all other things being equal. If there is a crop failure in Brazil then the price of coffee will go up and if there is a glut of a product then its price will fall, if no other factors are brought to bear on the equation. Of course, this relationship between demand and price is complicated by many other factors. For example, the utility of a product – that is, what we get out of it – is a consideration. One hundred people may pay £50 for an item, 75 people may pay £75, and only 50 people will pay £100. This is known as the demand curve, and can be seen in Figure 7.1.

One factor under consideration may be how much utility they can get out of the product, but there can be other factors, such as income, savings and other commitments. One author of this book would be happy to pay £100 for a Bob Dylan concert ticket, the other author would definitely not!

Demand is also affected by fashion, or tastes, which refers to how much a particular item is desirable beyond its mere practical usefulness. There can be few parents who have not felt the pressure of fashion from their children, who have demanded a designer labelled pair of trainers. Beyond the function that a pair of trainers are used for there is a collective value that brings forth a peer pressure to demand the trainers because they are fashionable. Advertisers understand this and know the power of peer group pressure to increase the demand for a product, and will attempt to influence how people feel about being in the in-group or the out-group (3:8, 4:10). Demand is also affected by *substitute goods* and the quantity and price of them. If the price

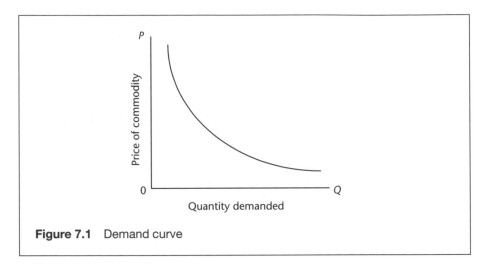

Figure 7.1 Demand curve

of the preferred item is too high then people are more likely to choose the second best. For example, if the price of coffee becomes too high for a coffee drinker they may switch to a substitute drink such as tea. This brings us to another factor affecting demand, and that is the quantity and price of *complementary goods*. These are items that are consumed together, or at least have a close relationship. They may include cars and petrol, shoes and polish, fish and chips, salt and pepper. If the price of one goes up, fewer will be bought and the demand for both will fall. Income is also a determinant of demand, and as people's wages increase there is also an increase of demand for what are known as *normal goods*. Normal goods are general items that most people would choose, and are contrasted with *inferior goods*, which are those that people buy when money is sparse. Another determinant of demand is the distribution of income. For example, 'if national income were redistributed from the poor to the rich, the demand for *luxury* goods would rise. At the same time, as the poor got poorer they might have to turn to buying inferior goods, whose demand would thus rise too' (Sloman 2001: 34, emphasis in the original). Finally, the expectations of future price changes are also determinants of demand and if people think that the price of a particular item is going to rise then they are more likely to buy more before the anticipated price increase. Taken in total, these factors make predicting demand a difficult task (Ison 2000; Sloman 2001).

Supply

Supply refers to the quantity of a particular commodity that producers will wish to sell at a particular price. If all other things remain equal then a greater quantity will be supplied at a lower cost. This occurs because a higher quantity will lower the costs of production per unit (2:2). According to Beardshaw *et al.* (1998) there are seven main determinants of supply.

- *Price*. This is the most important determinant of supply, and a change in price will usually cause a movement of supply up or down the supply curve.

- *Price of factors of production.* Producing a particular good usually involves numerous factors, such as cost of labour, resources, electricity and interest rates, and a shift in any of these costs will affect the supply.

- *The price of other commodities.* If there is an increase in the price paid for one item, say tomatoes, but not an increase in another related item, say onions, then economic theory suggests that there is a switch in farmers growing that product. However, in practice this is not always readily, or easily, undertaken.

- *Technology.* A technological advance usually means a more effective means of production, which can create an increase in supply and a reduction in price. Recent advances in production of the microchip have led to an increase in the supply of computers and a reduction in their price.

- *Tastes of producers.* Although we like to think that producers are objective beings who respond to the market forces of supply and demand to make profits, in reality they may make subjective decisions to produce what they prefer. This may be because it is challenging, stimulating, worthwhile or socially prestigious.

- *Entry to and exit from the industry.* New firms may not be able to enter the industry quickly, as it takes time to set up the production, and older established firms may leave the industry for numerous reasons. These factors will affect the supply of a product.

- *Exogenous factors.* There are numerous other factors that may affect the supply of a product, such as the weather, wars and disasters.

We can see that the determinants of supply are just as complicated as the determinants of demand, and in fact they affect each other considerably. If we also include in these determinants of supply such factors as organizational changes, government policies, eco-friendly lobbyists and greedy profit marketeers, for example, we can appreciate the relatively volatile environment of supply and demand (Beardshaw *et al.* 1998).

Markets

The term 'market' refers to the interaction between buyers and sellers (Sloman 2001), and the link between these two groups is the price of the goods that are being exchanged. There are a number of factors to this relationship and the first concerns the formation of an *equilibrium price*. Clearly there are differences in the motivations of buyers and sellers, in that the buyer wants to purchase as cheaply as possible and the seller wishes to sell for the maximum profit. The equilibrium price is the point at which the wishes of the buyer and seller coincide. The second factor is the issue of excesses in demand and supply. If there is an increase in the price above the equilibrium there will be more supplied than is demanded, and this surplus is called *excess supply*. On the other hand, if the price falls below the equilibrium then there will be more demand than is supplied, and this is termed *excess demand*. In these situations new equilibriums are formed (Griffiths and Wall 1999). Another factor is the uneven distribution of income. Some people are richer than others, which is determined by the extent to which their ability to work is rewarded, inheritance, chance and so on, and governments are forced to intervene in the market to protect the more vulnerable who cannot, or do not, work, such as is the case with pensions for the elderly and benefits for the unemployed. The market is also affected, albeit in a minor way, by government policies on dangerous products such as weapons or drugs. Finally, there is the lack of free competition. Free competition is needed in an open market system to keep the equilibrium between buyer and seller. Monopolies, subsidies and restrictions on free trade all serve to disturb the equilibrium and alter the market forces in favour of either the buyer or seller (Callon 1998).

Further reading

Callon, M. (1998) *The Laws of the Market*. Oxford: Blackwell.

7.4 Capitalism and its alternatives

Capitalism is a term that can evoke both negative and positive feelings, depending upon whether one agrees with its principles or not. This is further complicated by the fact that some may believe in the notion of capitalism as a model for the production of goods but do not feel that it is the most appropriate model for the delivery of health care services. By its very nature capitalism relies on competition, and in all competition there are winners and losers. However, when we move the semantics of the word competition away from the notion of a game and focus its meaning on life, including our living conditions, then the idea of winners and losers, or rich and poor, becomes more, poignant and profound. Capitalism equates with free enterprise and entrepreneurship, and in our society it is generally valued that people strive and work hard to better themselves or to provide for their family. These values are difficult to disagree with, but it should be remembered that if some get ahead, then others must fall behind, and in a finite world if some acquire more, then others must receive less. It is this particular point, among many others, that makes capitalism such anathema for some. The anti-capitalists, a growing lobby group, are vociferous, and sometimes riotous, at world trade conventions, World Bank summit meetings and intergovernmental economic assemblies. In this section we will attempt to outline the basic principles of capitalism, as well as two main alternatives to it.

The principles of capitalism

Capitalism refers to an economic, as well as a social, system in which individuals are free to acquire the means of production (2:2) and maximize profits. Capitalists are villains to Marxists (2:2) and heroes to Conservatives (Lipsey and Harbury 1988). Capitalism is founded on the notion of capital, which refers to assets that have the capacity to generate income, these assets themselves having been produced. Capital is the amalgam of raw materials and labour, and in one sense can be understood as holding the stored value of the item that has been produced. If a potter spends all day producing a vessel from clay he has not gained any utility from that vessel until he later uses it for carrying water. By making the vessel he has saved himself some future water-carrying labour and in this sense the capital represents deferred consumption. In another sense the potter can sell the vessel, thus generating income for him to purchase other goods that he desires. All other factors being equal, he is free to determine what he makes and what price he sells his product for. However, we can quickly see that the price is also determined by what the buyer will pay for it. Thus, the relationship between the seller and the buyer centres on the price of that particular item. This is clearly seen in a serious bargaining or haggling situation when the seller attempts to keep as high a price as possible and the buyer attempts to reduce it as much as they can. The agreed price is each's theoretical cut-off point.

Capitalism is also devoted to the notion of the free market, and this refers to the distribution and exchange of goods, or the allocation of resources, that are outside the control of the state. In short, it is a market based on private agreements between seller and buyer. The free market is based on the concept of free enterprise, in which individuals are allowed to produce, distribute or exchange goods, and this is usually accompanied by the right of ownership of private property in the means of production. In an ideal free market supply and demand govern the pricing system, and this extends to the availability of raw materials, the price of property, the wages given to workers, what the goods are sold for and so on. However, once there is interference in the free market, through either the state or the transfer of privately owned property to public or common ownership, the market can be said to be no longer free. Therefore, the nationalization of the coal mines and the railways in the UK during the twentieth century dismantled the notion of a free market for coal and rail travel.

Capitalism, as an economic system, like all other systems, has both advantages and disadvantages. The advantages of a free market system include the following:

- *Automatic adjustments.* Any intervention by governments require administration, which takes time and resources, while on the other hand a free market adjusts itself through the process of supply and demand. For example, take the crop failure in Brazil and the subsequent rise in coffee price mentioned above.

- *Dynamic advantages.* The chance of high profits encourages investments in new products, ideas and techniques, and although prices may initially be high the consumers will eventually gain through increased choice of products. Further, if profits are high then new firms will enter the market, increase competition and drive down prices.

- *A high degree of competition.* It is argued that even in monopolies and oligopolies certain competitive forces continue to take effect for a number of reasons: (a) there may be a fear that high profits will encourage other firms to break into the market; (b) other services may increase competition, such as bus services against rail travel; (c) there is a continuing, and increasing, threat of foreign competition as world markets open up; (d) the countervailing powers of large powerful producers to sell to large powerful buyers, with the former driving up prices and the latter driving them down; and (e) the competition for corporate control.

The advantages of the free market system are, of course, countered by a number of disadvantages, and these can be summarized as follows:

- *Lack of equity.* There is a lack of equity or fairness to a free market, as there are always some individuals with more than others, whether this be income or goods.

- *Inefficiency.* The market may over- or under-supply goods and services because of divergent interests, which makes the free market inefficient.

- *Sluggish.* Free markets may be sluggish in their response to changing demands.

Taken at face value we can see that these disadvantages may well prick the social conscience, and this leads many to argue against a totally free market system and offer some alternative approaches.

Alternatives to the free market system

The two main alternatives to the totally free market economic system involve an element of state intervention to one degree or another. The first alternative to be considered is what is termed a mixed economy, which is the most common approach in market-driven societies. A mixed economy involves some state intervention through laws, policies, directives, taxes and subsidies. Furthermore, in every country some production activities are organized and operated by governments (Lipsey and Harbury 1988). The extent to which the state does intervene is often critically debated and the issue of central planning is sometimes contentious. In periods of war central planning may be useful to bring about large structural changes, say in developing countries, which may require industrialization or modern agricultural expansion. What the state intervenes in will differ from country to country and industry to industry. States may intervene in the relative price of goods by taxing or subsidizing them, or by direct price controls. They may also affect the market by intervening in wage controls via taxes, rents, welfare payments and so on. States can also influence the patterns of production and consumption through legislation (unsafe goods) or by direct provision (education). Finally, governments may be concerned with the macroeconomic problems of unemployment, inflation, balance of payments etc., and may intervene in taxation, government expenditure, bank lending, interest rates and foreign exchange rates, to name but a few.

The second main alternative to the totally free market is the command economy, in which there is an all-powerful state-controlled planning authority. In this system the state determines the assortment of goods that will be produced and the basis on which they are distributed. The state, in effect, determines what the needs of the people are and then sets the means of production to meet those needs. This system has four main criticisms. First, determining the extent of satisfaction that people derive from consuming goods is impossible and control of consumption tends to make individuals angry. Second, by necessity, command economies require 'officials' to do the assessing, which increases bureaucracy, form-filling and red tape. Third, the dovetailing of the satisfaction of needs and wants by officials, politicians and administrators, who may be out of touch with the grass-root people, is difficult. Finally, state ownership of the means of production may lessen incentives and diminish effort, drive, enthusiasm and initiative. Command economies are arguably less efficient than systems in which private enterprise is allowed to flourish, which may account for the collapse of many communist economies.

Further reading

Lipsey, R. G. and Harbury, C. (1988) *First Principles of Economics*. London: Weidenfeld and Nicolson.

7.5 Global economics

Through the increase in communication technology and the speed of travel the world is now a 'smaller' place than ever before and with the advances in techniques of warfare through nuclear and biological methods the winds of the Earth ensure that we are all vulnerable and touched by world events. Furthermore, the expansion of capitalism through pioneering markets around the world and the McDonaldization of life (Ritzer 1997) make the relations between countries and individuals ever closer. World affairs, whether they be wars, stock markets, depletion of rain forests and so on, have a knock-on effect that involves all individuals around the globe, and just as a world famine may wipe out the human population so too may a change in the global climate. In focusing on global economics we are concerned with the stability of world markets, the need for international cooperation and the relationship between the developed and developing countries. We will not deal with the rights and wrongs of this expansion of capitalism through free trade, as they are outside the remit of this book.

Instead we will focus on the process and issues that underpin this growth. We will also outline the relationship between globalization and debt in developing countries, as this has serious consequences for ongoing poverty, disease and ill-health.

Globalization and stability

As we mentioned above, we are all affected by events in other countries and in this sense we can be said to live in an interdependent world. As Sloman (2001: 469) observed, 'countries are affected by the economic health of other countries and by their government's policies. Problems in one part of the world can spread like a contagion to other parts, with perhaps no country immune.' Sloman argues that there are two main ways in which this process of globalization affects individual countries' economies. The first is trade, and as long as one country trades with another there will be implications for both. If the government of one country feels that, say, its economy is growing too fast it may adopt deflationary policies to slow the growth down. The country will not consume as much, which will affect domestic products as well as imports, and this will affect other countries as well as the home country. The knock-on effect in the other countries may lead to a fall in outputs and a rise in unemployment. The process by which changes in imports, or exports, affect national income in other countries is known as the *international trade multiplier*. Open economies are particularly vulnerable to changes in economic activity in the rest of the world and this is likely to increase, as the World Trade Organization (WTO) is committed to dismantling trade barriers and encouraging freer trade among nations.

The second major way in which globalization affects individual countries is through financial markets. The flow of money between countries has grown rapidly over the past 25 years and according to Sloman (2001: 470), 'each day, over $1 trillion of assets are traded across the foreign exchanges'. Most of these transactions are short term and are aimed at making quick profits as exchange rates appreciate. If one country decides to raise interest rates because it is concerned with inflation it will attract an inflow of funds from other countries. The home country's currency will appreciate and speculators will try to buy the currency quickly before it has stopped appreciating and then sell at a profit. Thus, as one currency appreciates the others depreciate against it and, of course, the reverse can, and does, happen with changing events. This shows the interdependent relationship between the countries' currencies and if the globalization process is to maintain some degree of stability then there is a need for international policy coordination.

An economic crisis in one country can quickly lead to crises and collapse in another country and this economic 'contagion' is difficult to stop or even control. There has been a number of cases in which world leaders have been seriously concerned that the whole world would be plunged into recession with devastating consequences. In an attempt to counter this the leaders of the major industrial countries meet at least once a year with a remit of generating world economic growth while avoiding major currency fluctuations. In order to achieve this there is an attempt to 'harmonize' economic policies by endeavouring to get all the major countries to pursue consistent economic strategies aiming to achieve common international goals. However, despite the great efforts of the world leaders to achieve this harmonization it has proved difficult in practice, for a number of reasons.

- *Differing budget deficits and debt.* There is a considerable difference between countries' budget deficits and debt as a proportion of their national income, and this puts different pressures on interest rates.

- *Interest rate fluctuations.* If interest rates are allowed to fluctuate with the demand for money, without convergence the fluctuations could be very severe indeed.

- *Abandoning monetary and exchange rate targets.* To harmonize interest rates would entail abandoning monetary and exchange rate targets.

- *Internal structural relationships.* Countries have different internal structures and may react differently to harmonizing policies.

- *Products, investments and penetration.* Countries differ in terms of their productivity, the development of products, the investments that they make and the extent of market penetration.

- *Domestic versus international policies.* There may be an unwillingness for a country to change its domestic policies to those of the international community even though it may well agree with them.

It may well be that complete harmonization is impossible to achieve, but most world leaders are in agreement that some is better than none.

Globalization and debt

Most people are aware of the plight of many developing countries in terms of being trapped in paying debts owed to world banks. This situation came about in the 1970s as the world went into a recession following the oil crisis in 1973–4. As the oil price soared and the recession ensued the banks had plenty of money to lend and they readily set up massive loans to developing countries. The recession was short-lived and as world economies recovered the developing countries only just managed to service the debts. However, as oil prices soared again in 1979 and 1980 the developing countries found it much more difficult, if not impossible, to pay the required interest, let alone the capital repayments. Thus, they were trapped at three levels: (a) by being unable to pay the interest; (b) by a growing capital debt and increasing interest payments; and (c) by being unable to develop their country's economic infrastructure. In 1982 a number of countries declared that they would suspend payments completely, which created a debt crisis that threatened both the debtor countries and the world banking system.

Being trapped in debt means being trapped in poverty, and in terms of the developing countries this also means being trapped in starvation, disease, ignorance and ultimately death. To extricate the developing countries from this dire situation two approaches were adopted. The first approach was to reschedule official loans, which was done by the 'Paris Club', and usually involved delaying the date for repayments or spreading the payments over a longer period of time. There have been several attempts since the mid-1980s to reschedule these debts, with longer repayments, lower interest roles and moratoriums on when payments begin. However, the debtor countries had to agree to some internal structural adjustment programmes, which are overseen by the International Monetary Fund (IMF). Yet despite these efforts many debtor countries failed to meet the conditions and remained trapped in debt. The second approach involved dealing with the underlying causes of the debt and included the structural adjustment programmes as outlined by the IMF. These programmes frequently employed; (a) tight fiscal and monetary policies to reduce deficits, interest rates and inflation; (b) reforms to increase the use of markets and incentives for investments; and (c) strategies to increase trade exports and competition. However, these programmes can, especially in the short term, create hardship, unemployment and poverty as the country deflates. Despite the more positive longer-term development, in the short term the hardships may be too great to bear.

In 1996, 41 countries were identified as having substantial debt problems and the HIPC (heavily indebted poor countries) initiative was launched by the World Bank and the IMF. This initiative aimed to provide debt relief by reducing the debts to sustainable levels and in some cases involved cancelling the debts completely. Another initiative, the Jubilee 2000, was proposed to cancel Africa's debts, and was supported by almost 80 organizations from around the world. It called for the cancellation of all debts, no matter to whom they were owed, by 31 December 2000. The cancellation policy was to take account of the debtor's probity, economy, social policies and human rights record, with the released funds aimed at reducing poverty. However, by the end of 2000 only seven countries were receiving debt relief and at the time of writing many of the African countries originally identified as requiring debt relief remain trapped in poverty, with all its concomitant problems.

Further reading

Lee, K., Buse, K. and Fustukian, S. (2002) *Health Policy in a Globalising World.* Cambridge: Cambridge University Press.

PART TWO: APPLICATION TO PRACTICE

7.6 Economics and the NHS

Histories of our society will usually include an analysis of the relationship between sickness and health, and it is of no surprise that the care of the sick has long been associated with religious groups as representatives of the gatekeepers of the spirit world. In terms of ill-health, when a member of society becomes unwell for any reason they are reliant on others taking care of them and attempting to assist them in their recovery. Historically, there has always been some limitation to this assistance, which includes a limit to the skill of those doing the assisting and a limitation to the availability of drugs (e.g. plants) and equipment (e.g. bandages). However, in contemporary times there is a popularly held belief that such limitations are a thing of the past and an infinite amount of resources are now available to assist those in need. Of course, this is not the case and there is a growing awareness, albeit reluctantly, that resources are limited and that distribution of these resources is an important and difficult task if it is to be done both efficiently and effectively. In this section we outline the work of two economists, John Maynard Keynes and Sir William Beveridge, who both, in different ways, contributed to the post-Second World War societal structures in which economics and the NHS were fused together. They were both influenced by the Great Depression of 1929–39 and were concerned about the hardship that was suffered by so many in Britain, as well as others around the world.

Keynes

John Maynard Keynes (1883–1946) was educated at Eton and won prizes there for mathematics, English and classics. He went on to Cambridge University and graduated there with a first in mathematics. He eventually held numerous posts both at university and in government departments. Keynes varied his areas of work and publications but is best known for his 1936 treatise *The General Theory of Employment, Interest and Money*. We will look at the work of Keynes from two perspectives, first in relation to unemployment and second in terms of what became known as the Keynes plan.

Unemployment was the most serious problem facing Western societies during the inter-war years of 1918–39 as the world went into a long recession. This was further exacerbated by the 'Wall Street Crash' of 1929, which sent the world into the Great Depression. Prior to the 1920s economists generally agreed that there could be no such thing as mass unemployment and the classic economists of the time needed to explain what they believed to have been impossible. Their argument was that the growing unionization had priced the workers out of the market and that their wages were not flexible enough downwards. Workers, it was suggested, should take a wage cut to get themselves back into employment. Furthermore, savings were to be encouraged in order to provide a source of funds to support businesses. This, it was argued, would stimulate the economy again and create jobs. The classic economists further argued that there should not be an increase in government spending, as this would lead to an increase in government borrowing if a rise in taxation was to be avoided. This would lead to private businesses being starved of funds and thus to a further collapse and deepening recession.

Keynes criticized this analysis by the classical economists. He argued that full employment was not a natural state of affairs and that it was likely that the economy could slide into a depression and remain there indefinitely. In order to go some way towards a state of full employment it would be necessary for the government to intervene in the economy to ensure an adequate level of aggregate demand. With this government intervention a recession would become a short-term problem, Keynes argued, and classical economists seemed more focused on the long-term, which compounded the problem. He also dismissed the classical analysis that claimed a refusal of workers to accept wage cuts, and argued that workers are no more likely to accept wage cuts in a depression than they are in a boom. Moreover, Keynes also claimed that increasing savings in a recession would be counterproductive, as this would stifle spending. He argued that the solution to mass unemployment was for the government to spend more, not less, and that this could be funded by expanding the money supply. This government spending would stimulate businesses and increase employment, the employed would spend more and in turn stimulate more production and so on. In the post-Second World War era many governments of all parties claimed to be 'Keynesian' in their approach to economics.

In 1944 there was a conference held at Bretton Woods in the USA, which was to launch an international clearing union, and the UK government of the day requested that Keynes submit a proposal to effect this. This became known as the Keynes plan and it included the following points: (a) the same function as a domestic bank and clearing house; (b) international debts cleared on a unilateral basis; (c) overdraft facilities for member states; (d) own unit of currency called the BANCOR; and (e) a gold exchange rate. However, the proposal did not win approval at the conference as it was thought to be too radical and the more watered down IMF was established instead. Despite this, the principles of the original Keynes plan are now considered to be more plausible than the current IMF operations.

Beveridge

William Henry Beveridge (1879–1963) was the director of the London School of Economics (LSE) from 1919 to 1937. Like Keynes, Beveridge maintained a long-standing interest in the issue of unemployment and published a book of that title in 1931. In a later work, *Full Employment in a Free Society* (1944), he defined full employment as 3 per cent unemployed, which became a figure commonly adopted as a benchmark. He was also very influential in the setting up of labour exchanges, which are a precursor to the current Job Centres. However, the work for which he will always be remembered is his 1942 report *Social Insurance and Allied Services*, which became known as the Beveridge Report. The importance of this wartime report on social policy cannot be overstated and its influence on the post-war NHS is profound. As Berridge (1999: 14) noted, 'its [the Beveridge Report's] significance was less in the originality of the report's work than in its plans to rationalise the disjointed insurance schemes in existence before the war. The report's recommendation for a comprehensive social security system, based on subsistence rate benefits, assumed that among other benefits would be a national health service which would be free and comprehensive.' Remembering that this report was published in the middle of the Second World War, it must have reflected a future utopian dream while the German bombs rained down on the people of Britain. It received a rapturous welcome from the public and this gave an impetus to ministerial discussions throughout 1943, which culminated in an announced acceptance of its principles, a timetable for consultation and a programme for eventual legislation (Berridge 1999).

Although the Beveridge Report was wide ranging its central focus pivoted on the general practice service, in which the GPs would no longer have an independent status but would become paid employees of local authorities. They would work in health centres with other members of the health care team, the report suggested, and there would be a close liaison with other local authority workers (Webster 1998). The Minister of Health in 1943 put forth a White Paper, which turned out to be a modified version of the report and was rather vague on a number of issues. However, it claimed merely to be a consultative document that aimed to build on the pre-war platforms of voluntarism, local authority structures and health insurance. Its major revelation was the fact that certain elements of the medical profession were resistant to the idea of a national health service. Doctors working in wealthy areas were opposed to it, while those working in poorer areas supported it. Few liked the idea of being under the auspices of a local authority. Protracted negotiations ensued between the Minister of Health and the British Medical Association, which led to serious concessions being made by the government in 1945.

The power of the medical profession prevailed and as Berridge (1999: 14) reports, 'the administrative role of local government was weakened at the expense of the professional organisations; there was new financial provision for the voluntary hospitals; and doctors in health centres would not be local salaried employees'. In June 1945 the White Paper that was prepared on the basis of these negotiations had to be held back, as it was anticipated that there would be a bad reaction from the restless electorate. The concessions that were made to the medical profession and the private interests of the voluntary hospitals produced the worst possible basis on which to build a national health service and it did not receive popular support (Webster 1998). The National Health Service, and indeed the welfare state, were launched in an era in which social citizenship was changing. Although in the late 1940s the social basis remained one of class division and exclusion, society was changing and as the 1950s dawned there was a growing feeling that the National Health Service belonged to the people. There was a growing sense of ownership and 'the national health service did not conform to market principles; it was the seat of egalitarian collectivism and as a monopoly it necessarily had to be inefficient' (Hutton 1995: 211). Doctors maintained their position as gatekeepers between the sick who wished the best care at whatever the cost and the taxpayer who was perceived as an infinite source of money. The cost of the NHS soared to crisis point.

Further reading

Berridge, V. (1999) *Health and Society in Britain Since 1939*. Cambridge: Cambridge University Press.

7.7 Financing health care in contemporary society

The way in which a health care system is financed is crucial to the way that services are delivered, and as a corollary of this finances have a direct bearing on practice delivery. As best practice is central to nursing, as well as to the other disciplines, nurses at all levels must be concerned with the most cost-effective approach to both financing the service and delivering it. Therefore, an understanding of the basic principles of economics is important for all nurses. As Brosnan and Swint (2001: 13) claim, 'cost studies can be complex and difficult to conduct, but an understanding of the basic techniques allows nurses to fully participate in planning, implementing and evaluating programmes that greatly impact on the health of the community'. Furthermore, nurses are increasingly moving into managerial posts, or taking up clinical posts with a managerial component, and need to know how economics impact on practice, and how to manage resources efficiently and effectively. In this section we outline a number of methods by which a health care service might be financed and briefly set out a number of international comparisons.

Differing methods of financing healthcare services

In the UK, we are used to a health care service that is free at the point of delivery and financed by National Insurance payments that are deducted by employees from workers' wages before they receive them. Putting to one side for the moment the private medical insurance schemes that are available, but that only a few can afford, most people are familiar with the UK National Insurance structure. However, this is not the only system available to us, nor is it necessarily considered to be the most appropriate one. There are several methods, with all of them having both advantages and disadvantages, and Morris (1998) suggests that they can be grouped into six main types.

Direct out-of-pocket payments

In this system the individual directly pays for the care that they receive at the point of service use. The charge that is levied is governed by the service provider and in this sense the system reflects a free market component. If no one needs the service then there is no charge to be paid, unlike in our current National Insurance scheme, in which all those in employment pay irrespective of their health needs. In the direct out-of-pocket payment scheme health care can only be purchased by those who are able to afford it, and this highlights a major disadvantage. There may be many who do not have the finances to pay and there may also be some who run up enormous bills with long-term health care needs. However, this system does provide the consumer with the freedom to choose a provider if they have sufficient funds available.

Private health insurance

In this system a contract is formed between the insurance company and the individual concerned, in which there is an agreement that the latter will pay a premium and the company will agree to pay for any health care that may be needed. The individual assesses the extent to which they may be at risk of requiring future health care should they become ill and the company usually makes an assessment of the individual's health to establish the extent to which they may be at risk of having to pay the bill. There is competition between companies for the consumers' premiums and the individual can usually choose where they go for any health care that is needed. This system allows the individual to protect themselves from unexpected health care expenditure or large bills due to serious illnesses. Disadvantages to this system include the fact that only those who can afford it will insure themselves and some of those who are insured will take up treatment for minor conditions which they would not have done if they had not been insured. This latter action wastes valuable services.

Preferred provider organizations

Preferred provider organizations (PPOs) is a system that is derived from private health insurance and is similar in that: (a) there is a contract between the individual and the insurer; (b) there is an agreed premium to be paid by the individual; and (c) the insurance company agrees to pay for any health care costs that may be incurred. However, it differs because in this system there is less choice for the individual as to where the health care is received, as it is largely decided by the insurance company, i.e. the preferred provider. This is because agreements are made between insurance companies and health care providers so that premiums can be kept low and the providers receive a constant channelling of patients to their facilities. While the individual is protected against large health care bills they have less choice as to where they receive such care.

Health maintenance organizations

Health maintenance organizations (HMOs) also derive from private health insurance schemes but differ in that the insurance company and the health care provider merge to form what is in effect one organization. The individual agrees to pay a premium and, by contract, receives any health care that they may require should they become ill. Individuals continue to have a choice of HMOs but must receive the care from the designated provider. In the simplest terms the choice of insurer determines the choice of the provider. This system continues to protect the individual from large health care bills but severely limits the choice of provider. It has the disadvantages of uptake of health care for minor conditions as mentioned above, as do the other systems, and many may not be able to afford the premiums.

Public health insurance

A public health insurance scheme operates in a very similar manner to a private insurance scheme, as the individuals who consider themselves to be at risk of becoming ill pay premiums and receive treatment if needed, which is paid for by the insurer (the insurer in this scheme being the government). The difference here is that the individual may not have a great deal of choice of provider of health care, although they can move to another provider if needed, and there is no competition between providers in terms of prices charged. As the government is the only provider it has considerable power over providers and how much they will pay for such services. This system protects insured individuals against unexpected illnesses or large health care bills.

Direct taxation

This system is derived from public health insurance schemes and involves the compulsory payment of premiums by all individuals in employment through direct taxation. The government operates as the only insurer and there is no competition between providers. Providers have little say as to how much the government will pay them for their health care facilities. The individual has no choice as to the insurer, as the government is the only one in this system and they have no choice as to whether they wish to pay the premiums, as they are compulsory. However, the individual does have some choice as to health care provider as they are free to change this if they so wish.

We can see from the foregoing that there are strengths and limitations to the various systems of financing a health care service and that there may be a considerable overlap, with a number of these schemes operating at the same time.

International comparisons

We now briefly sketch four international comparisons to the UK system of health care delivery.

Canada

In Canada there is a public health insurance scheme, which involves 12 individual health insurance plans, i.e. one for each of the ten provinces and the two territories. While each of the provinces and territories can determine the level of service that they wish to provide, a basic provision is mandated by the federal government. This means that there are 12 separate insurance plans in Canada but they are very similar, due to the government setting the basic level of provision. There are also available in Canada private health insurance schemes, but these are not permitted for the services covered by the public scheme (Morris 1998). Health care services in Canada are in a state of flux due to the 'transformation of capitalism through the phases of entrepreneurial, monopoly, and global capitalism' (Coburn 1999: 833), but this is also likely to be reflected elsewhere around the developed world.

United States of America

The US system of financing their health care service represents one of the most mixed systems in existence. As Morris (1998: 168) notes, 'health care is financed [in the USA] by direct out-of-pocket payments, private health insurance, PPOs, HMOs and public health insurance'. Vulnerable individuals have some protection through *Medicare* and *Medicaid*. Medicare is a federal government health insurance system for those aged 65 years and over and Medicaid is a joint federal and state system protecting the poor. The majority of US citizens have some form of private health insurance or one of its derivatives. According to McCarthy and Minnis (1994), in 1990 there were approximately 14 per cent of the US population without health insurance cover, which represents 33 million individuals, and these must pay directly, go without health care or rely on charities.

Sweden

Sweden operates a national insurance scheme that is funded through compulsory taxation. However, the responsibility for health care provision is devolved to 26 authorities, called county councils, which are divided by geographical region. Each authority is responsible for its resident population and receives funding from the national scheme, with patients being able to choose their GP and their hospital. Furthermore, Swedes can refer themselves directly to hospital if they so wish. Sweden also has a small private health insurance market (Morris 1998).

Germany

Germany operates a public health insurance scheme, which is funded through compulsory taxation comprising equal payments from both employee and employer. Germany's health care system is subdivided into approximately 1000 decentralized funds that cover 90 per cent of the population. Private health insurance covers 8 per cent and the remaining 2 per cent are covered by a government administration. These decentralized funds are operated as private corporations but are under strict government regulations, and they must accept anyone who is eligible to join (Morris 1998).

Further reading

Hoffmeyer, U. K. and McCarthy, T. R. (1994) *Financing Health Care*. Dordrecht: Kluwer.

Morris, F. R. (1998) *Health Economics for Nurses: An Introductory Guide*. London: Prentice Hall Europe.

7.8 The NHS: changing expectations and demands

In 1948 the NHS had a very clear and simple remit, which was to provide free health care for all at the point of need. However, since then the NHS has gone through a series of restructurings, reorganizations and reshapings, alongside a growing awareness that it cannot solve all health-related problems and that resources supporting the service are finite. Governments, of all political persuasions, have influenced the NHS to one degree or another over the years and continue to do so today. The cost of providing health care is a contentious political issue and there is a growing urgency for all in the service to be aware of such issues as wastage, maximizing resources and cost containment (Strange and Ezzell 2000). Constant reforms of the health care service have taken their toll on staff as well as patients (Keddy *et al.* 1999), and there is an increasing shortage of personnel, particularly nurses (Dumpe *et al.* 1998). Staff shortages influence the quality of care that is delivered and are a worldwide problem, and not one that pertains to the UK alone. The demands that are placed on the NHS are considerable and increasing year on year. This makes the issue of supply and demand a central concern of health economics. Furthermore, the intricate relationship between supply and demand is constantly being tampered with in an effort to ensure economies of scale (Yafchak 2000).

Demand for health care

There are some who are convinced that the principles of the free market are most suited to governing the delivery of health care, while others are equally convinced that they are not. What is not at issue is the fact that there is a need for a health care system and, therefore, in terms of demand and supply this fundamental need requires some degree of satisfaction. How this may be achieved has been outlined above (7:7), and we now need to outline a number of the factors that may contribute to changing, or thwarting, this demand and supply relationship. According to Morris (1998) there are five main issues that influence the demand for health care. The first refers to whether consumers of health care are considered to be utility maximizers. The consumption of health care does not have the same utility as the consumption of other goods, as patients tend only to consume health care when necessitated by ill-health. Therefore, there is some element of disutility associated with the pain and anxiety of the illness (McGuire *et al.* 1988). On the other hand, Morris (1998: 53) has stated that 'health care may be treated as an investment, where short-term costs or disutility may be overshadowed by long-term returns. In this sense, it may be argued that consumers of health care do act in such a way so as to maximise their overall level of utility.' The second issue relates to the relationship between the cost of health care that is provided and the amount that is demanded. In economic theory it is accepted that as the price of a particular good rises the demand will fall, and vice versa. However, in terms of health care it is difficult to see this relationship taking effect, as, particularly in times of acute illnesses, patients will demand treatment because their need is great. Moreover, if health care is made cheaper then it is even more difficult to see that patients will demand more care. However, it may be a little more complicated than this, as the price that a person is willing to pay for treatment may well be governed by their income but we must also take into consideration the fact that some will pay beyond this level, say if they need a life-saving operation.

The third issue is concerned with the question of whether the quantity of health care that is demanded is actually affected by the level of income. The demand for goods generally rises as income levels rise, but usually for superior goods. When incomes go up and the demand for certain goods decreases then these goods are called inferior goods. In terms of health care it appears unlikely that income levels will affect health care demand either upwards or downwards to any great degree. The fourth issue concerns the extent to which the price of other goods affects the demand for health care. While we may appreciate that health may be related to other factors, such as diet, exercise and living conditions, it is difficult to think of another good that is directly influential on the demand for health care. Therefore, in a true economic sense the price of other goods does not influence health care demand. Finally, we need to address the issue of whether tastes and trends affect the amount of health care demand. Certainly, tastes and trends will affect the consumption of other goods. For example, fashion will influence a type of attire that is worn or a food that is eaten, and a social trend towards increased exercise will increase the consumption of sportswear and health foods. However, it is generally accepted that a trend towards health care, either for or against it, will not directly affect the quantity that is demanded.

Supply of health care

Again, in the economic theory of demand and supply it is assumed that the free market principles operate to balance this relationship and that the delivery of a health care service can function as an everyday business. This was summed up neatly by Rambur and Mooney (1998: 122): 'current wisdom holds that health care is a business and as such must abide by market principles . . . [and] most nurses are not well enough versed in economic theories to credibly critique health care delivery decisions based on economic theories'. However, applying the economic theory of supply to the delivery of health care requires several issues to be addressed (Morris 1998). The first issue refers to the extent to which providers of health care can be considered to be maximizers of profit. Maximizing profit is the main drive of most businesses yet it is hard to identify the main motivation in providing a health care service. It may well be that increasing patient welfare is the main drive, but the profit and income of the provider may well be another main concern. This may be the case because of the need to be efficient. Furthermore, individual doctors and nurses may not be motivated solely by maximizing their profits but the hospital that employs them may be motivated to maximize its profit margin in order to employ more doctors and nurses. The second issue concerns the question relating to whether there is a positive relationship between the price of health care delivery and the quantity that is supplied. If general economic theory were to be applied to the supply of health care then it is fair to say that when prices are low only the most efficient providers will make profits but when prices rise others could enter the market to compete. However, in real terms the delivery of health care is not strictly geared towards these assumptions, as the initial costs to providers are extremely high because hospitals are expensive to build and it is not acceptable for hospitals to close as many businesses do.

The third concern in the supply of health care focuses on the impact of the costs of production on the supply, and this is clearly an important issue. The costs of production are usually fixed and therefore are finite, so that if there is a rise in the cost of production then fewer health care services will be delivered. On the other hand, if the cost of production falls then more can be made available. The fourth issue revolves around the impact of technology on the quantity of health care that can be supplied. Advances in medical technology will usually enable more patients to be treated, more efficiently and with shorter inpatient admissions. Thus, in effect, technology does have an influence on the amount of health care that can be delivered. Finally, we must deal with the issue of whether the price of other goods affects the quantity of health care to be delivered. In the general market this relationship is well established, as the rise in the price of one good makes it relatively more expensive to purchase than other goods and producers can switch production to the more expensive items in order to maximize their profits. However, in health care delivery this is less likely to occur, as initial costs are high when building a hospital and health care staff tend to have specific expertise. Having said that, hospitals may change their focus by specializing in a more profitable type of internal hospital service; for example, moving from ophthalmic surgery to cardiac surgery.

We can see from the foregoing that the demand for and supply of health care services are complex affairs that do not, generally, adhere to the rules of the free market (Wilkinson 2001). However, we also note that an understanding of general economic principles is important to appreciating how the service operates in a capitalist society.

Further reading

Donaldson, C. and Gerard, K. (1993) *Economics of Health Care Financing: The Visible Hand.* Basingstoke: Macmillan.

▌7.9 Private sector health provision and vulnerable groups

We have seen above (7:7) that there are numerous ways in which a health care system might be financed and we should now be quite clear regarding the fact that resources are a finite entity. In the UK since the inception of the NHS we have become accustomed to the notion that all in our society are covered by this health care system irrespective of their ability to pay. This makes the system free at the point of delivery, but we also know that the system has to be paid for by someone – and that is the taxpayer through National Insurance contributions. The NHS, as we are all aware, had, and continues to have, many problems, and is often criticized for being inefficient, ineffective and wasteful, as well as having long waiting lists. In the 1980s the Conservative government undertook the privatization of many of the nationally owned industries, such as British Telecom, British Gas, British Airways and British Airports Authority, to name but a few. Furthermore, it employed numerous strategies to engage the private sector in competing for services, such as selling off state assets, opening up state monopolies and contracting out services (Harvey 1988). This policy drive included the NHS, which was restructured so that an element of competition for services could be undertaken, and one of the main developments of this was the increase in private sector provision. In this section we look at the private sector in relation to health insurance, the impact of the private sector and the creation of vulnerable groups.

Health insurance

The key element that drives the notion of health insurance is uncertainty. In a certain world – even in a certain NHS world – we would not require an alternative insurance system, as we would receive the best treatment, in the best service, immediately it was required. However, as this is not the case, we require access to alternative services to ensure our best chance of treatment, and ultimately survival, and various private health insurance schemes exist to make provision for this. Uncertainty involves two key elements and these are: (a) the *timing* of health care expenditure; and (b) the *amount* of expenditure that is required (Morris 1998). Let us look at these in a little more detail. Because, by its very nature, ill-health is largely unexpected and we are usually unable to predict when it will strike, the timing of when we might require health care services is uncertain. Although predictors, such as smoking, drug abuse and lack of exercise, are available to us, we cannot be specific as to when, or even if, we are going to become ill and in need of health care. In fact, even when we engage in unhealthy activities we tend to be 'surprised' when we become unwell. In cases where we become in need of health care services we are also uncertain as to the amount of expenditure that may be required. We do not know if we will need a small amount of care or require a large amount, which may be beyond our means to pay. Attempting to predict this is difficult and, furthermore, we are uncertain as to what we can do if the expenditure required is so great that we cannot afford to pay it.

Health insurance is a way of addressing the above tensions that are created through these uncertain elements, but it should be noted that it does not eradicate the uncertainly completely. Health insurance usually involves both a contract and a premium. The contract generally involves an agreement that should the insured require health care then the company will pay for it and the individual will make regular contributions to the company, which are known as premiums. Depending on the type of contract there may be a number of clauses that are included, such as a ceiling to the amount of payout by the company or a percentage to be paid by the individual. Differences in contractual arrangements make the health insurance market a competitive arena in which companies vie for consumers' premiums.

The impact of private sector health care

The impact of private health insurance can be seen in a number of main issues. First, adverse selection is a problem. Adverse selection is defined as 'the phenomenon under which exactly the wrong individuals from the point of view of the insurance company choose to buy health insurance' (Morris 1998: 144). This occurs because individuals who are insuring themselves tend to know if they consider themselves to be a high risk, while the insurance company generally does not. Those with a high risk of illness have a financial incentive to purchase insurance and those who expect to benefit will choose to buy it. The second major issue concerns a moral aspect, which involves the uptake of health care services that they would not have taken up had they not been insured. This is wasteful and may be considered a frivolous use of health care services, although it is understood that some consumers who have paid premiums would argue that they are entitled to it, having paid for it. Furthermore, the question of morality is also of concern in respect of the providers. As providers are focused on provision rather than the patient, they do not have the incentive to restrict the supply of health care services. This, again, is wasteful. Third is the question of non-price competition, and this pivots on the fact that as the insurer is paying the bill the consumer is no longer concerned as to the price of the treatment. This leads to patients choosing health care on the basis of non-price factors, which is antithetical to the notion of a free market.

Fourth, we cannot ignore the extent to which the private sector system has impacted on the UK. Morris (1998: 150) points out that 'relative to the NHS, the market for private health care is small. In 1995 health care expenditure on the NHS was £41,517 million, or 87.8 per cent of total UK health care expenditure. Expenditure on private health care was £2,536 million, or only 5.4 per cent of total UK health care expenditure.' Although these figures are for 1995 and there has been an increase in private health care services since then, there has also been an increase in the NHS expenditure and the gap is only a little narrower today. Finally, the affordability of private health insurance is a concern regarding the impact that it has on the UK health care system. In any fee-paying system there are going to be some who cannot afford the fee and in a system that involves premiums there are going to be some who cannot afford the contributions. This means that such groups as the unemployed, those on low incomes, the elderly, the disabled and the chronically ill may not be able to afford the private health care service. Given that it is morally unacceptable that they do not receive treatment, this means that the government must make provision or another method of financing the service should be developed. Thus, a private health care service, although providing an excellent service for some, will create a series of vulnerable groups who cannot afford it.

Vulnerable groups

As mentioned above, vulnerable groups are created by the inability to pay for private insurance, and there are two main groups: (a) those on low incomes who simply do not earn enough money to be able to afford the basic premiums; and (b) those who require high levels of health care. It should be remembered here that there may be some who belong to both (a) and (b). Members of the second group are those in the high risk group and once identified by insurance companies may not be covered by them, or they are set extremely high premiums, which they cannot afford. One such group is the elderly population, which is growing in numbers. Many elderly people are living longer on low state pensions and by the nature of their ageing years may be in need of high levels of health care. Insurance companies are reluctant to insure them and, if they do, they set very high premiums. Many vulnerable sections of society have lobby groups to attempt to persuade Members of Parliament to take up their cause and develop favourable policies that will raise the standard of living and health care. Reddy (2000: 43) argued that 'the quality of life can be improved if policy makers have a clear understanding of the factors that influence successful ageing, and develop appropriate economic policies accordingly'. However, this may be more difficult in practice, especially when it comes to changing government policies.

Fortunately, in the UK, as well as in many other countries, a 'social safety net' protects the most vulnerable in our society and provides a basic level of provision. However, in some other countries this may be set higher, or may be set lower, and in some it may be non-existent. Those left to the ravages of their illnesses or diseases, who must fend for themselves, or be cared for by family or friends, are a truly unfortunate group. Whatever criticisms may be levelled at a national health service, at the very least it operates to assist everyone in society, even those who cannot contribute towards paying for it.

Further reading

Morris, S. (1998) *Health Economics for Nurses: An Introductory Guide*. London: Prentice Hall Europe.

7.10 Global health

As we pointed out above (7:5), the globalization process ensures that the world is shrinking in time and space, as many cultures, creeds and races interact at a much closer and more frequent level than at any previous point in our history. Since the world trading system began we have taken Western diseases to foreign lands, such as plague, measles and smallpox. As these diseases were unknown in these foreign lands the locals suffered many deaths due to a lack of immunity against them. Similarly, the trading system brought foreign diseases to Westerners, who suffered the same fate. This basic historical example serves to show how the closer we interact globally the greater impact we have on each other, and in contemporary times this interaction is considerable. Furthermore, with global economics having an impact on all our lives and touching far-off peoples through cheap labour markets, capitalist expansion policy and international consumerism, there are few in the world who are not affected by this. In this section we outline the process whereby health care becomes a commodity, the impact of global economics, using a number of countries as examples, and the global concern about green issues as they impinge on the health of people.

Commodification

Health care in the majority of societies carries a subjective element, with a form of metaphysical component that involves selfless compassion in the care of others. This embroils the identification of those in some degree of need and others doing all in their power to help them within the notion that the reward for doing so is of a higher order than mere financial gain. Health care workers are thus respected above and beyond the salaries that they receive, and hold a high status for what they do. This can be seen as much in traditional cultures involving 'medicine men' as it is in our Western societies that employ what they like to consider to be 'scientific' principles. However, since the early development of the NHS in the UK we have noted a shift in thought relating to the status of health care, one that was influenced by the rationalization of the service throughout the 1980s. The focus in this period was on ensuring that health care resources were maximized to their greatest potential and wastage kept to a minimum. Of course, this was, and is, a laudable enterprise and one that is difficult to argue against. This focus also prioritized balance sheets, competition, cheapness, managerialism, accountancy and so on, with a clear emphasis on the marketization of health care and the entrepreneurialism of service delivery. This contributed to the overall McDonaldization of life (Ritzer 1997) in a postmodern (2:8) world.

Commodification refers to the process by which something that is not generally considered to be a commodity is managed and ultimately perceived as an item, and this both reduces the subjectivity attached to it and perforce increases its objectivity. If an aspect of life is objectified it can be treated in a certain way; that is, as an item that does not have feeling and, therefore, does not require compassion. Health care may be considered as having undergone some element of commodification, particularly since the 1980s, as the subjective element of the service has had to give way to an objective rationalization policy. The emphasis on limited resources, and maximizing them, has reinforced the notion that health care is a commodity similar to a car or hamburger. What underpins this is the idea that a commodity is a tangible good, or service, resulting from the process of production, and health care is a service that should be influenced by this production process. The production process, by its nature, is constantly striving for maximum efficiency in the quest for maximum profits. Health care, it is argued, should be equally efficient. However, as health care carries such an emotional content it cannot be completely commodified and this will always create a conflict in the production process.

Global health and the impact of globalization

We can deal with the impact of globalization on global health within two main areas. First, the impact of sanctions against certain countries has a direct bearing on the health of the people. When sanctions are applied, ratified by the United Nations (UN), it is not the direct intention of the sanction to affect the health of the population, but in effect it does. The intention of sanctions is to bring the government of the country under pressure, and this is applied through the discontent of the people. However, as the government of the sanctioned country holds the power in that country it is the people who tend to bear the brunt of the sanctions *before* the government feels under any great pressure. The first example to be drawn from is the case of Iraq – a particularly poignant example at the time of writing, following the overthrow of the Iraqi government. The sanctions against Iraq hit the Iraqi children the hardest, as Daponte and Garfield (2000: 546) reported: 'we found that after controlling for child and maternal characteristics, when economic sanctions were entered into the proportional hazards equation, the risk of dying increased dramatically'. The children of

Iraq have apparently suffered so badly from the sanctions, coupled to other economic events and the chemical legacy of the Gulf War, that they may never fully recover (Hall and Olahfimihan 1999). In Cuba, another sanction-hit country, Buxton (1998) found that despite immense difficulties health care continues to be a top priority. However, the fact that economic sanctions continue to exist against Cuba ensures that the poor, who are considerable in number, suffer the greatest. The final example is from Haiti, which underwent economic sanctions during 1991–4 and the impact of these included 'declining incomes, rising unemployment, poorer nutrition, declining infant mortality, rising mortality among 1–4 year olds, decreased attention to children's well-being and education, and family breakdown' (Gibbons and Garfield 1999: 1499). Even during such a relatively short time-frame the sanctions had a huge impact on Haitians' health, and the survival strategies that were employed including altered nutritional intake, black market activity, selling their household goods, decreased school attendance and indentured child servitude, which all affected the health and well-being of the poor.

Second, the health of a country's population is affected not only by sanctions from the UN but also by global economics in a general sense. There is much positive commentary regarding the impact of globalization, particularly from those who have gained from it. However, its negative impact by comparison receives less attention. Ganguly-Scrase (2000: 138) reports a negative effect in India: 'the major finding from this study reveals that there is a stark contradiction between the rhetoric and reality of globalisation, economic liberalisation and structural adjustment programs for the lower middle classes'. Although some in India have improved their living conditions and health, 'the vast majority of my informants have not benefited economically over the past nine years' (Ganguly-Scrase 2000: 138). The poor of India continue to be so, with the corollary of poor health for many. Research from Africa highlighted changes in health as a result of the devaluation of their currency. The research team noted changes in meal preparation and meal composition, with a depletion of fat and vegetable contents, the elimination of desserts and a reduction to one meal per day. 'These changes specifically affected economically disadvantaged and socially isolated households, and those headed by women' (Fouere *et al.* 2000: 293). A transition in nutritional intake was also observed in Korea as a result of modernization, with a greater consumption of animal food products and a fall in cereal intake. This produced a change in health status for many Koreans, particularly in the middle-income groups (Kim *et al.* 2000). These examples show the impact of global economics on individual lives, particularly in relation to health.

Environmental issues

It is, perhaps, the matter of the environment that coalesces all the issues of global economics, as a serious change in the global climate will affect everyone, from both developed and developing countries and from the poor to the wealthy. Global economics has contributed the most to the state of the environment, from the early traders to the current mass travel and from the destruction of the rainforests to the vagaries of the stock market. Most of us will be aware of the problems of climate change, global warming, resource depletion, ecotoxicity and reduced biodiversity as we, as humans, absorb the world's finite resources and produce toxic waste in the process. It is a fact of life that there is a limit to many of the world's resources and once used up they cannot be replaced, and this does have an impact on the world's environment. We can expect that certain warm regions will become cooler and cooler places become warmer; fertile areas may become desert and dry regions become flooded. This will have an impact on people's lives and health, and may even lead to some cultures becoming extinct. According to Hancock (1999: 68), 'we do not yet know the impact on longevity of lifetime exposure to a mix of persistent toxic chemicals in our environment, since it has only been widespread in the past 40–50 years. The health impacts of global warming are only just beginning to be understood and could be profound. But perhaps the most profound threat to population health is economic growth, to the extent that it undermines environmental and social sustainability.' In evolutionary terms we have evolved over millions of years in a close relationship with our environment, and we have dramatically changed this environment over the past 50 years. Therefore, we cannot be surprised if this sudden change affects our lives and our health.

Further reading

 Jamison, A. (2001) *The Making of Green Knowledge*. Cambridge: Cambridge University Press.

7.11 Conclusions

We have seen throughout this chapter that economics has a big impact on the practice of health care, from the delivery of the service to the bearing on people's lives and their health. The spread of capitalism and the free market has had major influences on the world's resources, with the consequences to the human species, as yet, not fully understood. We are undergoing a realization, albeit slowly, that just as the world's resources are finite so too are the resources supporting a health care service, no matter how that service is financed. Thinking economics is concerned with how nurses understand the underlying ideologies and subsequent economic practices that are implemented by various societies around the world. Nurses are increasingly being called upon to influence health care service delivery, whether through managerial approaches or through organizational policy development, and they must be knowledgeable regarding economic theory and its impact on health.

8

Thinking politics

8.1 Introduction

Previous generations of health care workers, policy-makers and financial managers were fond of attempting to separate politics from the delivery of care. This probably had its basis in the commonly held notion that the NHS was a 'free' service at its inception in the post-Second World War era and that it was just reward for previous hardships. However, some decades later, particularly through the 1980s and 1990s, it became abundantly clear that health care was not an infinite commodity with limitless resources, and the view was taken that health care *is* politics. Each successive parliamentary opposition since the birth of the NHS has accused the standing government of attempting to dismantle, reorganize or under-fund the health service, as it is held so dear by the majority of people in the UK, and thus to do so is an easy vote winner. However, in contemporary times the majority of people appreciate that the NHS is limited by funding and by political ideologies. Thus, there is a growing awareness that politics and health care are inextricably linked and that political theory has a practical impact on health.

In this chapter we are concerned with politics as theory, in relation to health care, and we set out some of the central political positions as they impact on social welfare. These perspectives are based on how they perceive that their particular society binds together and how members of the community ought to behave towards each other. They carry interpretations of social and individual responsibilities and pivot on the perceived values that each holds regarding the relationship between human nature and a social contract. Politics in relation to health care is concerned with the relationship between the individual, the society, ill-health and power. Thus, we are as much interested with politics *in* health care as we are with the politics *of* health care. To understand the political structure of our society as a welfare state we are attempting to appreciate how the sick and diseased, the disordered and the disabled, are cared for at a societal level. Thus, the focus of analysis is in relation to political theory from various perspectives and how these may impact on the health of the society, and world at large.

PART ONE: THEORY

8.2 Ideology

The term ideology has several layers of meaning, and it is useful to work through these in order to arrive at the relevant political definitions, but we should also note that each layer has areas of overlap with the others to provide an overall rich understanding of its usage. The first layer concerns a lay understanding of what ideology means and this is highly relevant, as we will discuss below the importance of the transition of ideas between lay knowledge and 'scientific' knowledge. A lay definition of ideology would refer to a manner of thinking based on a set of ideas, which may be rooted in a particular class, religion or political persuasion. From a sociological (see Chapter 2) perspective the term ideology has been used in three important senses. The first involves a very specific kind of belief organized around a few central values, usually opposed to dominant institutions. The second refers to beliefs that may be considered to be in some sense distorted, or false, and this usage is usually associated with Marxist (2:2) literature. The third involves any set of beliefs embracing a wide range of domains, including science, religion and proper conduct, and these are usually socially determined rather than having a true or false status (Abercrombie *et al.* 1980).

From a philosophical perspective the term ideology refers to a set of ideas, beliefs and attitudes that may be consciously or unconsciously held. It serves to recommend, justify or endorse a collective response that is geared towards maintaining one's own ideology or changing someone else's. In these terms the word ideology can be used pejoratively as a criticism of someone or something, or non-pejoratively to represent the diversity of cultural differences of belief systems (Freeden 2000). Finally, in political terms ideology refers to any systematic and all-embracing doctrine that gives an overall theory of humanity and society, or at least claims to do so, and provides a platform for political action. This perspective embraces everything that is relevant to the human political and economic condition and provides the rationale for changing that condition. Thus, we can now see that there are areas of overlap between these various definitional frameworks, and we can highlight the main points to an ideology:

- a set of beliefs, ideas, opinions and attitudes that may be consciously or unconsciously held;
- regarding a particular perspective such as science, religion, politics or behaviour;
- that may be considered by some to be true or false;
- that serves to recommend, justify or endorse a particular course of action.

Informal and formal ideologies

From the foregoing, it can be said that 'ideology refers to a set of ideas which interpret the world according to the point of view (the interests, values, and assumptions) of a particular social group' (Winter 1989: 186). These social groups may include being a member of lay clubs and social circles of friends, as well as a scientific community or professional body. Thus, we all share a number of ideologies. In fact, it is hardly possible not to belong to one ideology or another. Therefore, we are likely to hold ideologies from our lay worlds as well as ideologies from our professional one, which may well create tensions between them. These ideological dilemmas are part and parcel of being thinking human beings in a world of bigotry and prejudice. A major argument in Billig *et al.*'s (1988) approach to ideological dilemmas is that the contrary elements may not only arise *within* ideologies themselves but also exist *between* them. These authors argue that contrary elements 'could be represented by the contradiction between possessing a theoretical ideology and at the same time living within a society whose everyday life seems to negate that ideology' (Billig *et al.* 1988: 27).

Let us now draw a distinction between formal ideological systems (intellectual) and informal or lived ideology of ordinary life (common sense). Within this distinction there is an accepted transformation of concepts, a passage both from formal ideology to informal ideology and the converse (Moscovici 1984). The distinction between informal ideology and formal ideology can be briefly explained. Informal ideology refers to 'the ideology of an age or of a concrete historico-social group, e.g. of a class, when we are concerned with the characteristics and composition of the total structure of the mind of this epoch or of this group' (Mannheim 1960: 49–50). This brings the concept of culture and informal ideology into very close proximity. Formal ideology, or intellectual ideology, is more akin to a philosophy. Aron (1977: 309) wrote: 'an ideology presupposes an apparently systematic formalization of facts, interpretations, desires and prediction'. This brings it close to the notion of 'science' (see Chapter 9). If we accept the existence of ideologies from both informal and formal settings then we can begin to appreciate that they must influence each other in some way. In fact, Billig *et al.* (1988) suggested that there is a movement of informal ideological concepts through to formal ones and vice versa, and this usually occurs with the use of the language pertaining to a particular concept. For example, we may employ the formal (scientific) term of paranoia in our everyday use to express our feelings regarding our perception of someone, or in the formal system of physics we may use the term 'wormhole' to express the theoretical mechanism of transferring from one dimension of the universe to another.

Political influences on health care

In the UK, politics plays a significant part in the delivery of health care and in this subsection we briefly outline the major political forces that impinge on the service. Until recently we could locate the right, centre and left political parties as Conservative, Liberal and Labour respectively. However, the political spectrum is a constantly changing dynamic and one that attempts to respond to the changing society and the needs of the people. This makes such polarizations as right and left somewhat inaccurate, and this is particularly so at the time of writing, as the Labour government appears to be more at the centre of politics than at any other time in its history. The spectrum of right, centre and left is also unhelpful unless we begin to define what the criteria are that denote these positions.

Conservatism is considered to be on the right of British politics and there are said to be three distinct parts to this political position. First, its attitude to society is based on the idea that society is an achievement that, although far from perfect, is preferable to the pre-social state. It also suggests that society in one sense is an antecedent to the individuals that compose it. Society holds the values and customs without which the individual is considered damaged. Second is the idea of government, predominantly through the power of institutions. Power should be vested in offices and departments, and in individuals only as holders of those offices and departments. These institutions are set to conserve the customs and values of civil society. Third is the idea of political practice that is pragmatic and local. It wishes to resolve conflicts through the inherited institutions and rule of law, via the exercise of power. Conservatism emphasizes natural social relations and the defence of private property and the free market.

Labour is considered to be on the left of British politics and is a movement that seeks to better the conditions of the working class, usually through gaining political power. It has a number of main features that are rooted in history:

- explicit appeal to the working class;
- affiliation with the trade unions;
- representational government through democratic elections;
- belief in a welfare state;
- belief in the redistribution of wealth through taxation;
- commitment to democracy.

The Labour Party tends to be constitutionalist in its main activities and relatively conventional in its economic policy. It is often viewed as the party of the people.

Liberalism is considered to be at the centre of British politics and has a number of main features.

- belief in the value of the individual and his rights;
- belief that the individual has inherent rights, which are independent of the government;
- belief in individualism, ensuring that individual needs take precedence over collectives and groups;
- belief in human potential and achievement as the main values;
- belief in the value of freedom;
- belief in universalism, which suggests that rights and duties stem from the human condition;
- belief in toleration regarding morality and religion.

Liberalism is concerned with limited government, and considers itself to be open and corrigible.

There are other groups in the British system of politics that have, at one level or another, an impact on the delivery of health care services through political persuasion. First are those groups that may be brought under the umbrella term of ecology politics. These groups are concerned with the relationship between the human being and the environment, and they are involved with conservation, depletion of the ozone, pollution and so on. Second are those groups that fall under the term nationalist politics, and these are based in the identity of the nation. This involves territorial integrity, and common language, customs and culture. Third are the numerous religious groups that have an impact on political parties. British politics has a close relationship with the church, and many political ceremonies involve members of the clergy. All the foregoing contribute to the cauldron of society, in which health care is but one feature.

Further reading

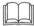

George, V. and Wilding, P. (1985) *Ideology and Social Welfare*. London: Routledge and Kegan Paul.
Leach, R. (1991) *British Political Ideologies*. London: Philip Allan.

8.3 Society and the state

The concepts of society and the state are inextricably entwined in advanced capitalist societies, but so too are the problems that emanate from them, and the social policies that are geared towards resolving them. A society can be viewed as any number of individuals who interact in an organized and systematic way and who determine their criteria for membership. There is no agreed definition of society, as there are as many ways of determining societies as there are forms of social interaction (see Chapter 2). For our purposes a society forms a set of rules that its members must recognize and abide by, or face a set of sanctions. Members of a society recognize each other not as individuals, but as belonging to a set of cultural norms and values (see Chapter 4). To contrast the idea of society with that of state is recognized as indeed difficult, as, again, there is no clearly accepted defined distinction. However, for the purposes of political thought an attempt must be made.

It is often said that a society can precede a state, but not the other way round, and this suggests that as a group of people become organized via a set of systems, they form a society, which then may develop a state, in order to control them. Thus, the notion of power often features in definitions of the state. For example, Weber (1968) (2:2, 2:9, 2:12) viewed the state as the organization that monopolizes legitimate power over a given territory. Furthermore, Marxists (2:2) conclude that the state is a product of a society in terms of a stage of its development. In contrast to the 'power' theory of state is the 'rights' theory of politics, but they have a considerable number of overlaps that make a distinction difficult, especially given the short space available here. Both theories employ legal frameworks derived from laws, certain liberties and certain powers to rule. Both centre on the notion of social conflict.

Theories of order and social conflict

Theories of order and social conflict stem from the world of sociology (see Chapter 2), as well as economics (see Chapter 7), and here they are grounded in politics. There is such a wide range of approaches and emphases in dealing with these ideas that we can only focus on the main view here, and that is concerned with the work of Parsons. From the early functionalist (2:3) perspective every part of society is seen as having a specific role to fulfil in order to ensure the smooth running of the society as a whole (Ryan 1970). Although modern functionalists have abandoned this analogy, it is still useful in highlighting the relationship between subsystems and the society at large. Within these types of theories the functional nature of a subsystem maintains order. However, other theorists suggest that it is not the functional necessity alone that maintains order but the consensus of values that underscore the society. As Parsons (1969: 6) noted, 'the set of normative judgements held by members of society who define, with specific reference to their own society, what to them is a good society . . . With all these qualifications, it is still true to say that values held in common constitute the primary reference point for the analysis of a social system as an empirical system.' Thus, for Parsons, these consensual values of a society are passed on from generation to generation and are dependent on the socialization of the young generation and the social control of all (Parsons 1951a). However, focusing on conflict, an apparently ubiquitous condition in modern societies, Lockwood (1956: 222) observed that 'the two major threats to a given system are infants who have not been socialised and individuals who are motivated to deviance or non-conformity'. Although this debate is set in the 1950s it appears to resonate today with the political concerns regarding youth crime, truancy, bullying, illicit drugs and so on, resulting in the social exclusion of a growing number of young people.

There are numerous approaches to understanding the nature of conflict, from a political perspective, in society and we can briefly mention two. Conflict is closely associated with deviance and deviance can cover both non-conformist behaviour and aberrant behaviour. Non-conformist behaviour refers to actions that are visible, unselfish and highly esteemed by other members of that group (for example, Greenpeace action), while aberrant behaviour refers to invisible actions, for personal gain, and known to be stigmatizing by the practitioners themselves (for example, drug addiction). It is this latter group of behaviours that are considered to be the basis of social problems. The second theory, or group of theories, argues that it is not the individual that causes social problems but the society in general. In the institutional model the root of social problems lies in the economic and social conditions in which people find themselves trapped. Poverty, ill-health, unemployment, poor housing and so on are considered to be the contributing factors to the creation of social problems. Ryan (1971: 7) put it succinctly: 'it is a brilliant ideology [blaming individuals] for justifying a perverse form of social action designed to change, not society, as one might expect, but rather society's victim'. These approaches see society as conflict-ridden and are more prone to accept a wider diversity of cultural forms of behaviour. Conflict theorists would prefer not to use the term 'social problems', as it tends to have a clinical semantic, whereby the individual is held responsible, and prefer instead to use the term 'social conflict' to locate the 'problem' as society's.

Class theories and the health problems of class

We have outlined class in Chapter 2 (2:2, 2:9) and here we focus a little more on class from a political perspective. Class can be seen as a political or theoretical term, which is employed as a form of explanation of a system of inequalities. When it is employed in this manner it is necessary to identify the observable features that enable people to determine what class they believe a particular person belongs to. In British society a person may be allocated to a particular class on the basis of overt factors, such as their dress, manners, accent, deportment and so on. Other, less overt, signs of class include wealth, type of employment and leisure activities. In many societies a person is born into a class and there is no movement between them, in other class structures movement is possible, but always extremely difficult to undertake and to maintain.

The functionalist view of class in modern society is related to the development of the social services as a series of subsystems contributing to the overall functioning of the society. This subsystem development emerged, it is argued, as a result of the increased differentiation and specialization that were brought about by industrialization. The function of the social services is to promote social integration and reinforce the basic values of society. The conflict theory of the development of social policy results from functionalists' view that society is made up of classes and groups with conflicting interests. Their theories pivot on the notion of power, particularly in relation to the struggle for it and the fight against it. The Marxist theory of class is covered above (2:2) but, briefly, class is considered to be a result of the conflict between the means of production and the needs of the capitalist system. Whatever the theory of class, the corollary of this hierarchical structuring is that health problems tend to ensue.

There are many differences in health-related problems in terms of the class divisions in society. If we take the basic class structure of lower, middle and higher classes (2:2, 2:9), we note that historically the lower classes tend to have higher rates of birth but this is accompanied by higher rates of infant mortality. Furthermore, childbirth was a significant hazard to women with frequent births. Access to health care facilities is proportionately greater in the higher classes, and they tend to receive more specialist attention. There are also class inequalities relating to housing tenure, with increased illnesses in those in poorer quality housing accommodation. Other problems that occur in the lower classes are that they have increased rates of unemployment and occupational injuries, and die earlier. It should be noted that there are many more that the discerning student should follow up. Although the explanations for all these statements are highly complex they none the less show that class divisions in society do impact on health-related matters (Townsend and Davidson 1988). This is of continuing political concern today.

Further reading

d'Entreves, A. P. (1969) *The Notion of the State: An Introduction to Political Theory.* Oxford: Clarendon Press.

Hoffman, J. (1995) *Beyond the State: An Introductory Critique.* Cambridge: Polity Press.

8.4 Collectivism

Collectivism, as the name suggests, is concerned with the political theory and practice that advocates the overall 'collective' as the economic, social and political unit, rather than the individual or the state. The collective is not a private group, such as the family, but a wide and variable membership, which is partly determined by local attachments. It is an autonomous association of individuals and a central theme is the right of the collective over the individual, but it should be noted that there is a healthy debate both within collectivist political parties and also from anti-collectivists regarding this.

Collectivism is said to have three distinct meanings. First, in a Marxist (2:2) sense collectivism refers to the theory that the means of production, distribution and exchange should be owned and controlled by the collective. This means that the major decisions are a collective choice. Second, in a broader sense collectivism refers to any socio-political system in which individuals act in accordance with the collective wishes, under the directives of the collective or in the name of it. This includes all matters of social, cultural or productive activity. Third, and in a still broader sense, the term collectivism is used to denote any views that allow the collective to have rights that can override the individual. These collectives might include the state or institutions of education, religion or sport. We can see from these broad meanings that the term collectivism may be interpreted differently, and indeed there are numerous political parties that would fall under this term. In short, we may say that the term collectivism is loosely defined but may be employed to describe those thinkers who believe in the necessity of a government-managed economy, albeit reluctantly. We can outline the collectivist position through a brief analysis of their underlying social values, the relationship that they maintain between the society and the state and their view on the welfare state.

Collectivist social values

It should be stressed that there are no absolutes in many political persuasions, there is often debate regarding various interpretations and indeed there is often a good deal of overlap with other political perspectives. Thus, the values of the collectivists are a belief in liberty, individualism and competitive private enterprise (George and Wilding 1985). However, they are also pragmatists at heart and this pragmatism is based on the conviction that capitalism is not a self-regulatory system – it needs some element of adjustment. This pragmatic approach is set not in abstract intellectual debate but in the necessary conditions at hand. Freedom is central to the collectivist ethic. However, this again has a pragmatic flavour, as for the collectivists 'liberty means more than freedom from the arbitrary power of governments. It means freedom from economic servitude to Want and Squalor and other social evils' (Beveridge 1945: 9). Again, their core values of individualism and private enterprise receive a dose of practical grounding as they are rooted in the notion of self-help. Thus the core values are all tied to each other: 'above all, individualism, if it can be purged of its defects and its abuses, is the best safeguard of personal liberty in the sense that, compared with any other system, it greatly widens the field for the exercise of personal choice' (Keynes 1936: 380). Although this may seem at odds with the earlier statements regarding the subordination of the individual's rights to that of the collective, the focus on the individual is seen as important *in relation* to the overall collective.

Collectivism, society and the state

As we are ultimately concerned with health care, and in particular the role of nursing in this service, we must understand how political parties see the relationship between the society and the state (as they would should they form a government). The reluctant collectivists, as George and Wilding (1985) call them, have a critique of capitalism that can be identified under four headings.

- *Capitalism is not self-regulatory.* It is considered to be wasteful and inefficient. It misallocates resources and in itself will not abolish injustices, unemployment or poverty. It is ultimately threatening to political stability. It is dependent upon the relationship between spending and production, and if one fails, then the system fails.

- *Unregulated capitalism is uneconomical.* This is based on the social imbalance between private affluence and public squalor. Poverty means that the poor do not have the resources to engage in capitalism and thus 'an austere community is free from temptation. It can be austere in its public services. Not so a rich one' (Galbraith 1970: 212). It is common knowledge that in times of poverty problems of crime, vandalism, violence and drug abuse are more likely to proliferate (George and Wilding 1985).

- *Economic development will not, by itself, abolish poverty and injustice.* They believe that capitalism will benefit some, even possibly many, but that it will always, if left unregulated, leave a marginalized group in poverty. There will always be the 'haves' and the 'have-nots'. Therefore, reluctant collectivists believe that some form of regulation is needed in managing the economy.

- *Sectional interests come to be equated with the public interests.* This is likely, they argue, to result in the creation of conditions that threaten political stability. Capitalism requires the consumption of products, and production becomes the sacred. Thus, production is planned by the powerful and the affluent and their views on public policy will dominate. This is not a good recipe, they argue, for the loyalty of the poor.

We can see that the reluctant collectivists feel that some form of government involvement is necessary in order to improve the conditions of the society's members, and this stretches to the delivery of welfare.

Collectivist governments and the welfare state

We saw in the previous section that the reluctant collectivists acknowledged that some government involvement was necessary in a free market, and this extends to the welfare state. They accept the welfare state as a mechanism for making good the faults of the market in order to protect the vulnerable from its ravages, rather than as an instrument to promote economic and social changes for the good of all. As early as 1943 Beveridge was to highlight the major common social enemies of Want, Disease, Ignorance, Squalor and Idleness, and the responsibility to tackle them was not the individual's alone but part of our social conscience (collective) (Beveridge 1943). Galbraith (1963), in a critique of American capitalism, argued that it does not serve individual welfare or the public interest *per se*, and that the 'aim is for a state concerned for welfare, the public interest and the good life – a welfare state' (George and Wilding 1985: 63). Again, there is a pragmatic approach to the delivery of a welfare state, and it is to be reactive rather than promotional, thus making it problem-orientated. It will cover what private enterprise cannot, and will provide a 'social safety net' for the poverty and disease that the affluent state has created.

The reluctant collectivists, at an individual level, are concerned with a national minimum standard of protection. There is a minimum for all in terms of housing, health, education, nutrition and so on. However, this minimum is at a subsistence level only and it is not the responsibility of the government to provide any more than this. The funding source for the provision of these minimum standards is through the idea of insurance. Although initially it was thought that the insurance payments were to be made voluntarily, they soon became compulsory for all those in employment. In all the reluctant collectivist thinking the ultimate concern is the benefit of the collective, through some form of protection of the individual. For example, expenditure on education is considered a communal investment that is likely to bring good returns for the community, and a health service can make people better so that they can continue to work and contribute to the overall society on whatever level they are in the process of capital production.

Further reading

George, V. and Wilding, P. (1985) *Ideology and Social Welfare*. London: Routledge and Kegan Paul.

8.5 Anti-collectivism

Anti-collectivism was the dominant ideology in nineteenth-century Britain but became increasingly challenged in the twentieth century, and it lapsed into relative obscurity until the recession of the 1970s. From then it has had a resurgence, particularly with the work of Hayek, Friedman and the Institute of Economic Affairs, and it has now gained a new eminence and influence (George and Wilding 1985). It shares a close relationship with philosophical concerns with the morals and ethics of the individual (6:2) and the rights of the individual. It sees the individual person, their rights and needs, as taking precedence over all collectives in moral and political decisions. The individual takes precedence over the family, institutions, corporations, civil society and even the state. This is based on the idea that only individuals have natural rights and that collectives only comprise an aggregate number of individuals. A collective does not exist in itself outside of the individuals and thus, it is argued, cannot have rights above the individual. For example, although we understand on one level that the law exists, it does not have an independent reality outside of the individuals that constitute its operational functioning. Anti-collectivist political groups vary in their thinking but we deal with the same three central components as in the previous section on the collectivists (8:4).

Anti-collectivist social values

The main social values of the anti-collectivist group of political parties are freedom, individualism and inequality (note that the first two values are also central to the collectivist group: 8:4). Friedman (1962: 12) wrote: 'as liberals we take freedom of the individual, or perhaps the family, as our ultimate goal in judging social arrangements'. Note here that in contrast to the collectivist group, who hold the collective as supreme, the anti-collectivists hold the individual as paramount. However, also note that both perspectives hold freedom as a central core value; therefore, it is a matter of belief how best this might be achieved. Freedom, of course, is a complex concept and the anti-collectivists are aware of this. Freedom can be viewed as a negative state, simply as the absence of coercion, as Hayek (1960: 20–1) defined it: 'such control of the environment or circumstances of a person by another that . . . he is forced to act not according to a coherent plan of his own but to serve the ends of another'. However, freedom becomes obscure when we ask such questions as: to what extent do people have freedom if they do not have the freedom of opportunity? Furthermore, what of freedom if this means the freedom to do undesirable things (6:2)?

The second core value, individualism, concerns two elements. The first refers to a theory of society in which social phenomena can only be understood through an appreciation of the role and function of individuals. This suggests that society as an overall concept cannot be understood independently of the individuals that compose it. Thus, the individual is vital, in fact central, to an analysis of economic and social development. The second element concerns a set of political maxims that relate to the way that society ought to be organized, derived from and contributing towards a particular view of the role of the state. The main maxim would be that much of what the state currently does would be better undertaken by individuals, but individuals are fallible and we need certain social processes to ensure that mistakes are corrected. These processes include an interaction with others. As Hayek (1949: 22) puts it, 'the spontaneous collaboration of free men often creates things which are greater than their individual minds can ever comprehend'. This almost seems a collectivist position, but differs somewhat as it is grounded in the notion of competition. The third core value is that of inequality. This is based on the notion that the pursuit of egalitarian policies is incompatible with freedom, as it would necessitate the imposition of a form of coercion. The freedom to which the anti-collectivists refer is so strong that it means the freedom not to be equal to all the others in society.

Although there is a huge philosophical and political debate regarding this position, suffice it to say here that inequality lies at the very heart of anti-collectivism as a corollary of both freedom and individualism.

Anti-collectivism, society and the state

As the anti-collectivists focus so heavily on the individual, they tend not to have an overall consensus regarding social structures and their conflict model is primarily a question of conflict between individuals. This takes the form of competition, which they believe is desirable for both individuals and society. Any emphasis that anti-collectivists place on conflict tends to be based on groups rather than on class interests. Their focus on the individual extends to their economic system and lies at the heart of their philosophy. Liberalism, it is argued, emanates from 'the discovery of a self generating or spontaneous order in social affairs . . . an order which made it possible to utilise the knowledge and skill of all members of society to a much greater extent than would be possible in any order created by central direction' (Hayek 1967: 162). Their view of economic forces is essentially competition in the free market, which they argue is far more complex than anything that could be created through central strategy, planning or direction (George and Wilding 1985). As Friedman (1962: 15) argued, 'by removing the organisation of economic activity from the control of political authority, the market eliminates this source of coercive power. It enables economic strength to be a check to political power, rather than a reinforcement.'

In terms of the state, the anti-collectivists view democracy as the best way of resolving conflicts and have three central arguments for this. First, democracy is the only way of resolving differences in a peaceful manner, and this has led to the abandonment of the belief that the sphere of government should be unrestricted. Spontaneous order depends not on strategy, planning or design, but on the free decision-making of a number of individuals. Democratic governments, from the anti-collectivist point of view, need to show considerable restraint in their desire to govern. The second argument for democracy is that it is an important safeguard of individual liberty. If governments make a claim to be able to change the world then they will become the target for all manner of pressure groups, conglomerates and other interest groups, which would result in an ever-expanding web of government. This, they argue, would strangle the growth of civilization, which rests on individual freedom. The third argument for democracy is that it is considered to be the best way of educating people about public affairs. The 'state' is a disparaging term in anti-collectivist thought and in the wrong hands can be used to fool the people. Democracy, used appropriately, can reveal the true nature of regulatory governments.

Anti-collectivist governments and the welfare state

George and Wilding (1985: 35) clearly stated the anti-collectivist position to the welfare state: 'as might be anticipated from the values of the anti-collectivists, their faith in the spontaneous order of the market system, and their suspicion of government activity, their attitude to the welfare state is fundamentally hostile'. However, this is not to deny some role of government in the provision of welfare, but this role, in their view, should be minimal. The anti-collectivists believe that state welfare policies are threatening or damaging to the family, work incentives, the economy, individual freedom and so on; in fact they see welfare as damaging to the central social values and social institutions of our society. The minimum standards that should be provided by governments are compatible with anti-collectivist principles as long as three conditions are met: first, that government should not maintain a monopoly on the provision; second, that resources to provide the welfare are raised by taxation that is based on uniform principles and the taxation is not used as a means of redistributing wealth; and, third, that the needs to be satisfied are collective needs of the community as a whole and not the needs of particular groups. If governments go beyond these minimum standards based on these principles then the anti-collectivists' anxieties increase considerably. They argue that if people have paid taxes they are then not in a position to provide private means of welfare. The anti-collectivists also argue against any welfare above the minimum standard on the basis of it destabilizing the economic and social system due to the implications of the politicization of issues of resource provision, use and distribution. Furthermore, it is paternalistic, in that it suggests that a welfare state provides what officials and politicians believe others need. Finally, they argue that it is inefficient, as it is less responsive to individual needs than a market-driven service would be. There can be little doubt that the anti-collectivists would prefer a market-led welfare service rather than one provided by the state.

Further reading

George, V. and Wilding, P. (1985) *Ideology and Social Welfare*. London: Routledge and Kegan Paul.

8.6 Unionism

At a basic level a trade union is a body of people who have joined together in an attempt to protect themselves and to improve pay and conditions at work. These trade unions are wide and varied in terms of the types of employment that they represent, and they are also specific in terms of the specialist areas that they cover. They claim to represent the workers' interests and will engage with employers to negotiate pay and conditions, but some have also argued that they develop into oligarchies that have their own agendas and fail to act in the best interests of their members (Michels 1962). Trade unions develop an organizational structure that is hierarchically based but the positions within the unions are generally elected ones.

Modern research suggests that although oligarchic tendencies may exist they generally maintain member representativeness under certain conditions, namely when they have strong workplace rank-and-file organizations with shop stewards (Crouch 1982). It is often asked if unions have sufficient power to operate effectively with employers, and it is generally agreed that the power imbalance tends to vary with economic conditions and changes within the law. Whatever their current status of power they have historically had a significant impact on society as a whole. We focus on two areas of social life that have been, and continue to be, influenced by trade unions: social and economic change, and the health-care service.

Unions and social and economic change

As much as unions may have had an impact on society they have also had to adapt themselves in response to changes in social circumstances. The more that this occurs the more that 'trade unions are inseparable from the society in which they are created and recreated' (McIlroy 1995: 1–2). Membership of the trade unions in the UK peaked in 1979 at 55 per cent as a proportion of the employed workforce in union membership, which represented a total of 13 million members (Marsh *et al.* 1996). However, this figure has been drastically reduced as the industries have contracted, for example, in mining, engineering and shipbuilding, although it should be noted that membership has remained constant in some other areas, such as that of the National Association of Local Government Officers (NALGO, now UNISON) and women's presence in unions is on the increase (Marsh *et al.* 1996). Trade unions are having to adjust to the new labour market environments, which have a huge female input, and given that the traditional union formation was in the masculine work environments this has meant a shift in perspective. Union reorganization must now take account of the demands of a post-industrial society, a workforce that is increasingly fragmented, a decrease in full-time male employment, diffuse working environments and the dispersal of factories away from urban bases.

The unions' power was severely curtailed through the efforts of the Thatcher government, which was hostile to unionism. Sweeping legislation throughout the 1980s and the 1990s was passed in order to limit the unions' ability to defend their members' interests. These curtailments included the limitation of what constitutes a 'lawful' dispute, a reduction in the time off work for union representatives, the banning of all secondary action and the requirement of seven days' notice for industrial action to take place. The unions have also had to make adjustments in the face of the expansion of multinational corporations that can move production plants from one country to another. This enables the corporations to undermine national agreements and places pressures on unions to accept pay and conditions or special practices, or face unemployment. However, despite their waning power the unions continue to enjoy support from workers, with eight out of ten employees seeing them as being essential in protecting their workers' rights (McIlroy 1995).

Unions and health care

The union movement has a long tradition in the health care service in the UK and has been influential in improving the working conditions of health care staff and contributing towards an improved service. The unions in health care services have a dual master: first, the workers that they must represent; second, the patients that are the recipients of care. This relationship is a difficult one to balance, and to maintain, and should always be viewed with some caution. For example, in disputes between unions and health care services concerning pay and conditions it is customary for both sides to claim an overriding concern regarding the care that is delivered to the patient. The unions will assert that an improvement in pay and conditions will lead to an improvement in patient care, while the service managers will argue that an improvement in staff pay and conditions will detract from the ability to deliver an effective service and thus patient care will suffer. These bargaining positions are usually displayed publicly to elicit the desired emotional response from society, who is ultimately concerned with patient care. The unions hold a strong card in this bargaining position, which is the fact that the public hold health care staff in such high esteem and it is easy for the unions to make a claim for an improvement in their pay and conditions. While service managers find it difficult to make statements to the effect that doctors, nurses, paramedics and so on should not be granted improvements in their pay and conditions. The social tension is created through the attempt to balance the high esteem that health care staff are held in with the desire to have the highest level of patient care, and the fact that resources are limited.

Another area in which unions are involved in health care development is in terms of their role in parliamentary, rather than industrial, action. Many health care professionals are extremely reluctant to be involved in industrial action, especially strike action, which may have a negative impact on patient care. This is the case even in situations in which the industrial action may be indirect; that is, it does not directly affect patient care. The unions have a long traditional association with the Labour Party and act as important, and significant, lobbyists in the development of parliamentary policies. Although at the time of writing this traditional association with the Labour Party is under severe strain, with the unions reducing their financial support to the government, it none the less remains a powerful force. The unions have also been influential in the privatization debate concerning health care, and have taken up a very strong opposition to any moves to privatize the NHS. The main thrust of their concerns with private health care facilities revolves around the twin issues of the quality of patient care for those who cannot afford the large sums of money needed for private health and the minimalist approaches that most private employers have towards staff pay and conditions. They argue that if the *raison d'être* of health care is financial profit then clearly patient care, let alone staff conditions, cannot be the paramount concern that it ought to be. Currently, private facilities in the UK tend not to provide for the chronic (nursing homes apart), or serious, conditions and will turn to the NHS for this type of provision. Many people in the UK are not covered by medical insurance, although this is changing, and we deal with this below (8:9).

Further reading

Crouch, C. (1982) *Trade Unions: The Logic of Collective Action*. Glasgow: Fontana.
McIlroy, J. (1995) *Trade Unions in Britain Today*, 2nd edn. Manchester: Manchester University Press.

PART TWO: APPLICATION TO PRACTICE

8.7 Structural politics

We have begun to see in the first part of this chapter that a particular political perspective may have an impact on the delivery of health care and that this impact differs between political views irrespective of the fact that each political party may hold similar values. For example, we saw that the collectivists and the anti-collectivists both hold the social value of freedom as central to their philosophy, but they differ in how they believe that this freedom should be achieved. Thus, when they are in power as a government their policies on delivering freedom will differ, and the way in which they exercise their policies will affect the people differently. This is the same in health care and, although each political party may hold the belief that a healthy society is a desirable state of affairs, how they feel that this is best achieved will be different. It is the relationship between the policies, their implementation and the felt impact that is the concern of structural politics. To have a structure, an object must have parts that are in some way united under ordered relations. In this sense the structure of health care services will be the determinant of the impact that health care has on society's members.

International, national and local politics

The relationship between political ideologies and political parties concerns how members implement their policies, and some element of power is needed to undertake this. Thus, there is a practical impact from political thinking and this takes place at international, national and local levels. For example, in the USA there is some concern regarding the apolitical stance of many nurses and the detrimental impact that this might have on the development of patient care. As Des Jardin (2001: 613) noted, 'political-ethical conflicts can mean choosing between job, patient care, and professional ideals. Many nurses never have considered it their place to challenge the structure of the health care system or the rules guiding that system.' Furthermore, as the UK is now a member of the European Union, European politics have an impact on the British health care services. For example, when comparing average lengths of stay for certain health-related conditions, we can note some political disquiet between countries, as we observe with childbirth in hospitals and mothers' length of stay (Hasseler 2001). At a national level each general election brings a flurry of attention to the state of the NHS and the relationship between professional values and political activity is highlighted. Munro (2001: 14) outlined this: 'as New Labour continues to court favour with nurses . . . [it is suggested] that the profession may be a pawn in the ongoing battle between the government and doctors for control of the health service'. Without becoming too cynical, each political party's commitment to the NHS is questioned, particularly at election time (Mahony 2001). Finally, at a local level politics can have an impact on local services, as Elliott (2001: 413) noted: 'the election of . . . [an independent candidate] was one of the biggest upsets of last June's general election. But, by the autumn the tide appeared to be turning . . . [his] way as a government report recommended improvements for patient services at Kidderminster.' This can also be seen within a US example, as a nurse ran for office in Delaware state: 'the chronicle of campaign activists illustrates the great value of nursing experience as well as the benefits of other nurses' assistance and leadership when campaigning' (Hall-Long 2001: 149). Therefore, we can see that at all levels of political activity there is the potential to impact on the practical aspects of health care delivery.

Feminist politics

Feminist politics, for the sake of this subsection, takes the form of two different perspectives, which when viewed together provide a rich source of insight. The first approach is to understand the relationship between the sexes as fundamentally a political one (Millett 1970). Millett outlines a sophisticated feminist argument in which she defines politics as the 'power-structured relationship, arrangements whereby one group of persons is controlled by another' (Millett 1970: 23). This power-structured relationship, she argues, forms the basis of eight theoretical trajectories, which underscore sexual politics. The first concerns an ideological (Chapter 2) view in which sexual politics obtains consent through both sexes being fundamentally socialized to basic patriarchal polities in relation to temperament, role and status. From this perspective males and females learn to exercise their stereotypical temperaments through role and status. Second, there is the biological view that traditionally has seen the psychosocial differences between the sexes as being due to biological distinctions (Chapter 3). The third concern is with the sociological forces, beginning with the patriarchal family as a mirror of, and connection to, the wider society. The family must interact with the wider society and all its institutions, such as religions, law and the state, all of which tend to be patriarchal in their structure. The fourth trajectory is class (2:2, 2:9), which concerns the status of women in patriarchal families that employ such terms as 'manhood' to affirm males' dominant status and 'romantic love' to subjugate females by emotional manipulation.

The fifth perspective concerns economic and educational factors as forms of patriarchal government within the agency of the family. Men traditionally control the family's finances and are better educated than women. Sixth is the element of force. This force is enacted through families and society, via the legal system, which can be explicitly seen in strict religions where women's punishments for sexual transgressions are disproportionate to their male counterparts'. The seventh trajectory employs an anthropological (Chapter 4) approach through myth (4:2, 4:8) and religion, in which women are viewed as inferior in any number of dimensions. Finally, there is the psychological (Chapter 3) perspective, in which it is suggested that male and female psyches are fundamentally different, outside of a learnt explanatory framework. Thus, sexual politics is rooted in the relationship between the sexes, the patriarchal family, the institutions of society and the state (Millett 1970), and the health care system is but one part of the societal structures that contributes to the politics of sex (Durham 1991).

The second approach is to understand the feminist critique of health care services in relation to an overall social policy framework (Pascall 1997). This form of feminist critique is about analysing how the various structures of social policy – health, housing, education, the family and so on – deal with women. However, 'if the mainstream of social policy writing has failed to appreciate the special connection of social policy with the domestic world, and with women's lives, this is not so of women themselves' (Pascall 1997: 3). The main thrust of this feminist argument is that all mainstream approaches in social policy have, in practice, marginalized women, but women now see this and can begin to fight back. In terms of health, feminists have perceived medicine as controlling women especially through reproduction, childbirth, contraception, abortion and new reproductive technologies. Furthermore, it is not only as recipients of health care services that they are subjugated. As Pascall (1997: 180) noted, 'the focus on women as reproducers is limiting and potentially damaging. Women are not only "consumers" of medicine's miracles. They are also major providers in health labour, both unpaid and paid, private and public.' In many countries, particularly in the developing ones, women hold the key responsibility for the provision of care, and this provision is often unpaid. Even in paid health care provision women often provide the majority of the workforce, the exception being in medicine. Thus, we have two approaches to the feminist critique of health care services: first, indirectly from a relationship between the sexes and society; second, from a focus on the relationship between women and health-care services directly.

Further reading

Allsop, J. (1995) *Health Policy and the NHS Towards 2000*, 2nd edn. London: Longman.
Millett, K. (1970) *Sexual Politics*. London: Virago Press.

8.8 The National Health Service

In 1911 the then Liberal government introduced the National Health Insurance Act, which was designed to protect some workers from the medical costs of illness. It provided a limited access to medical care for those working men who earned less than £2 per week and the scheme had contributions from the state, the employer and the employee. However, at this stage hospital services were not included and the scheme was administered by 'approved societies' that consisted of people with previous experience of running sickness clubs and friendly societies' private and commercial schemes. It was an inchoate service that, despite alterations during the years between the First and Second World Wars, remained limited in its coverage (Day and Klein 1991). Having said that, at least it was a start at government attempting to provide some health services, for some of the people, and was a significant factor leading towards the NHS as we know it today.

A second major factor was the two world wars themselves. War usually brings into focus the health of the nation, in terms of providing healthy soldiers to fight, and also the country's ability to take care of the injured on their return home from war. The massive number of soldiers killed and wounded in the First World War was only surpassed by the number killed in the Second, with the Second World War also claiming huge civilian casualties as well. War also produces great hardships and focuses attention on one's own mortality and the need to protect future generations from such hardships. People tend to want 'better' for their offspring as well as for themselves following a war (Webster 1988). Furthermore, between the wars there were large-scale economic and financial hardships, with massive unemployment and poverty for many. Thus, going into the Second World War, things had been very hard for the British people (as well as for many in other countries) for a very long time. Conditions were, thus, ripe for a change in thinking. In preparing for the impending emergency of the Second World War 'the first survey of hospitals undertaken since 1863 was carried out. It revealed that there were 78,000 beds in voluntary hospitals, 32,000 in local authority hospitals and 35,000 in isolation and tuberculosis sanitoria' (Allsop 1995: 24).

Historical background

The NHS came into operation on 5 July 1948 following the passing of the NHS Act some two years earlier in 1946, and six years after discussions had begun in 1942. As the early discussions began there was a general agreement over the main principles of the NHS, but as the war came closer to an end divisions and differences began to appear in many interested groups and this was most apparent in the medical profession (Allsop 1995). The Minister of Health for the Labour government at the time, Aneurin Bevan, steered the Bill through Parliament, with great effort and skill, with the eventual agreement of most doctors. It was a rare moment when politics, professional values and public opinion were generally in agreement, and this probably accounts, at least in part, for why the NHS is such a valued service within our society. The basis of the NHS was grounded in the principle of a collective responsibility of the state to provide a comprehensive health service for all, free at the point of delivery. The finances to support such a service, and a very expensive one at that, were to be raised through taxation based on the principles of collectivism, comprehensiveness, equality and universality. This had the effect of 'a redistribution of resource to the less healthy and poorer sections of society – unskilled manual workers, women and their children – who stood to gain the most from the changes' (Allsop 1995: 15). The whole population now had equal access to specialist medical services throughout the country.

Let us look a little more closely at the principles on which the NHS was founded. The first is the collective principle, which concerns the state providing access to health care, free at the point of service, as required by those in need. This is rooted in the collectivist view that the state should be responsible for the provision of health services for its citizens. The collectivists argue that society becomes more wholesome, better adjusted and more mature with a health service that society believes should be provided for all its citizens who become ill (Bevan 1961). The second is the comprehensive principle, at least comprehensive for its time, which was to ensure that the health service was geared to providing treatment and promoting physical and mental health. However, health for school children was excluded and left in the hands of local education authorities. The third is the universal principle, which focuses on the real needs of the people irrespective of an individual's ability to pay. It also dismisses race, colour and creed as determinants in the provision of health care and ensures that the full resources of the country should be brought to bear on providing advice, early diagnosis and speedy treatment for its citizens. The fourth principle, that of equality, was based on the notion of a uniform standard of service for everyone throughout the country. This led to the tripartite structuring of the early NHS, based on regional hospital boards, hospital management committees and boards of governors. Access to health care did not have boundaries and patients could be referred to anywhere in the country. The final principle is that of professional autonomy. In this view it is argued that the medical profession (and presumably the other professions) is founded on the values of delivering the best practice to the patients in their care. Given this, it was argued that the medical profession should be given the best and most modern apparatus by which they could exercise their practice. This also involves the decision-making in, and the running of, the health service.

The organization of the NHS

At its inception in 1948 the NHS was organized as a tripartite structure, with England divided into 13 regions, and Wales functioning as one, which unified the hospitals within each region under one central control. Hospitals within each of these regions were managed by hospital management committees (HMCs) and the teaching hospitals were run by boards of governors. These latter boards were composed of lay and professional members, often drawn from very different walks of life and experiences. The third part of the structure had two main elements to it: (a) local health authorities covering maternity, child welfare and so on; and (b) executive councils covering family doctors, dentists and so on. Figure 8.1 shows the outline structure of the NHS in England and Wales between 1948 and 1974.

Throughout the foregoing period, concerns developed regarding the nature of this tripartite structure and the extent to which resources were being effectively used. However, although reforms were being debated they required the agreement of the medical profession and in 1962 the Medical Services Review Committee agreed that reforms should be, at least, considered. The 1960s evidenced an economic boom and a growing optimism that good times were here, and here to stay, and several major commissions and committees were given the task of assessing what changes were needed to reform the structure of health services. The major proposed changes included the restructuring of local government, the establishment of social service departments, social work to be part of local government, the creation of a social service ministry to cover personal social services, health and social security and the devolution of power to regions. In short, the reforms of the NHS were being planned alongside reforms in other government structures (Allsop 1995). April 1974 saw the restructuring of these services and the organization of the NHS from 1974 to 1982 can be seen in Figure 8.2.

This restructuring had several strands to it: (a) administrative unification with the retention of the 14 regional health authorities and the implementation of 90 area health authorities providing a new administrative tier; (b) management changes focusing on consensus decision-making from multidisciplinary teams; (c) planning strategy, to provide for better resource management; (d) centralization to reduce inequalities and encourage the development of community care; and (e) increased accountability through the NHS by the establishment of community health councils to operate as watchdogs.

The managing director of Sainsbury's, Roy Griffiths, was commissioned to inquire into the cost containment issue of the ever-spiralling finances of the NHS, and the main thrust of his report called for a rigorous management restructuring (Griffiths 1983). 'Although far reaching for its day, the Griffiths report was clearly not enough to placate the then prime minister, Margaret Thatcher, who caught the world unprepared when she announced her far-reaching health service reforms live on prime-time BBC, during an interview on *Panorama*' (Sweeney 2001: 1). The main areas for these reforms were: (a) the internal market; (b) dividing the purchaser from the provider; and (c) the introduction of fundholding services. Therefore, the changes already introduced in 1982 through the development of 192 district health authorities and nine special health authorities were already under pressure. The responsibility for spending decisions and cuts to the service were rooted at a local level and therefore any blame for a reduction in services lay with

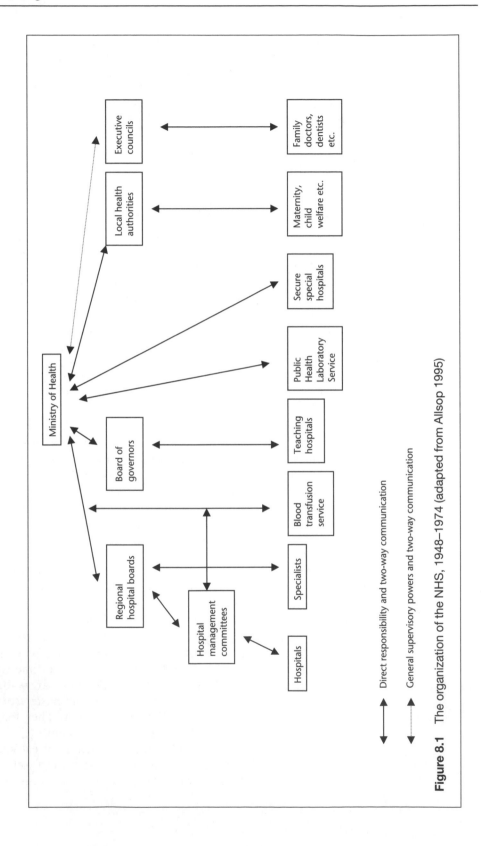

Figure 8.1 The organization of the NHS, 1948–1974 (adapted from Allsop 1995)

Direct responsibility and two-way communication

General supervisory powers and two-way communication

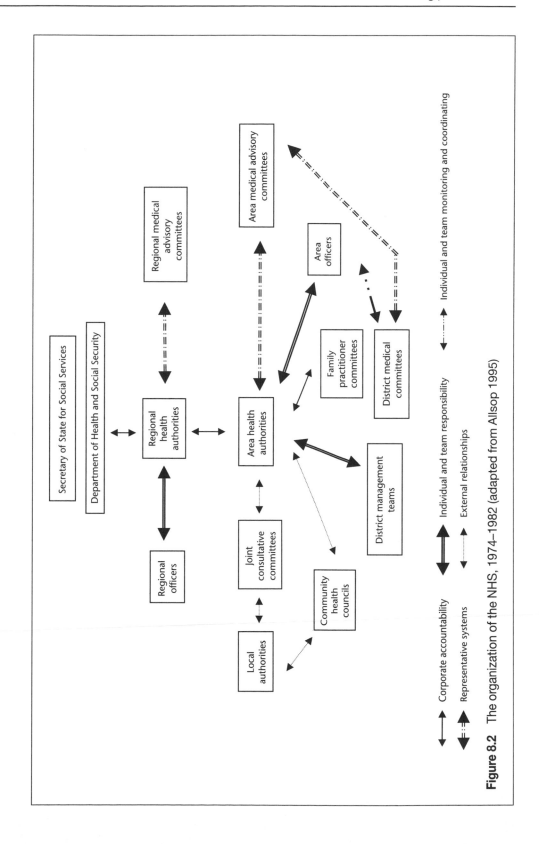

Figure 8.2 The organization of the NHS, 1974–1982 (adapted from Allsop 1995)

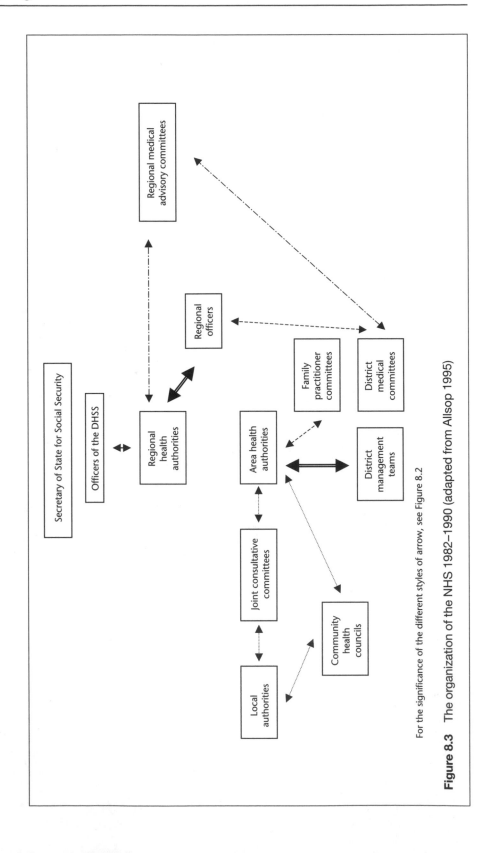

For the significance of the different styles of arrow, see Figure 8.2

Figure 8.3   The organization of the NHS 1982–1990 (adapted from Allsop 1995)

the districts and not central government. The organization of the NHS from 1982 to 1990 can be seen in Figure 8.3.

Since 1990 there have been a series of strategic and significant developments rather than any major restructuring, not least because of a change in government in 1997. We conclude this section with a brief overview of these developments.

- *Internal market.* Large hospitals could become trusts, although remaining publicly owned. They would be free to operate to their strengths and could raise income and capital without the permission of the Department of Health. They would be free to choose their pay scales and conditions of service.
- *The introduction of primary care groups (PCGs).* These consist of GPs, community nurses, social services and some lay members. They take responsibility for assessing community needs and commissioning

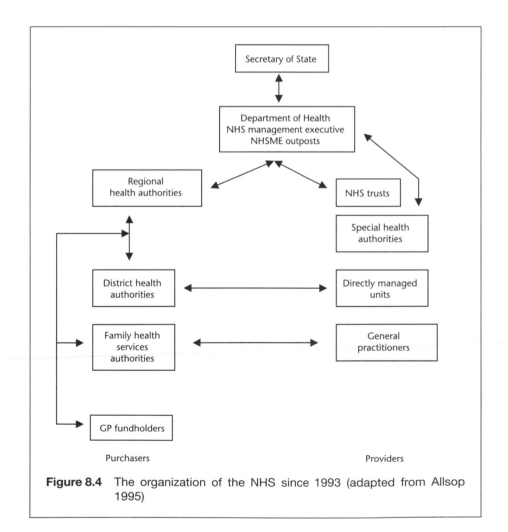

Figure 8.4   The organization of the NHS since 1993 (adapted from Allsop 1995)

services. They function to undertake primary and community health service developments and make decisions on resource allocation.

- *Clinical governance.* This is a broad approach with a wide remit to undertake clinical audit and to combine this with evidence-based practice. Risk management is also a significant feature: learning from complaints, recording adverse incidents and reducing medical and legal implications of error. Workforce appraisals and improving professional practice are also important aspects.

- *National Institute of Clinical Excellence (NICE).* This was introduced to produce and disseminate clinical guidelines that are grounded in sound evidence. Its members advise on clinical audit methods and on best practices. They appraise new and existing interventions. Their remit is to focus on the major enquiries into perioperative deaths, stillbirths, maternal deaths and suicides and homicides by those with mental health problems.

- *Commission for Health Improvement (CHI).* This body has the responsibility to oversee the implementation of clinical governance. It undertakes visits to hospitals and PCGs to assess arrangements to support and develop high quality services. It has a vast array of networks and links with many departments and offices.

Although there are many more developments, these serve to give a flavour of the main developments over the past decade or so. As we pointed out above, the NHS is an ever-changing dynamic organization that is set to continue to evolve over the coming years, particularly through the influence of politics. It is worth concluding this section with an illustration of the organization of the NHS in the 1990s, which brings us relatively up to date (see Figure 8.4).

Further reading

Allsop, J. (1995) *Health Policy and the NHS towards 2000*, 2nd edn. London: Longman.

Dixon, M. and Sweeney, K. (2001) *A Practical Guide to Primary Care Groups and Trusts*. Oxford: Radcliffe Medical Press.

Scott, C. (2001) *Public and Private Roles in Health Care Systems: Experiences from Seven OECD Countries*. Buckingham: Open University Press.

8.9 Private health service

Drawing on the theoretical components of the political ideologies in Part One of this chapter, we are now in a position to analyse how they may impinge on practice in relation to private health care. Briefly stated, in a traditional sense, the political left have considered that the best approach to the delivery of health care is through the state, via government legislation, in order that all can access it according to need, whereas the political right focus on the free market and the idea of open competition between services as the best way of achieving an increase in the standards of health care delivery. However, as we have seen, there are problems with both these polarized, and now probably unrealistic, extreme positions. Notwithstanding this, they do serve to highlight a difference of opinion, and policy, and we discuss this further below. Ideologically, in political thought, the distinction between private and public denotes separate but overlapping spheres of activity in which the private refers to personal affection, antipathy and satisfaction and the public concerns civil society and the state. Clearly, this involves a question of human relations focusing on self, society or both. Although this distinction between private and public can be defined in these terms it is, as we have seen, a question of ideological (8:2) belief as to which we would tend to lean towards. However, private enterprise itself can be understood in relation to the undertaking of economic activity using privately owned capital. Of course, it also has to be accompanied by private gain through profit. In private enterprise risk must be undertaken, with the possibilities of profit or loss in order for people to engage in that risk. Furthermore, in private enterprise ownership is more intense and individually located, whereas in public funded services the interests of individuals are diffused throughout society. Contemporary, mainstream thought on both sides of the political spectrum now incorporates a number of perspectives regarding the provision of health care, which leads to a mixed economy approach. We now highlight a number of these elements.

The social safety net

In an ideal world everyone would receive the best possible care according to their needs, immediately they require such treatment. Unfortunately, health care costs money, and finances lie at the heart of service delivery (Epsing-Anderson 1990). Financing health care is also an ideological and political concern and tax-based systems 'at best . . . seem to be capable of supplying good quality health care according to clinical need, financed at a reasonable cost. However, they are frequently attended by waiting lists and seem to encourage a brisk and impersonal style of service. At worst, the result is overloaded and low-quality services which are supplied by ill motivated staff in shabby premises' (OECD 1992: 16). If these comments are accepted today, in the early twenty-first century, more than a decade after they were first published, then we must be concerned as to the level, or standard, of service delivery, given the point that the OECD report says that *at best* this is what a tax-based system can produce. Questions must be raised as to those patients who are not receiving the highest standard of care that can be delivered. The policy delivered under a tax-based system would suggest that as long as it is equitable for all concerned, and therefore it is fair and just, then it is a better system than a privately delivered service. In these circumstances the social safety net for those who cannot afford a private service appears to have a relative strength and a wide catchment area, although it would appear, from the foregoing comments, that the net is of a low quality standard.

Private health care, in ideological terms, is less concerned with a social safety net, but it clearly is a big political issue, even in democratic capitalist societies that believe in a free market economy. This concern may be rooted in a social conscience that accepts that there are always likely to be some in society who will not be able to contribute towards paying for health care services. Allsop (1995: 73) commented that 'private insurances gives the greatest choice to individuals to consume healthcare once they are accepted as subscribers. However, the take-up of insurance depends on the willingness and the ability to pay . . . Those with the least ability to pay premiums are often at the highest risk.' Furthermore, private insurers may engage in 'cream skimming', in which they exclude vulnerable individuals who do not appear to adopt a healthy lifestyle or those with histories of predispositions to certain conditions. Individuals may not see themselves as at risk or ignore the necessity of contributing to an insurance scheme. It has also been noted that, once privately insured, there is a tendency for patients to over-consume, as they then consider it is their right and that they have paid for it (Allsop 1995). Thus, as we have said, most capitalist societies now have a mixture of private and public health care services to ensure that the least affluent members of their societies have, at least, some health care service coverage.

Private medical insurance

Over the past 25 years or so private medical insurance has increased dramatically, not least because of the 18-year reign of the Conservative government from 1979 to 1997. Without going into intricate detail regarding the reasons for this increase, we focus on several factors that contributed towards setting health care services along business-like lines. The first factor that we mention is the move in the 1980s towards competitive tendering. Health Circular HC(83)18 made it necessary for health authorities to put their catering, domestic and laundry services out to tender, so that private businesses in these areas could compete to provide these facilities in the NHS. This would test the public services against market prices to see if they could deliver a cost-effective and competitive service against private businesses. Irrespective of the advantages and disadvantages of this tendering process, it was reported that after a settling period approximately 55 per cent of catering contracts were awarded to external tenders and about three-quarters of the domestic and laundry services (Milne 1992).

The second factor was the move towards encouraging the private sector. Since its inception in 1948 the NHS had not precluded private health care, although the relationship had often been tense. However, in the 1980s the Conservative government adopted a number of aspects in order to encourage private health facilities. The first was to ensure that anyone could receive private treatment in a private facility, paid for by private means, which meant that there was an increase in the overall number of private beds available. Many businesses, including those from the USA and Europe, were able to expand their companies into the British private medical sector. Second, since the beginning of the NHS, consultants could treat private patients in NHS hospitals, and although the number of such pay-beds had decreased since 1948, they were again encouraged by the Conservative government. However, pay-beds remain politically contentious and despite this authorization they have tended to decline in favour of private hospitals. A third factor in the expansion of private health care concerns the agreement that consultants could hold part-time contracts with the NHS, so that they could maintain some private practice. Labour governments tended to discourage this but the Conservative government in the 1980s reversed this trend and encouraged more private practice. It was reported that this led to some consultants having shares in the private hospitals that were being developed at this time (Mohan and Woods 1985). This was a clear indication that the government of the time was actively encouraging private practice and these sorts of encouragements were influencing the ethos of the medics in practice. Fourth, NHS patients 'could be treated in private hospitals, nursing homes and residential institutions . . . In the 10 years between 1979 and 1989, there was a four-fold increase in private residential homes and nursing home beds' (Allsop 1995: 167). Waiting lists were tackled by this route, as was the testing of NHS facilities against market forces. At the time of writing, under a Labour government, the waiting lists are again under attack, this time by treating British patients in hospitals in Europe, and there is an acceptance, albeit reluctantly, that there is some need for private medical facilities. This shows the earlier tensions between these ideological positions.

Further reading

Higgins, J. (1988) *The Business of Medicine: Private Health Care in Britain*. London: Macmillan Education.

Mossialos, E., Dixon, A. and Figueras, J. (2002) *Funding Health Care: Options for Europe*. Buckingham: Open University Press.

Strong, P. and Robinson, J. (1990) *The NHS: Under New Management*. Milton Keynes: Open University Press.

8.10 Resource limitations

All health care systems, either public or private, are limited by the skills and competencies of the staff operating within them, as well as by the financial support that is given to the service. Given that the former limitations, those of the skills of the professionals, are an ongoing professional issue, the latter financial limitations are a political or economic matter. Private systems that rely on insurance schemes tend to have limitations placed on them by the insurer through upper expenditure limits or through exclusion criteria. Public systems that rely on taxation have limited financial support *per se*. In this section we are concerned with the political ramifications of the impact on the public health care system of limitations on resources. We are probably familiar with the numerous stories in the press regarding the limitations of private facilities that transfer patients to the NHS when things go wrong and they are unable to provide the level of sophisticated facilities that the NHS can. Furthermore, we are also probably aware of the stories in the press regarding NHS facilities that refuse to treat someone, or operate on someone, because of the expense. There are also frequent examples of patients waiting for many months for operations and some waiting for many hours on trolleys for admission to a ward. Expensive drugs and bed shortages are but two of the most frequently occurring concerns in the NHS. Resource limitations are, of course, a major concern at a philosophical level (Chapter 6), as well as a practical one in terms of a person's right to life (6:11) (Honigsbaum 1992). However, on a day-to-day basis the politics of resource limitations must be dealt with through the process of balancing and allocating resources in relation to the provision of a quality service.

Balancing and allocating resources

Within the NHS resources are first allocated to the regions and then from there they are redistributed to the districts. This has been the case since 1975 when the resource allocation working party (RAWP) was set up to ensure that resources were distributed appropriately and on a more equitable basis than was previously the case. The distribution formula was based on weighted capitation reflecting healthy needs as measured by age, sex, mortality rates, fertility and marital status. This was then adjusted according to two factors: (a) the number of patients that were treated across regional boundaries; and (b) a special increment for teaching (SIFT) if appropriate. Although this system was heavily criticized in the late 1970s, particularly by those who had lost out under the formula, it was applied to the regional budgets and by the mid-1980s it had achieved its objectives. Now, with the vast array of changes within the NHS structure and the implementation of such things as GP fundholding, increased competition and the raising of capital through trusts, the funding system is highly complex. However, what tends to remain a standing issue is the complaint that the NHS is under-funded (Berridge 1999). Given this, the main questions that emerge refer to how to balance the limited resources and who should get what, and why.

There are several factors that must be considered in the political process of resource allocation, and the first concerns the size of the population. Although this is a simple consideration if it stood alone, as it would be a relatively simple matter to divide the resources by the number of people in the region, it does not take into account the make-up of the population, which is the second factor. The make-up of the population will include the number of elderly, the gender rates (women have different needs to men), the number of children (high users of health services) and so on. The third factor is the morbidity rates, the reasons for which are difficult to quantify but can be simply stated as being caused by the type of environment, social circumstances, heredity, occupations etc. The fourth factor is the cost of treatment, which can be variable between regions. For example, the London weighting that is paid to staff will increase the cost of health care provision, and some conditions are more expensive to treat than others, with the rates of these conditions differing between regions. The fifth factor is the extent of administration costs that occur when patients are treated across regional boundaries. This may be through choice or necessity but the financial adjustments need to be taken into consideration. The sixth factor concerns the responsibility of the NHS to provide medical and dental education, which are expensive services to provide, and increase the costs considerably within the regions that provide them. Finally, there is the need for capital investment, which again varies between regions, but buildings and equipment do need to be replaced eventually. Thus, balancing resources is a complex affair with no easy solution, irrespective of political ideology.

Information on how resources are allocated, other than identifying the balancing of the above factors, is sparse. However, there is some general consensus that the 'creation of competition between those supplying health services is an effective method of financial control because it limits expenditure within fixed budgets and pushes down costs within them' (Allsop 1995: 266). The main thrust of decision-making in relation to the allocation of resources refers to maximizing treatments available to the greatest number of people, which is a utilitarian (6:4) approach. However, this is often complicated by two main factors. First, some individuals need more resources in terms of health care costs than others, and this brings into focus the issue of quality of life for some individuals in relation to the quantity of life (6:11, 6:12) for others. Second, there is the question of the efficacy of treatments that are available. As the World Bank (1993: 60) noted, 'only a small share of the thousands of known medical procedures has been analysed, but approximately fifty studied would be able to deal with more than half of the world's disease burden. Just implementing the twenty most cost effective interventions could eliminate more than 40 per cent of the total burden and three quarters of the health loss among children.' This brings us back to the issue of cost-effectiveness in relation to the allocation of resources, and systems have been developed in an attempt to ensure that the quality of service delivery is maintained to as high a standard as is possible.

QALYs and DALYs

Cost benefits of treatments have been measured with varying techniques, and two will be mentioned here. The first is the QALYs (quality adjusted life years), which is a measure to assess which forms of interventions are the 'best buy' in relation to health care. This measure can be used to assess two alternative approaches to the delivery of care; for example, receiving inpatient treatment as opposed to receiving treatment at home. It can also be employed to assist in determining priorities in a health programme. QALYs, as a measurement tool, have technical problems and do not overcome the unease regarding the moral issues. However, this is a popular approach as it offers a quantitative assessment, which gives it a scientific credence, and takes the personal element out of the decision-making, or at least pretends to do so. It is used to ration resources and helps people to make decisions regarding priorities. Another approach is the DALYs (disability adjusted life years) measuring instrument, which 'is a measure to assess the extent of "health" in terms of a reduction in disabilities incurred through illness and added years of life through particular interventions' (Allsop 1995: 84). However, difficulties are encountered with the definitional components of this measure, as it is difficult to define what 'health', 'disability' and 'illness' are likely to mean to different people. Furthermore, these measures are not sensitive to the individual nuances of health and disability and cannot gauge the qualitative element of the human condition. Proponents would argue, of course, that they are not intended to; they take the subjectivity out of the equation and provide a more objective approach to the cost–benefit assessment of health care delivery.

Further reading

Davey, B. and Popay, J. (1993) *Dilemmas in Health Care*. Buckingham: Open University Press.

Klein, R., Day, P. and Redmayne, S. (1996) *Managing Scarcity: Priority Setting and Rationing in the NHS*. Buckingham: Open University Press.

Robinson, R. and Steiner, A. (1998) *Managed Health Care: US Evidence and Lessons for the NHS*. Buckingham: Open University Press.

8.11 Global citizenship

The expansion of technology, particularly since the Second World War, has led to what is now termed the globalization process. Technology has enabled faster communication and travel, with many areas of the world in touch with one another that were previously isolated. Communication can cover telephones, televisions and newspapers, as well as surveillance satellites and spy planes. In any event it has allowed the mass insurgence of, usually Western, values throughout the world. Globalization has led to what is termed a shrinking time and space (Giddens 1999), as most areas of the globe can be reached in a relatively short space of time. Although there are resistances to this globalization process, from anti-capitalist (8:3, 8:4, 8:5) groups and countries, it is a system that is currently dominating global politics. We are very quickly aware of disasters, wars and famines around the world and pictures and words are beamed into our living rooms around the clock. Events in one part of the world can have a direct or indirect effect on another part of the world, either immediately or later. This can be seen in terms of war, disease, terrorism, pollution and so on, and distance is no longer a safeguard against events in other countries. Global politics is often concerned with national interests played out on the world stage, which is testimony to the fact that global events affect individuals in each country and therefore the country itself (Held *et al.* 1999). Despite its problems the globalization process has made us citizens of the world, and this citizenship brings with it global responsibilities for ourselves and our neighbours around the globe, and health care is only one of the many concerns.

Some effects of globalization

There are many aspects to the process of globalization and, of course, many consequences of it. Some of these are said to be positive and others are believed to be negative (Hirst and Thompson 1996). We will briefly outline two aspects of globalization that have an impact on global health, but the reader should note that there are many more. The first aspect to mention is commercialization. Commerce has a long tradition in the history of mankind and it has brought individuals and communities together in the process of exchange. However, in contemporary times it is associated with power and influence through the operations of large-scale business corporations. We only need to take the expansion of McDonald's as an example, a simple fast food outlet on one level and a much more sophisticated McDonaldization of life on another (Ritzer 1997). Explicit levels of commerce are readily seen throughout the world but behind the scenes are the implicit aspects that revolve around power, control and domination. Commerce, of course, can be honest and legal, but it can also be dishonest and illegal. Commercialization extends from food, clothing and building materials, which are the basic requirements of survival, to weapons, cars and electronic games. However, it is also a process that includes the commercialization of drugs both licit and illicit, sex in the forms of pornography, prostitution and human slavery, and labour in terms of low wages and child workers. Industries may move their plants to underdeveloped countries to capitalize on cheap labour and slack laws relating to health, safety and pollution. Therefore, the goods that we consume may well be affecting not only the health and welfare of individuals at the manufacturing end of the commercial process but also ourselves as global citizens.

The second aspect to mention in relation to globalization is the notion of trust. We note in Chapter 2 (2:8) that we are reliant on many others around the world as we traverse our daily lives. For example, we are reliant on miners to extract the metals, factory workers to make the component parts to the correct specifications and the manufacturers to put the parts together correctly so that a car works safely for us to drive (Giddens 1999). This trust extends to many areas of our lives through the rules, regulations, standards and values of all the countries of the world, and it is in relation to health and welfare that we are here concerned with. Whether it be in the manufacture of medicines or medical equipment, the transfusion of blood and blood products or the skills and competencies of health care workers around the world, we need an element of trust. Furthermore, this trust extends to the health care systems that embrace the fundamentals of caring for the sick and injured of any race, colour or creed. Unfortunately, this trust is not always upheld, but none the less it is an expanding aspect of the globalization of health care, and one that we all contribute to at one level or another.

Aid

Like most other aspects of human life, the idea of providing aid to someone in need can have different levels of interpretation. First, it can be viewed as a kind, compassionate and benevolent action that is rooted in the best possible of intentions. However, it also has a negative aspect, which is politically and/ or economically driven, and although it offers help in the short term it can have long-term damaging consequences. To understand the politics of aid we have to make an assumption about the world that is based on a division between 'developed' and 'developing' nations. Furthermore, we must assume that it is better to be developed than undeveloped. For a country to become developed certain conditions must be met; for example, 'it has been argued before the UN Conference on Trade and Development that growth in real terms in nations recognized as "developing" can be secured only by a level of imports which exceeds their capacity to export' (Scruton 1982: 10). One argument that is relatively well accepted is that if left to market forces alone the rich countries become richer and the poor ones poorer. Therefore, aid is needed for the 'developing' countries in order to give them the boost needed to compete with 'developed' nations. However, one dissenting voice against this argument was Bauer (1971), who claimed that aid removes real incentives to exploit natural resources, leads to a deeply entrenched impoverishment and merely ends up in the hands of a ruling elite.

Most 'developed' countries have policies relating to aid. However, they are not always as overtly benevolent as at first appears. For example, one developed country had a huge glut of wheat that the farmers would have been unable to dispose of unless their government intervened. The politicians offered the wheat as 'aid' to a famine-ridden African country but insisted that it had to be shipped by the home country's merchant fleet, for which the African country had to pay. Thus, it employed the developed country's shipping merchants for some considerable time. Another example is that aid is often given with certain conditions applied, such as the receiving country having to grow produce that is used by the home country. When equipment is given as aid, such as tractors, there is usually no infrastructure to service them or provide spare parts, and these must be purchased from the home country. Thus, the politics of aid usually ensures a pay-back for the country that is giving the aid, but questions must be raised as to how effective that aid is in helping the country to develop in the longer term. Clearly, in cases of disasters, either through natural events or through man-made ones, there is an immediate need for the better off countries to provide emergency aid in whatever form is needed. However, in the case of planning political policies for the delivery of aid it would appear to us that there is a greater need for altruism.

Further reading

Coulter, A. and Ham, C. (2000) *The Global Challenge of Health Care Rationing.* Buckingham: Open University Press.

Giddens, A. (1999) *Runaway World: How Globalisation is Reshaping our Lives.* London: Profile Books.

Gray, A. and Payne, P. (2001) *World Health and Disease.* Buckingham: Open University Press.

8.12 Professional politics

It should be clear by now that politics, at all levels, has an impact on everyone's lives, either directly or indirectly, and politics has had a huge influence on the way in which individuals are treated in society. This has taken place in terms of both the relationship between individuals and the relationship between employers and employees. Politics is partly concerned with passing legislation regarding the treatment of individuals in society, but also influences organizations by granting them the powers to set their own regulatory frameworks. This ensures that there is a considerable amount of regulation that governs our lives, although it is fair to say that some consider that we have too much regulation in our society, while others believe that we need more. In any event, it is important to understand that politics has an influence on nurses as individuals as well as on the nursing profession itself. In this section we briefly mention equal opportunities, race relations and employment issues as these impact on nurses as employees, and then discuss the role of the Nursing and Midwifery Council (NMC) and the Royal College of Nursing (RCN) in terms of their impact on the nursing profession.

Equal opportunities, race relations and employment issues

There are a number of overlapping terms that are often used in politics and social policy arenas, but each one has a distinct usage that sets it apart from the others in definitional terms. Some of these terms include equality, equity and, justice and, although we can appreciate some areas of overlap, in popular usage they refer to different ideas in political forums. Equal opportunities is a refinement of the concept of equality and refers to the removal of 'barriers of discrimination, improving access to jobs, education and training' (Blakemore 1998: 25–6). Although we are probably familiar with the idea of equal opportunities in relation to employment we should also remember that its principles can be applied to improving access to, and use of, welfare services such as benefits, social security and health services, as well as other areas. There are usually political differences of opinion regarding equality of opportunity, with some stressing *opportunity* and others emphasizing *equality*. The different emphases have very substantial differences in terms of policy formulation and practical outcomes. Blakemore (1998) suggests that it is better to consider equal opportunity policies on a spectrum of 'modest' to 'tough', or minimalist to maximalist. For example, he would argue that 'minimalist principles fit best with liberal or conservative principles and values [while] maximalist principles fit best with social democratic or egalitarian principles' (Blakemore 1998: 27).

The term race relations has two perspectives to it. First, it is a term used in academic circles to refer to a form of social relations and in sociology it has become a distinctive analytical subdiscipline. It is based on the idea that *Homo sapiens* is one species and any controversy regarding differences in genetic variations are socially constructed as differences in 'race'. Second, the term race relations can be understood in terms of how people predicate their relationships with others based on their beliefs regarding differences between 'races'. In this sense people will act according to their beliefs about a particular 'race' and this action can be both positive or negative, but forms the basis of discrimination. Political moves to combat discrimination in our society have included the passing of the Race Relations Act 1965, which 'established conciliation machinery to deal with complaints of discrimination which was to be unlawful on grounds of race, colour, ethnic or nations origin in public places such as hotels, restaurants and transport' (Jones 1987: 217). However, it was criticized on three main counts: first, that it did not cover housing or employment; second, that it was not easy to enforce it; and, third, it did not have much of an impact. The later Race Relations Act 1976 built on this and extended both its coverage and its powers. Complainants can now proceed directly to an industrial tribunal or a county court without awaiting decisions from the Commission for Racial Equality. Race relations have also been supplemented by a range of measures, which are aimed at urban deprivation, particularly where there is racial tensions and active racial discrimination. However, legislation and policy formulation alone will not eliminate racial discrimination – it will also require an attitude change in racists through growth and maturity.

There are numerous employment issues, which are grounded in politics, and may lead to health problems. Employment carries a high status in our society and unemployment can have deeply stigmatizing aspects to it. (2:12) Just as employment can make a person feel good, unemployment can make someone feel bad. Becoming employed is related to issues such as equal opportunities and race relations as mentioned above, but it is also related to issues of equal pay, gender, motherhood, single parents, part-time work, segregation and policy formulation, for example. Health and illness are also closely related to employment, both directly in terms of being fit to work and indirectly, as the foregoing issues can impinge on employment and problems in these areas can lead to unemployment and ill-health. It is not surprising that a professional health discipline has developed in the area of employment, and that is occupational therapy. Furthermore, politicians have been concerned to pass legislation in the area of employment in the form of the Sex Discrimination Act 1975 and the Employment Protection Act 1978. Employment theory is concerned with questions relating to what constitutes full employment, how the workforce is defined, how many hours constitute full-time employment, what the function of that work is and so on. Employment issues also include the relationship between voluntary work and society, and the role that it plays in the economy of the country (Pascall 1997).

The Nursing and Midwifery Council and the Royal College of Nursing

For some it may seem strange that nursing as a profession has a political dimension to it, but it is in our opinion naive to think otherwise. Any large organization will have some element of politics to its functioning, both in terms of its internal politics and in relation to its influence on the larger macropolitics of the country. At the time of writing there is a new organization that is replacing the United Kingdom Central Council and this is the Nursing and Midwifery Council (NMC). The NMC 'is an organisation set up by Parliament to ensure nurses, midwives and health visitors provide high standards of care to their patients and clients' (www.num-uk.org, 2002). In order to achieve this the NMC:

- maintains a register of qualified nurses, midwives and health visitors;
- sets standards of education, practice and conduct;
- provides advice for nurses, midwives and health visitors;
- considers allegations of misconduct or unfitness to practise due to ill-health.

This gives the NMC the power to strike a nurse, midwife or health visitor off the register in the case of misconduct, which means that they cannot practise in their profession. The NMC must be accountable to the government and must ensure that best practices are encouraged and developed. Therefore, it is keen to ensure that nurses, midwives and health visitors are developing their professional practice through research and the production of evidence (Chapter 9). It holds a certain number of values that commits it to:

- being informed and accountable to the public;
- openness, transparency and accessibility;
- fairness and equitable treatment;
- respect for individual and group differences;
- flexibility and openness to change;
- mutual respect and collaboration;
- integrity and loyalty.

The NMC has developed an action plan by which it is judged, and this working document covers a wide range of activities, which are designed to help the organization to fulfil its objectives. Quality assurance lies at the heart of this organization and it is employed to ensure that students meet the required standards to enter the register, and then to remain on it through professional development. It is a regulatory buffer between the patients and the public and therefore is political by nature.

The Royal College of Nursing (RCN) is the largest union of nurses in the UK and one of the largest in the world. It received its 'Royal' status from King George VI in 1928. It offers indemnity insurance to the tune of £3,000,000 and provides advice and guidance on many aspects of nursing geared towards promoting the interests of nurses and patients through improving standards. The RCN offers practical advice and the latest information on nursing practice on a 24-hour basis and is involved in negotiating pay and conditions for nurses. The RCN's charter is

- to promote the science and art of nursing and the better education and training of nurses in the profession of nursing;
- to promote the professional standing and interests of members of the nursing profession;
- to promote the above aims in both the UK and other countries through the medium of information and other means;
- to assist nurses who, by reason of ill-health or other adversity, are in need of assistance;
- to institute and conduct examinations, and to grant certificates and diplomas to those who have met the requirements laid down by the Council of the College.

The RCN is divided up into a number of sections, which focus on specific areas of nursing practice, and it has many branches throughout the UK. It is a political organization in that it is accountable to Parliament and engages politicians (through civil servants) in negotiations regarding pay and conditions, which is a vital role, as these can very easily be eroded (Armstrong 2001). Midwives have their own organization in the form of the Royal College of Midwives (RCM).

Further reading

Ham, C. (1997) *Health Care Reform: Learning from International Experience.* Buckingham: Open University Press.

▌8.13 Conclusions

We have seen throughout the chapter that politics is extremely important in the delivery of health care services and this importance is recognized through the relationship that exists between members of the society that become ill or injured and the provision of help by those that are in good health. There are numerous political ideologies that are concerned with how best to deliver such a service and these are often in conflict with each other. Politics can be employed positively to develop health care services but also can be employed negatively when used for personal reasons, and as a corollary services are disrupted. It is also important that nurses become more politically aware and involved in the politics of health care, both through being informed and through becoming active in the various organizations surrounding the nursing profession (Ferguson 2001).

Thinking science

9.1 Introduction

It might seem odd that a chapter on science is necessary in a book that is concerned with thinking and nursing. However, it is necessary for a number of reasons. First, medicine has a long developmental history of attempting to apply scientific principles to the study of the human body, and although some early practices were a little dubious, to say the least, over the past 200 years or so medicine has been guided more by science than serendipity. The other professions allied to medicine – psychology, physiotherapy, radiology and so on – although having a shorter history, also founded their developmental practice on scientific principles. Nursing, on the other hand, largely developed its early practices based on personal theories and grounded experience. It is predominantly in the post-war era, and particularly over the past two decades, that science has featured larger in the development of nursing care. Second, over the past two decades there has been a rationalization process in the NHS, which has brought attention to the limited resources that are available, an increase in consumerism that involves higher standards of care and an increase in public expectations (Chapters 7 and 8). This has led to a focus on evidence-based practices in all aspects of health care delivery, and nursing is no exception. We can no longer justify the personalized approaches to delivering nursing care, such as the diverse treatments for pressure sores that used to range from the application of egg whites to blowing oxygen on them. At least these practices are no longer acceptable without the underlying scientific evidence for them, and a rigorous examination as to their efficacy. Thus, science has a role to play in providing evidence for practice as well as balancing expensive resources. Third, we are living in a world that is becoming more litigious, and professionals, including nurses, are being made more accountable for their practices. Thus, it is paramount that nursing practice is examined, investigated and underpinned by science. Finally, science is central to progress, as a species, as individuals and as professions. In our quest to understand the nature of the human condition, and how best to assist those in a state of ill-health, however we define that, we must understand the role of science in the progress of nursing care.

The notion of science, or something being scientific, has a lay appreciation of a knowledge that is considered to be of a higher order, and brings with it a suggestion of credibility and credence. However, before we explore some of the components that constitute science we should point out that there is considerable debate as to how convincing the scientific method actually is. We will not dwell on this here but the reader should be aware of this debate and appreciate that there are other ways in which the world, and the humans within it, can be understood. Here we focus on the traditional process of the scientific method by, first, outlining some of the major theoretical components and, second, examining the practical elements of this process.

PART ONE: THEORY

9.2 What is science?

As we note above, it is generally accepted that science is respected in our society, and we are all familiar with comments such as 'that's not a very scientific approach' or 'scientists have proved that this washing powder is better than all the rest'. These comments serve to inform us that something considered to be scientific is held in higher regard than something that is not. We hear these types of comments from newsreaders, politicians and even advertisements. However, we must be clear as to what we are referring to when we evoke such merit by employing the term 'science'. Definitions of science differ considerably depending upon who is doing the defining, and this remains the case from lay persons as well as from scientists themselves. For example, Robinson and Reed (1998: 102) stated that the everyday use of science was defined as: '(1) the process of gaining knowledge by systematic study; (2) a body of accumulated expert knowledge'. From two scientists we note the definition to be 'generally, *science* refers to the pursuit of objective knowledge gleaned from observation' (Neale and Liebert 1986: 6, emphasis in the original). What is clear from these two definitions is that science is related to knowledge, and indeed etymologically the word science is derived from the Latin word *scientia*, which refers to knowledge. However, this is not particularly helpful as there can be several types of 'knowledge'.

Types of knowledge

According to Nachmias and Nachmias (1981) there are three types, or modes, of knowledge. The first is the *authoritarian mode*, in which persons in authority are perceived as qualified to produce knowledge, and this knowledge is rarely questioned. For example, in religious circles what archbishops or the Pope say is taken as knowledge on religious matters and is largely undisputed by believers of those faiths. However, the authoritarian mode can also exist in tribal societies through the chieftain or medicine man, and in monarchical societies through the reigning king or queen. Furthermore, we should point out that it may also exist in technocratic societies when we view the knowledge of scientists as a form of supreme authority that is rarely questioned. We should note that in the authoritarian mode the person who is seeking the knowledge attributes to the authoritarian person the power and ability to produce the knowledge, and with each solicitation it reinforces the relationship between the knowledge-seeker and the knowledge-producer.

The second type of knowledge is the *mystical mode*, which is similar to the authoritarian mode but differs in its requirement on the manifestation of supernatural signs and the reliance on the bio-psychological state of the person seeking the knowledge. It may be knowledge that is implored from gods, prophets, mediums, divines, psychics, spiritualists and so on, and is usually accompanied by some form of ritual and ceremony involving the seeker of the knowledge. Nachmias and Nachmias (1981: 5) point out that 'the confidence in the knowledge produced in this manner decreases as the number of disconfirmations increases, or as the educational level of a society advances'. However, despite this, this type of belief system in the mystic mode of knowledge usually employs strategies by which any contradictions are absorbed by the seeker.

The third type of knowledge is the *rationalistic mode*. This type of knowledge emanates from the rational philosophers, who claim that knowledge can be produced by adherence to the forms and the rules of logic. It is based on the belief that, as humans, we can apprehend the world independently of observation of it and that types of knowledge exist outside of our experience of it. This means that in this mode we can understand the world through logic and mathematics and apply categories that we create, which form the knowledge of the phenomena that existed before we studied them. However, this pure form of rationalism, which was predominantly concerned with the physical sciences, has been 'softened' somewhat in the social sciences by the suggestion that pure mathematics and formal logic 'should be applied, as complex tools always should, only when and where they can help and do not hinder progress' (Lewin 1951: 12). Now, glancing back at our definitions of science above we can recap that although science may be related to knowledge it is not the only semantic. What we mean when we use the word science is more to do with *how* that knowledge is produced. In short, science is about the process or method of producing knowledge.

Underlying principles and assumptions of science

If we accept that science is concerned with the method of producing knowledge then we should appreciate that there are a number of ways by which this can be achieved. Of course, proponents of one method do not always agree with proponents of another. A basic distinction between methods is usually drawn between quantitative and qualitative approaches. Quantitative approaches are largely concerned with the collection of data in the form of numbers collected via various measures and indices. They then employ various statistical methods to analyse and describe the data. These quantitative approaches are influenced by the methods of the natural sciences and Box 9.1 shows some methods of collecting quantitative data and some statistical tests that are commonly used.

Box 9.1   Some quantitative data collection methods and statistical tests

Some data collection approaches

- Questionnaires
- Thurstone scales
- Likert scales
- Guttman scale
- Time sampling

Some statistical tests

Non-parametric tests
- Wilcoxon signed-ranks test
- Mann–Whitney test
- Friedman test
- Page's *L* trend test
- Kruskal–Wallis test
- Jonckheere trend test
- Chi-square test

Parametric tests
- The *t* test (unrelated)
- The *t* test (related)
- One-way ANOVA (unrelated)
- One-way ANOVA (related)
- Two-way ANOVA (unrelated)
- Two-way ANOVA (related)
- Two-way ANOVA (mixed)

Correlational tests
- Spearman rank correlation coefficient
- Pearson product moment correlation

Qualitative approaches, on the other hand, are concerned with collecting data about human social contexts and tend not to employ numerical data. They usually collect data through questioning and observations, and analyse the information through a number of methods, which rely on very different assumptions about the world. These approaches are influenced by the methods of the social sciences, and it is this contrast of assumptions between the natural and social sciences that causes the continual debate regarding which approach to science is more credible. Box 9.2 highlights some qualitative research methods.

The fact that both quantitative and qualitative approaches are based on different assumptions about the world makes them, on one level, *belief systems*, and with all belief systems one is either a believer or a non-believer. However, having said that, there are a number of principles that underscore all scientific methods, or at least there should be, and the first is *the importance of precision and reliability*. In all sciences propositions, hypotheses, aims, research questions or objectives should be expressed in clear, precise and logical terms. They should have a high precision of meaning, which is why science employs technical definitions and specialized terminology. It is this precision that allows accurate testability and this is undertaken through measurement and observation. The second principle is *the critical perspective of science*. Science is concerned with a higher level of confidence and certainty of knowledge beyond belief, faith or reason. This means that the scientist must be a sceptic, cynic and doubter, and leads them to believe that they are being deceived by confounding variables (Frank 1977). The third principle is that of *cause and effect*. All scientific research involves the

---

Box 9.2   Some qualitative research methods

Participant observation
Ethnography
Ethnomethodology
Action research
Symbol theorizing
Heuristic research
Social network analysis
Field decision research
Organizational analysis
Comparative methodology
Collaborative enquiry
Experiential research
Illuminative evaluation
Endogenous research
Participative research
Educational research
Phenomenology
Grounded theory

empirical search for the logical relationships between variables, actions or events. This involves observation or measurement of something, applying an intervention or waiting for an event to happen, and then observing or measuring the consequences. This, then, gives us an idea of the relationship between these happenings.

These principles are reliant on a number of assumptions that we hold, but that are unprovable. The first refers to the assumption that the natural world is orderly and regular. That is, even within the constantly changing environment there are patterns that can be understood, and these patterns do not occur haphazardly. In science the natural world refers to all the empirically observable phenomena, events and conditions that occur, which includes the human being as one biological subsystem of that world. The second assumption concerns our belief that we can know the laws of the natural world. This includes the conviction that we can know the natural objects of the world and also ourselves within it. The third assumption refers to a belief that knowing the world is better than not knowing it. In short, knowledge is superior to ignorance. Of course, not everything can, or will, be known, and knowledge may always be modified, but the assumption concerns the *quest* to know. Fourth, in science it is assumed that all natural phenomena have natural causes, and it is this cause and effect relationship that is the focus for testing. This assumption stands in opposition to fundamental religious beliefs, spiritualism, magic and so on, and does not accept that supernatural causes can have effects in the natural world. Fifth, in science nothing is self-evident. Thus, truth is sought through objectivity, and tradition, personal beliefs and common sense cannot be relied upon in the scientific endeavour. Finally, it is assumed that knowledge is derived from the acquisition of experience; that is, it must be empirical. This involves perceptions and observations through our senses. However, it is not merely through our five senses of sight, touch, sound, smell and taste (3:7) but also from an interpretation of the experience of the physical, biological and social world having an impact on our senses (Nachmias and Nachmias 1981).

Further reading

Chalmers, A. F. (1999) *What Is This Thing Called Science?* Buckingham: Open University Press.
Grbich, C. (1998) *Qualitative Research in Health: An Introduction*. London: Sage.

9.3 Explanation

One of the most interesting, some may say irritating, periods of a child's development is that time of a toddler's life when they repeatedly ask 'why?' 'Why is that bus red, Mum?' 'Because that is the town's colours.' 'Why?' 'Because the company decided so.' 'Why?' 'Because they thought it meant something to the town.' 'Why?' 'Well, erm, because it's tradition.' 'Why?' 'Oh, I don't know, eat your sweets.' In the quest to know something we need not only information, but also explanation – even at 3 years old. However, the concept of explanation is a complex one indeed. If we take the word at face value, as we employ it in everyday use, we can understand it as simply to make something known in detail or to give meaning in order to make something intelligible. However, explanation is a concept that has been studied closely in many academic circles. For example, philosophical reflections concerning explanation are common in this traditional discipline, and the subject has been covered by no lesser philosophers than Aristotle, Hume, Kant and Mill, to name but a few. Furthermore, historians have a long-standing interest in the idea of explanation as they strive to provide meaning to historical events. Historians deal with, basically, two types of explanation: (a) individual human actions that have had a significant impact on a society, e.g. Stalin; and (b) large-scale social events that have had a significant impact on many societies, e.g. wars (Ryan 1973). In science, explanation is concerned with the production of knowledge about some thing or event, but also has, at least, three other elements to it. The first is concerned with *understanding*, which in this context refers to establishing the causal relationships between events or variables. The second relates to the ability to formulate accurately a *prediction* that if one thing happens then another will follow. Third, explanation in science is concerned with *reasoning*, which involves how we employ research in the development of theory. Let us now look at each of these in a little more detail.

Understanding and prediction

Understanding is yet another term that can be both simple and complex. Simply stated, we know it to be a perception of the significance of a fact, or a series of facts. However, in science it is more complex than this, as we begin to question what perception is, what significance might be and what constitutes a fact. In science there is considerable disagreement as to the meaning of understanding and it is often applied in two distinct ways. The first is usually called *Verstehen* (empathic understanding), while the second is termed *predictive*. These different usages are said to exist because social sciences are humanistic as well as scientific, and we should also note that researchers in the social sciences are both observers and participants in the world (Nachmias and Nachmias 1981). In empathic understanding the view is that the natural and social sciences are different and, therefore, require different methods of investigation. In the natural sciences molecules, gases, planets etc. act according to the laws of physics, as defined at any given time, and they do not have a level of consciousness, and so cannot alter their actions. On the other hand, the social sciences must take account of the ability of humans to change their course of action in response to perceptions of self and others. Humans have a historical dimension to their behaviour as well as a subjective element to their experience. Weber (1922) argued that social scientists, in order to understand human behaviour, must put themselves in the place of the subject of enquiry. This involves gaining an appreciation of the subject's reality and this is achieved by understanding their values, attitudes, symbols and so on. The *Verstehen* tradition of understanding produced an off-shoot, the symbolic interactionist (2:6) approach, which suggested that humans continually remake their social environment and, therefore, their social order is in a constant state of flux. This makes the establishment of universal human laws, or fixed explanations, pointless, as societies are constantly changing.

Predictive understanding, on the other hand, has its roots in the logical empiricists, who take the view that objective knowledge can be achieved in both the natural and social sciences. From this they argue that both sciences can employ the same method of investigation and that all discoveries should be verified before they are incorporated into our body of knowledge. However, there are some scientists who believe that there is no logic of discovery and no totally rational single scientific method (Kuhn 1970). Kuhn argues that one scientific paradigm will be dominant until it is overthrown by a crisis, which he calls a scientific revolution. Verification is concerned not with method, but with whether scientists are justified in making the claims that they do. This is often referred to as the logic of justification.

Inductive and deductive reasoning

Induction is concerned with reasoning from particular facts to a general conclusion. Popper (1980: 27) made the claim that 'it is usual to call an inference "inductive" if it passes from *singular statements* (sometimes also called "particular" statements), such as accounts of the results of observations or experiments, to *universal statements*, such as hypotheses or theories'. This is based on making a number of observations of a particular phenomenon and then drawing a conclusion regarding the prediction of the next observation. Popper gives us the example of white swans. Say we observe all the swans on a lake and identify the fact that they are all white. Would we then be in a position to state that our theory is that all swans are white? We may be challenged regarding this and decide to make more observations and investigate all the rivers and lakes throughout the UK. If all the observed swans were white could we then theorize that all swans are white and no black swans exist? We can see that there may be problems with this method of producing knowledge. We cannot make this theoretical claim that all swans are white unless we have observed all existing swans. Even if we do that, how can we say that a black swan did not exist in the past or that one will not exist in the future? We can see here that we have problems with the number of observations to be made in order to verify our theory, and in effect that the observations can only serve to support a theory and cannot prove it. It is clear that a single observation of one black swan will falsify the theory completely. However, Chalmers (1999) has argued that while these types of inductive theories can never be proven, in the sense of being logically deduced from that type of evidence, we can construct good inductive arguments. He states that if an inductive inference from observable facts to laws is to be justified they must meet certain conditions. These conditions are:

- the number of observations forming the basis of a generalization must be large;
- the observations must be repeated under a wide variety of conditions;
- no accepted observation statement should conflict with the derived law (Chalmers 1999: 46).

Although Chalmers is at pains to point out that there are numerous problems with inductivism, he shows how it has some appeal when seen in relation to deductive reasoning. This is achieved by facts acquired through observation inductively producing laws and theories, and then deductively leading to predictions and explanations. For example, if we make many observations that pure water freezes at 0 °C if given sufficient time, we can then inductively produce the law/theory that all pure water freezes at 0 °C, given sufficient time. If my car radiator contains pure water then we can deductively predict that the water in my car radiator will freeze if the temperature falls below 0 °C for a sufficient time (Chalmers 1999).

In contrast to inductive reasoning is deductive reasoning as a form of scientific explanation, and the foremost advocate of this approach is probably Karl Popper, who termed it the hypothetico-deductive model. According to Nachmias and Nachmias (1981: 10), 'a deductive explanation calls for a universal generalization, a statement of the conditions under which the generalization holds true, an event to be explained, and the rules of formal logic'. Thus, a phenomenon can be explained by showing that it may be deduced from the universal generalization. With a universal law or generalization, testing of the phenomenon can be undertaken. In Popper's (1980: 32) words, 'from a new idea, put up tentatively, and not yet justified in any way – an anticipation, a hypothesis, a theoretical system, or what you will – conclusions are drawn by means of logical deduction'. An example of this would be a scientist's explanation of items falling to Earth as being caused by the law of gravitation. This can be deduced from observing that all objects fall to Earth, in all natural conditions, and encompasses the past, present and future.

Further reading

Braithwaite, R. B. (1960) *Scientific Explanation*. New York: Harper.
Pitt, J. (1989) *Theories of Explanation*. Oxford: Oxford University Press.

9.4 Evidence, proof and falsifiability

We briefly mentioned above (9:1) the importance of evidence-based practices in the modern health care setting, and as resources become more limited we will need to rationalize our practices even more. Evidence is important both in providing information to support a particular theory or point of view and in providing information to falsify a particular theory or point of view. Therefore, the central issue is that we need to have the ability to produce reliable evidence for what we do in providing nursing care. However, what constitutes evidence needs careful consideration, particularly in relation to the issue of cause and effect. This is concerned with ensuring that the effect is a result of the cause, and is not a result of a confounding variable. For example, we may wish to obtain evidence that a particular cream improves the healing of leg ulcers. We may then design a research strategy to gather evidence for this and, assuming that the data that we collected support the use of the cream, we may conclude that the use of the cream is the cause that produced the effect of improved leg ulcer healing. However, supposing that we discovered that, unbeknown to us at the time of doing our research, the patient had an unusually high nutrition diet, which they do not usually have. Then, this too may have contributed to our patient's improved leg ulcer healing. It is a confounding variable and weakens our evidence in terms of the cause (cream) and the effect (healing). These problems in scientific research, particularly that which deals with humans and animals, are often difficult to overcome and research designers spend some considerable time trying to ensure that they surmount these difficulties by controlling for these variables. We are now in a position to consider what constitutes evidence in more detail and to outline its relationship to proof and falsifiability.

Evidence

In dealing with what constitutes good evidence we must address the issues of prediction, control, causality and weight. Neale and Liebert (1986: 10) argued that 'it is often said that the social sciences deal with the prediction and control of behaviour through the understanding of related physical and mental processes'. In scientific research we are attempting accurately to anticipate future, or unobserved, events through a causal relationship. We expect, in science, that knowledge should result in accurate predictions based on the logic that if we know that A causes B, if A is present then we can predict that B will occur. The underlying assumption here is that if the generalization or universal law is both known and true then the causal conditions are adequate for predicting the effect. If the prediction is incorrect then this can only be because: (a) the universal law or generalization is not true; or (b) the causal conditions were not satisfied. Take, for example, the freezing water and car radiator in section 9:3 above. If the temperature of 0 °C and the presence of pure water are the conditions, then freezing of the water is the effect. Thus, if the antecedent conditions are satisfied we can accurately predict the freezing of the water.

Control has two basic meanings in science. The first refers to the ability of the investigator to influence, or bring about, alterations in particular phenomena. This may also refer to the ability of the researcher to control certain factors in a particular situation and to be able to state what these are, or it may be having the knowledge of what may need to be done to achieve a certain outcome (Neale and Liebert 1986). The second is concerned with controlling for other factors, or variables, that may contribute to producing the effect (as in our cream/nutrition equals healing of leg ulcers above). They are, in short, rival explanations and need to be controlled for in order to produce sound evidence. This element of control will influence the internal validity of the research, which refers to the extent to which the independent variable is actually responsible for the dependent variable. Internal validity of research designs can be affected by both extrinsic and intrinsic factors. Extrinsic factors are usually related to the possible biases that result from the recruitment of subjects to the experimental and control groups. If the two groups of subjects are not matched appropriately this can result in skewed results and the production of unsound evidence. Intrinsic factors affecting the internal validity of a research design are usually related to changes in the subjects during the course of the study, alterations in the measuring instrument or in the way that it is applied or changes in the way in which the observations are made (Campbell and Stanley 1963).

The establishment of causal relationships has a philosophical history stretching back to early Greek times, and remains a central issue today. The basis of a causal relationship is that X causes Y, and if a change in X occurs then this will bring about a change in Y. The demonstration of causality is said to involve three distinct procedures. The first is the demonstration of covariation, which refers to two, or more, phenomena varying together. For example, alcohol intake may covary with aggression, but if the causal relationship cannot be established we cannot say that alcohol causes aggression. In science covariations between two, or more, phenomena are usually expressed as measures of correlations or associations. The second procedure involves eliminating spurious relations. As we saw above in our example of the cream/nutrition and leg ulcer healing, one of the variables (cream or nutrition) may well be a spurious relation. Unless we control for one of the variables we cannot make a reliable claim that it is either the cream or the nutrition that causes the improved healing process (it may well be a combination of both). The third procedure is to establish the time order of the occurrences, which simply stated means to ensure that the events occur in the correct sequence before claiming a causal relationship (Simon 1978).

There are said to be four broad types of causal relationships (Neale and Liebert 1986). The first is a *necessary and sufficient* relationship in which a factor, X, is required to produce an effect, Y. For example, a gene may be both necessary and sufficient to cause a certain disease. Second, there may be *necessary but not sufficient* causal relationships; that is, X is necessary but not sufficient to cause Y. For example, a writing instrument may be necessary to take notes in a lecture but not sufficient for doing so. Third, there are *sufficient but not necessary* causal relationships in which X is one of many causes of Y. For example, a barking dog may be sufficient to stop us from walking into a dark alley late at night but may not be necessary, as other factors may stop us as well, e.g. fear of being mugged. Finally, there are *contributory* causal relationships, in which X is neither necessary nor sufficient to cause Y, but does have some contribution in that it increases the likelihood of it occurring. For example, a bad day at the office is neither necessary nor sufficient to cause an argument at home but may well contribute to it. The establishment of causal relationships in the production of evidence now allows us to deal with the two issues of proof and falsifiability.

Proof and falsifiability

When we use the term proof we are referring to the establishment of a fact through the production of logical causal relations between events. Put another way, in a non-formal context, a proof is a demonstration of a proposition X, which is valid from true premises with X as a conclusion. However, depending on which view of science one holds to be more effective, it can be seen that proving something has serious philosophical flaws. Take, for example, the case of Popper's white swans, as outlined above, and consider whether the observation of another white swan proves the theory that all swans are white. Clearly, it does not. According to Popper the observation of a white swan can only serve to *support* the theory that all swans are white. Therefore, it is safer, in social science circles, to make claims that research findings support a particular theory rather than prove it.

Again, according to Popper, the observation of one black swan clearly falsifies the theory that all swans are white. However, he cautions us that 'we say that a theory is falsified only if we have accepted basic statements which contradict it' (Popper 1980: 86). Some theories are difficult to support or falsify and no amount of observation can serve to establish either. For example, Freudian psychoanalytic theory or Marxist theory of capital cannot be falsified, in any scientific sense, and Popper would argue that this excludes them as sciences. Falsificationism is closely related to scientific progress. Science begins with some identifiable problem associated with the explanation of some aspect of the world, or universe. Solutions are then proposed by scientists, in the form of hypotheses, and these are then tested and criticized. Some hypotheses may be helpful and others eliminated. Even when theories have been rigorously tested and withstood a wide range of approaches they may eventually be falsified, providing another problem to be tested. Thus, according to Popper, science progresses.

Further reading

Bowling, A. (1997) *Measuring Health: A Review of Quality of Life Measuring Scales.* Buckingham: Open University Press.

Punch, K. F. (1998) *Introduction to Social Research: Quantitative and Qualitative Approaches.* London: Sage.

9.5 Ideas, concepts, theories and models

Many people will tend to use ideas, concepts, theories and models interchangeably, and while in everyday usage this may well be fine, in science we must be able to distinguish between them. As we have noted above (9:2), in science we strive for precision and reliability of meaning and go to some length to establish the constructs of a particular notion. This may employ technical language as well as some element of mental gymnastics, but is necessary in order to achieve the standard of precision that is required. Furthermore, precision is required so that other scientists will understand what is meant by the terms and will be able to use them in a normative way in their research. In this way they will know what we mean and we will know what they mean, even if there is disagreement.

Ideas

The word ideas has two basic meanings, with the first being equivalent to the Greek term *eidos* (form) and the second to the Greek word *idein* (to see). Both of these meanings are connected to give us an early stab at a definition; that is, an idea is something that is seen by some form of intellectual vision. However, what it is that is actually seen is open to philosophical, as well as psychological, speculation. In fact, Plato considered ideas to be real and objective, and appeared to claim that there exist objective standards that are not dependent on a person's decision to think about something. On the other hand, Descartes, in the seventeenth century, gave the word idea a new sense. He claimed that an idea is whatever the mind directly perceives irrespective of the external objective that is represented. Popper's (1980) reading of Descartes's work argued that ideas can be clear and distinct, and thought to be true, but, alas, they can be wrong. Thus, he argued, ideas alone as a source of authority of the senses, as a source of knowledge, were not reliable. They need to be built upon by testing them out.

Ideas, in scientific research terms, can be understood as an intellectual process of *thinking through* the causal relations between the events of the idea. In relation to the ideas we need to ask questions such as 'If this happens, then what will be the result?' and 'If we do that what is likely to happen?' Once we have undertaken this intellectual process of thinking through we then need to write down certain elements of the idea as a series of statements. First, we should establish whether there are any axioms – that is, self-evident generally held truths – that can be made regarding the idea. Acceptable axioms can be of two types in science: (a) *conventions*, which fix the meaning of the fundamental ideas that are introduced by the axiom, and determine an agreement about what can be said about the idea; and (b) *hypotheses*, which are empirical or scientific statements that are open to testability. The second group of statements to be established are *propositions*; that is, assertions that can be made consisting of subject and predicate. From thinking through our idea and establishing if we can arrive at some axioms and propositions we are now in a position to deal with concepts.

Concepts

When we think, we think in a language, which is a communicative system comprising symbols and a set of rules for how we can combine these symbols. The concept is one of the most important symbols in this language, which allows us to begin a description of the world. Nachmias and Nachmias (1981: 27) define a concept as 'an abstraction representing an object, a property of an object, or a certain phenomenon'. Such concepts as 'social status', 'roles', 'power' and 'bureaucracy' are often used in the social sciences, and concepts such as 'intelligence', 'perception', 'learning' and 'forgetting' are the stuff of the psychological sciences.

Concepts are useful to scientists for a number of reasons. First, they allow communication of ideas and thoughts at an intersubjective level and can 'hold' a large amount of information regarding a specific subject. As they are abstractions they do not really exist as empirical phenomena, and they are representations of something in the real world, but they are not the phenomena themselves. Too frequently concepts are ascribed as having dynamic qualities as if they are 'alive', such as the concept of power having drives or needs. This is termed the *fallacy of reification*. Second, concepts are used to offer particular points of view regarding empirical phenomena in the external world. They are useful tools to allow individual experiences to be shared among others and they can be either rejected or accepted to form a consensus (Denzin 1970). Third, concepts are helpful to us in classifying and generalizing, and in science it is a common activity to order, structure and categorize experiences and observations in terms of concepts. For example, we can take a pig, sheep, cow and chicken and ignore their differences while focusing upon their generic resemblances with the use of the concept 'animal'. We can take the general concept of 'animal' and appreciate the multivariate aspects that can be comprehended, and ordered, within it. However, within the concept of 'animal' we can also lose the sense of the specific differences between a pig, sheep, cow and chicken. Thus, the concept allows us to abstract and generalize to delineate the essential features of empirical phenomena in the external world. Fourth, concepts are essential building blocks for theory development and lead to explanations and predictions. Concepts are extremely important, as they will be significant in defining the structure and content of theories in a systematic way.

Concepts are used to define things in the real world and they may be concrete things such as planets or they may be abstract things such as perception. However, they are extremely useful and concepts may be used to define other concepts. When this occurs they are seen as developing a basic language relating to the area being defined and are known as *conceptual definitions*. It must be remembered that conceptual definitions are neither true nor false, and that they are merely symbols permitting communication and as such are either useful or not. What we must now do is establish how we can relate the concepts to the things or events in the real, or empirical, world. The real world may contain directly observable properties, such as planetary orbits. However, it also contains properties, which are represented by the concepts, that cannot be directly observed. For example, the idea of 'perception' or 'role' cannot be directly observed and we are left with inferring the empirical existence of them through *operational definitions*. These are sets of procedures that we need to perform, to establish empirically the extent to which the concepts exist. Thus, if we were studying someone's response to a 'role' we would need to define operationally what behaviours we would expect them to be performing.

Theory

Theory means different things to different people, and while some would use concepts as theory, others look for logical relations between concepts that comprise a theory. In this latter sense, sometimes known as logico-deductive theorizing, there is an emphasis on the logical relations and testable propositions. However, attempting to define theory in these narrow terms does not take into account the variety of ways in which social scientists employ the term. For example, Easton (1966) argued that theories can be defined according to their *scope* in terms of macro or micro; they may be defined according to their *function* in terms of static–dynamic and structure–process; they may be defined according to their *structure* in terms of their tight logical interrelations or loose propositions; or, finally, they may be defined according to their *level* in terms of relations of behaviour and how this is hierarchically scaled.

Nachmias and Nachmias (1981) usefully employed Parsons and Shils's (1962) work to provide a good classification of four levels of theory.

- *First level:* ad hoc *classificatory systems*. This refers to the many ways in which we arbitrarily group and categorize many items, events and statements. This categorization is of our own construction, such as 'like–dislike', 'agree–disagree', and is undertaken in order to summarize empirical observation.

- *Second level: taxonomies*. This again is a categorical system that is constructed to establish empirical observations in order to describe the relationships between certain categories. Taxonomies ought to bear a close relationship between their concepts and the empirical world. Their importance is threefold in social science research: (a) they specify the empirical unit that is to be analysed; (b) they provide description; and (c) they provide inspiration.

- *Third level: conceptual frameworks*. At this level the descriptive categories are set within a framework of explicit, as well as assumed, propositions, which provide both explanatory power for empirical observations and predictions of them.

- *Fourth level: theoretical systems*. From the other levels, we now combine descriptions, explanations and predictions in a systematic way. Relationships are clearly established and there is 'a system of propositions that are interrelated in a way that permits some to be derived from others' (Nachmias and Nachmias 1981: 41).

Models

Models are often used interchangeably with theory, but for social scientists they have distinctive qualities, although they remain closely related to each other. A model is often viewed as something that has a likeness to something or as a representation of reality, but it should be emphasized that a model is not reality itself. For example, one may hold up a model of the aeroplane Concorde and most people would agree that it represents the real thing – but only in certain respects. The model will have the main, and basic, features that will distinguish it from other aeroplanes, but it will not have other aspects such as the electronics and other intricate features. The distinguishing point is that the basic features may be tested (i.e. in a wind tunnel) and the intricate features are not (if the electronics needed to be tested then it is likely that engineers would build a model of them). Thus, we can delineate certain aspects of a model: (a) it establishes a relationship between an aspect of the real world and a specific problem under investigation; (b) it highlights the relations between the identified elements; and (c) it allows for the formulation of empirically testable propositions regarding these relations. Models are important in allowing us to formulate a representation of abstractions that may not be empirically attainable in the physical world, but irrespective of this a model should be testable, or have testable elements within it.

Further reading

Laurence, S. and Margolis, E. (1998) *Concepts*. Cambridge, MA: MIT Press.

9.6 Research process, testability and generalizability

From the foregoing sections in this chapter on science we are now in a position to consider some elements of the research process. We note from the above that we have considered the notion of science in health care settings and highlighted the importance of logical explanation. To begin a scientific approach to understanding our world we need evidence, and this is used in order to support or falsify our beliefs. We have shown how we use ideas, concepts, theories and models to give us a framework for establishing propositions about the world, which should now be tested, with generalizations being made. Testing and testability, however, must be treated with caution, as this involves the study of method (methodology) and this is very different between the physical and social sciences. Testing the reaction of molecules and testing the reaction of human subjects is clearly very different, yet both are very important if we wish to understand our world. If a particular theory, or idea, cannot be tested then it will remain what it is, an abstraction. Generalizability, again, differs in importance between the physical and social sciences. In the former, generalization lies at the heart of this science, establishing universal laws, while in the latter its importance is somewhat diminished. However, before we deal with these two central issues we outline the research process and locate both testability and generalizability in relation to this.

The research process

All sciences are concerned with the production of knowledge that is established through both reason and observation. Claims to knowledge must be verifiable by other scientists and this is achieved by undertaking a generally recognized process of research. The stages of this process may differ slightly in relation to particular scientific paradigms but overall this process remains generally the same. The first stage usually begins with the formulation of a problem: something is seen as needing attention, or an issue is identified that needs to be addressed. It may be stated as a general query or as a simple question, such as 'I wonder why that happens.' The second stage involves amassing background information on the problem. This may involve undertaking a literature review, and obtaining published and unpublished material such as official reports, letters, files and any other documentary evidence. This then needs reading (9:8, 9:9) and synthesizing into the next stage, which is Stage 3, and this includes formulating hypotheses, aims, objectives or research questions. These should be clear and concise and should emanate logically from the documentary evidence. The next stage is to design the research strategy, which should be appropriate to satisfy the demands of Stage 3. Designing the correct method is crucial to the research process.

Stage Five is to outline the measurement instruments or observational

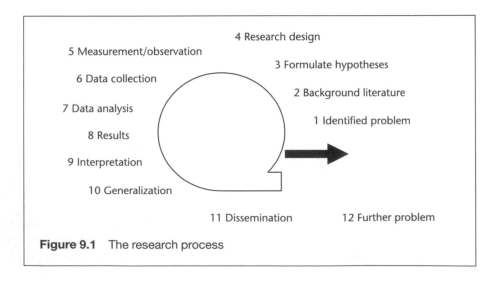

Figure 9.1 The research process

techniques that you are going to employ, which is closely related to your research method. Stage 6 involves outlining what data you are going to collect, how it will be done and how the data will be both managed and stored safely. Stage 7 is to explain what data analysis will be undertaken, whether it is statistical or qualitative and who will be supervising it. This is often a difficult stage and advice should be sought early. The next stage, Stage 8, is to organize your results in a clear and systematic manner. Stage 9 involves undertaking the interpretation of your findings and establishing what they mean to you. In Stage 10 you establish the strength of generalization and if this is not achieved then you will need to explain why this is the case. Dissemination is Stage 11, which means to publish your research widely through journals, seminars, workshops and conferences. It may involve writing a research report. Finally, further problems may be highlighted or areas for further research may be identified. This shows the cyclical nature of the research process and indicates its self-correcting element as it constantly refines problem areas.

Testability

This is concerned with how we can establish both how and to what extent the independent and the dependent variable are causally related. As we have noted above (9:3), this is a complex area but one that is crucial to the advancement of science. Popper (1980: 53–4), setting out the methodological rules as conventions for a logic of scientific discovery, stated: 'once a hypothesis has been proposed and tested, and has proved its mettle, it may not be allowed to drop out without "good reason". A "good reason" may be, for instance: replacement of the hypothesis by another which is better testable; or the falsification of one of the consequences of the hypothesis.' Thus, Popper is placing testability at the heart of theory building and claiming that this 'logic' is central to the advancement of science. This highlights the research process as a mechanistic progression in which testability is central and involves the three main components of comparison, manipulation and control. This reflects the traditional research design of testability, and it should be noted that qualitative approaches may differ in this.

Comparison is concerned with establishing an association between two or more variables. This association is also known as covariation and correlation, and all these terms are concerned with the strength of the causal relationship. An example of this is a relationship between a particular teaching method and the achievement of students, with students having a higher degree of success if they have been exposed to the particular teaching method. It follows that students who have not been exposed to the particular teaching method would show a lower achievement level. If research were to be undertaken to study this we would need a group of students who were exposed to the particular teaching method and a group who were not, so that a comparison could be made. This would also involve assessing both groups of students' achievement levels *before* one group is exposed to the teaching method and then assessing both groups' achievement levels *after* the exposure. Of course, there are a number of variations to this design but we can see the basic principle of comparison between groups of subjects. Furthermore, it should be noted that we have mentioned matching the groups for certain variables: as age, gender, educational background and so on (Peat 2001).

Like so many other things in science, manipulation is concerned with causality. If X causes Y, then a change in X will result in a change in Y. From this we deduce that the relations between X and Y are asymmetrical; that is, that one variable (X) is the determining force and the other variable (Y) is the determined response. Clearly, in logical terms, the response must come after the changing force, as otherwise the latter would not be the influencing power. In our example above, regarding the influence of a particular teaching method on achievement levels, the teaching method must come before the achievement levels rise, as otherwise it cannot be claimed that the teaching method *caused* the rise in achievement. Therefore, the manipulation of the independent variable, i.e. the teaching method, is crucial in terms of when it is applied in the sequence of events if cause and effect is to be claimed. We can achieve some control over this by measuring achievement levels before the teaching method is applied and again afterwards. However, in the social sciences there are difficulties with ensuring the control of variables. For example, the measurement of achievement levels would need to be undertaken close to the introduction of the teaching method and closely following it in order to reduce the possibility that something else affected the rise in achievement. But how do we know that it was the teaching method and not some other variable, say the charismatic nature of the teacher, or the increased enthusiasm for the teaching method, rather than the method itself that caused the rise in achievement? Of course, there are ways of controlling for these variables, but they serve to show how careful we need to be before we make cause and effect claims. This brings us to the issue of control.

To establish causality we need to control for dependent and independent variables under investigation. In the physical sciences this is more easily established, particularly in laboratory settings where the experimenter can introduce the independent variable when the other variables are controlled for. However, in natural settings, and particularly when dealing with human subjects, it is often difficult to control these other variables. The central issue is a question of the internal validity of the research design, which refers to whether the independent variable did actually cause the dependent variable, and this can be jeopardized by extrinsic and intrinsic factors. Extrinsic factors were mentioned in 9:4 above and here we briefly outline the intrinsic factors. Nachmias and Nachmias (1981) outline seven major intrinsic factors affecting the internal validity of research designs.

- *History*. This refers to the fact that as the research is under way, life events continue to occur and can influence the subject and confound the causal relationship being studied. As we mentioned above, the longer the time lapse between pre-test and post-test the greater the possibility for other factors to affect the causal relationship between the independent and dependent variables.

- *Maturation.* Subjects under study grow and mature as time goes by and therefore their bio-psychological systems may produce the changes rather than the independent variable.

- *Experimental mortality.* Being a research participant is a voluntary decision and experimental mortality refers to those who decide to drop out of the research and thus affect the research findings.

- *Instrumentation.* This refers to the question of whether the measuring devices being used (e.g. scales, questionnaires, indexes) in pre- and post-tests are the same, and being used under the same conditions.

- *Testing.* This refers to the fact that, unlike atoms, molecules and planets, humans react when they know they are being studied. They may become sensitive to the tests, improve with frequent taking of them and respond as they think they ought to rather than as they really want to.

- *Regression artefact.* This occurs when individuals have been selected to experimental groups on the basis of their scores on the dependent variable, which are unreliable. For example, they may have had an 'off day', not reflecting their true ability, and later improvements are wrongly attributed to the independent variable.

- *Interactions with selection.* This refers to the selection of research participants from different settings, with some being affected by other processes, or events, causing the changes that the research makes a claim for.

The problems associated with controlling for all these intrinsic factors are considerable. However, we attempt to overcome them by two main approaches. The first concerns matching, which means ensuring that the subjects in the experimental and control groups are as similar as possible. The second refers to randomization, which means that subjects are randomly allocated to either the experimental or the controlled research group.

Generalizability

Generalizability is concerned with the extent to which research findings can be related to larger populations. For example, it would be important to understand if research findings on a particular new drug would be the same for the general population as for the research subjects. This is called the *external validity* of research designs, and involves the two central issues of: (a) representativeness of the sample; and (b) reactive arrangements. Representativeness of the sample is not necessarily guaranteed by randomization alone, as the results of a study might be specific to that group only. To take an extreme example, if you were studying height ranges and took a sample from basketball players then the results might well be generalizable to the overall population of basketball players but not to the population in general. To ensure generalization to the overall population we need to select a sampling method that takes account of this. Probability sampling from various sections of the population would increase the generalizability of the research design. However, there are often difficulties with recruitment in these approaches (Gomm and Davies 2000).

Reactive arrangements are concerned with the extent to which research findings are generalizable outside the research setting. Research, particularly that which is undertaken in social laboratories, may be relevant only to that setting, especially when social situations are contrived. This may make the research setting artificial and cause reactions within the design, which results in reducing the external validity of the study.

Further reading

Burton, D. (2000) *Research Training for Social Scientists: A Handbook for Post-graduate Researchers*. London: Sage.

9.7 Probability

Probability is a term that carries many different interpretations. In everyday use we employ it in a wide range of settings, generally referring to events or actions that are 'likely' to occur, but even these general statements appear to carry other semantic factors. For example, if someone asks 'are you going to the cinema this weekend?' and your response is 'probably' then this suggests that it is likely that you will be going to the cinema. However, if we think a little more deeply about this, it also suggests that in your response of 'probably' you have considered many other factors, weighing them carefully and arriving at some form of chance measurement that you are more likely than not to go to the cinema this weekend. This may have involved such factors as: (a) you have not been to the cinema for some time; (b) there is a good film on that you wish to see; (c) your friends wish to go; (d) there is little else that you want to do. The result of this is a likelihood that you will go to the cinema this weekend. We can see from this that the 'likelihood', or probability, has a certain 'strength', but of course it is dependent on whether other factors influence this 'strength', such as a huge lottery win (what is the probability of this?).

In this everyday use the outcome of the probability is not a serious matter; however, in science it may well be a life and death issue. Who would fly on a plane that had a 50 per cent chance of landing safely? Furthermore, in health care settings we often use probability as a gauge of success in decision making for patients. For example, there may be a 60:40 chance of survival for an operation or a 90 per cent chance that a particular drug will work, and so on. Thus, we can appreciate that probability is concerned with uncertainty, and in science we attempt to give this uncertainty a numerical value to provide us with some indication as to the likelihood of something happening or not, as the case may be (Sim and Wright 2000).

Probability is traditionally categorized into *objective probability*, which is subcategorized into classical probability and relative frequency probability, and *subjective probability* (Daniel 1991; Sim and Wright 2000). Classical probability is concerned with the chance occurrence of, say, rolling a dice with the six uppermost, and in these events all factors are controlled for, and the desired effect, a six uppermost, is always a one in six chance. However, real life is rarely like throwing a dice. Relative frequency is based on empirical observations and defines probability as 'the proportion of occasions, under certain circumstances, on which some specified event occurs in the long term' (Sim and Wright 2000: 189). This requires the occasions to be countable and repeatable, and the desired outcome to be clearly identifiable. For example, low back pain is said to affect 14 per cent of the UK population, and therefore the probability of its occurrence in a randomly selected sample of people would be 0.14 (Rose *et al.* 1997). Subjective probability is based not on empirical observations but on a personal belief in the probability of some event occurring. In this section we are predominantly concerned with objective probability.

Properties of probabilities

According to Sim and Wright (2000) there are three features of probability: (a) the numerical representation; (b) the probability of independent events; and (c) the idea of conditional probability. Let us look at these in a little more detail. The numerical representation of probability is located between zero and one (Hodges and Lehmann 1964). The closer the probability number is to zero, the less likely is the occurrence of an event, and the closer the probability number is to one, the more likely is the occurrence of an event (Sim and Wright 2000). In real terms the numbers zero and one do not represent probability, or uncertainty, as they would technically indicate that zero represents an event that can never occur, and the number one an event that is certain to occur. Therefore, when reading probability figures, such as $p < 0.001$, we can see that this is closer to zero than it is to one, which means that it is less likely that the event occurs.

The probability of independent events refers to the fact that two events can occur in which one provides no information about the occurrence, or non-occurrence, of another event. For example, someone fracturing their arm and winning the lottery are two events that are unrelated; that is, they are independent. In establishing the probability that both events will occur we need to multiply both the independent probabilities. For example, the probability of fracturing your arm may be a thousand to one (0.001) and that of winning the lottery may be a million to one (0.000001). Therefore, multiplying these probabilities gives us the probability of both fracturing our arm and winning the lottery as 0.000000001. This indicates that both events are unlikely to occur at the same time. The probability of independent events is important in many statistical tests.

The idea of conditional, or dependent, events is concerned with one event providing information about another event. In these situations the probability of one event is conditional on the other. For example, the probability of having blue eyes is conditional upon having blond hair (predominantly). Again, conditional probability is important in hypothesis testing when strengths of associations need to be established, and it is important in establishing positive or negative predictive values for diagnostic tests.

Probability uses

Probability is used for a number of purposes in science and here we outline a few of the major applications. The first concerns probabilistic explanations. In health care policy it may be argued that an increase in government spending may result in improved health care services. In these situations the improvement in services is causally linked to the increased spending. This cannot be expressed as a universal law, as there are cases where increased spending does not result in an improvement in services. However, we suggest that there is a high probability that an improvement will follow an increase in spending. This probabilistic explanation can be expressed as an arithmetical ratio between the tendencies of these events. These probabilistic explanations do have limitations, in that certain conclusions cannot be drawn from one part of the overall set of properties.

The second major application of probability refers to prediction. In science, whether health care science or otherwise, we are mainly concerned with predicting what will be the result of doing something. In the words of Nachmias and Nachmias (1981: 12), 'the expectation that scientific knowledge should lead to accurate predictions is based upon the argument that if it is known that X causes Y, and that X is present, *then* the prediction that Y will occur can be made' (emphasis in the original). The process of prediction is, in real terms, the reverse of explanation, in that in the latter we may say that Y was the result of X occurring and in the former we are saying if we do X then we predict that Y will occur. Here we are concerned with the *predictive validity* of our claim. Take, for example, the use of a psychological test to predict who will best perform in a particular job. We may apply the tests and see whether the future course of events actually bears out our predictions.

The third major application of probability relates to its use in sampling. The interpretation of results in scientific research pivots on the extent to which the sampling of subjects was undertaken. In probability sampling the concern is with ensuring that each population element has a specifiable chance of being included in the research sample. However, this is more difficult in practice than it is in theory. For example, in a street survey it may be theoretically possible that everyone stands the chance of being selected for the survey. However, in reality a research surveyor is less likely to approach a couple who are in discussions or a busy parent with heavy bags and a difficult toddler. This introduces sampling bias. Although we employ randomization in an attempt to overcome this bias it remains problematic. We may sample every tenth person in the telephone directory, and clearly this does not give every person the chance of being selected, as we have eliminated nine of every ten, but it is an attempt to randomize selection. But problems remain. What of those who are ex-directory, those who do not have a telephone and those who only use mobiles?

Finally, probability theory lies at the heart of many statistical tests. Statistics can be usefully divided into:

- *Descriptive statistics.* These include the presentation of data in tables, charts, diagrams and so on, as well as calculating percentages, means, medians and modes, and measures of dispersion and correlation. They are used to highlight the salient features of the data and reduce them to manageable proportions (9:11).
- *Inductive statistics.* These involve tests to infer properties of a population based on known sample results, and these tests rely directly on probability.

Remember that what is being attempted in probability theory is the prediction that an event will occur, or not occur, based on the causal relationship between X and Y. Although we can look backwards in time and use statistics to give us an inference about the relationship between events, most work in the statistical field is about looking forward and predicting what may or may not occur. The most commonly used statistical test that we see in the literature on healthcare is probably the chi-square test (pronounced Ki) and we see it represented as χ^2. This test is used when the data are nominal, which means that we have allocated subjects to categories. However, because subjects cannot be allocated to more than one category, the chi-square test is only appropriate when we wish to make predictions concerning how many different subjects are likely to fall into each category.

We have seen from the above that science is of growing concern in the delivery of health care services and its emphasis cannot be over-expressed for us in nursing. Scientific thinking is about logic, structure, planning and predicting, and no matter whether one is a follower of quantitative approaches, qualitative approaches or both, it is important that we become proficient in undertaking the *method* appropriately and applying the principles accurately. We now move from the theoretical perspective of science to the more everyday practical requirements of becoming scientific nurses.

Further reading

Feller, W. (1968) *An Introduction to Probability Theory and Its Applications.* New York: John Wiley & Sons.
Fielding, J. and Gilbert, N. (2000) *Understanding Social Statistics.* London: Sage.

PART TWO: APPLICATION TO PRACTICE

9.8 Literature reviews

In most research it is important to write some form of written report, journal article, thesis or conference paper so that the findings can be shared with the rest of the interested public. In the construction of writing about research on a topic it is always of central importance to demonstrate that you have a command of the existing literature, and a firm understanding of what related research has been carried out. Researchers, both experienced and students, are required to show that their current research emanates from existing literature on the topic and to demonstrate that it fills a gap in the knowledge, is relevant to the field or is appropriate for it to be replicated. In this way the researcher can demonstrate that the skills of reviewing the literature have been attained. The skill of reviewing the literature involves being able to make an accurate summary of other research that has been undertaken in this field, being able to demonstrate the skill of searching, being able to compile accurate and consistent reference lists and bibliographies and being able to summarize key ideas in a critical way.

Reviewing the literature is a skill, and as such can be broken down into individual parts, practised and reconstituted as one smooth overall process. This is not too dissimilar to driving a car, which has the separate parts of gears, brakes, accelerator, mirrors, steering and so on, and when learnt and brought together produces a smooth journey from A to B (it is hoped). Furthermore, like driving a car in contemporary times, reviewing the literature is becoming more difficult with the volume of 'traffic' and the extent of congestion. In this section we discuss the growth of this literature, which is constantly expanding, ways in which this literature can be accessed and how to read and critique the literature, and offer some practical suggestions for managing it.

Growth of literature

Since writing began manuscripts have been constructed to pass on information regarding an account, event or idea, and since the invention of the printing press we have traditionally stored this information in the form of books and journals. Year on year, the shelves on which to store these books and journals have grown, leading to the huge university libraries that we see today. However, since the advent of the microchip the capacity to store vast amounts of printed words on computer disks is now almost infinite. Many books and journals are now available electronically and it is likely that this trend will continue. Journals, in particular, have grown in number since the Second World War and in the health care field alone the number of journals is immense. If we take nursing specifically, the number of journals 50 years ago would number only a few, but there are now well over 100 nursing journals to be drawn upon. It should also be noted that some journals cease being published, are taken over by other publishing houses, are renamed or refocused, but those editions that have been published are always available for reviewing or referencing. Thus, the literature continues to expand.

This growth, however, also continues in other areas that are highly relevant for nursing students. The impetus for many disciplines to publish has increased significantly over the past decade or so, as it is linked into what is known as the Research Assessment Exercise (RAE). This exercise is undertaken every few years, and universities in the UK are judged against, among other things, the number of research publications produced by university staff. This, in turn, is linked into the way that the university is funded. So all disciplines are urged to publish, which is why we have witnessed a growth in publications from, for example, psychology, sociology, medicine and public health. Therefore, the student of nursing today has not only all the relevant publications from nursing journals to contend with but also the related material from the other health care disciplines. While it cannot be expected that everyone in health care studies can cover all the aspects of health care, the corollary of this is that there is more material available in specialist areas. This is leading to ever-expanding areas of specialist expertise in all areas of health care, including nursing. Finally, we ought to point out that while this growth in literature is at its apogee for today's student it is going to be even higher for tomorrow's.

Accessing the literature

Fortunately, the expansion of technology has enabled many of the sources of published material to be listed in electronic databases. Prior to this, a student had to access the literature via library index cards or by tracking down references by searching reference lists at the end of relevant articles. However, the majority of the search can now be done at the computer. There are databases covering most disciplines, but clearly we will focus on those referring to health care. What the databases do is to scan literally thousands of journals in the relevant field and index the articles for bibliographic information and abstract details. The information includes the author's name, date of publication, title of the paper, journal source, volume number, issue number, page numbers and in many cases an abstract. The databases not only cover published journal articles but may also cover books, dissertations, conference papers and other source material. The two most popularly used databases for nurses are *CINAHL* and *Medline*.

- *CINAHL* (Cumulative Index to Nursing and Allied Health). This database claims an authoritative coverage of nearly all English language nursing publications and many from allied professions. It indexes over 500 journals, as well as accessing books, standards of practice, conferences and dissertations.

- *Medline*. This database claims to cover information from *Index Medicus*, dental literature and international nursing. It focuses on medical literature and many other areas of health care delivery, from biological and physical sciences as well as humanities in relation to health. It advertises that it currently has 9.5 million records from more than 3900 journals and other source material (Whitehead and Mason 2003).

As we note above, there are many such databases covering many areas of health care delivery, which brings problems of overlap. Clearly, if both *CINAHL* and *Medline* are covering international nursing journals then both will cover, at least, some of the same material. Therefore, when searching the literature one needs to be aware of this, and with the growing wealth of publications we need to be skilled in narrowing our searches to those that are most relevant. We undertake this through the idea of search strategies. Search strategies are a way of cross-referencing searches of specific terms, which in turn can be cross-referenced with each other. Search strategies can usually be learnt in university, college or hospital libraries, and rather than absorbing space here with this, we conclude this section on accessing the literature with two useful tips. The first is to search the databases for 'review' papers in the specific topic that you are searching, as these ought to have covered many aspects of the field of study that you are interested in, and they should provide a good overall summary. Second, search for seminal papers that have changed theory, or developed it significantly, and identify both the main points and the line of argument.

Reading and critiquing the literature

The search strategy ought to have identified the main papers that you will need for your study, and they will now need to be acquired, read and critiqued. We deal with each of these in turn. It is wise to begin acquiring the literature as early as possible in your study as they can take some considerable time to arrive when ordered. Although we are concentrating on journal articles this also remains the case for books. Check with your own library to see if they carry the journals or books, and if they do, then it is a simple matter of tracking them down via the library referencing system. You may need to photocopy the articles, ensuring that you comply with copyright laws. If your library does not take the journal or the book that you require then you will need to order them, which usually involves filling in a short form and may incur a small payment. It is advisable to acquire primary sources wherever possible, and this refers to published material by the original author(s) rather than secondary sources, which refers to secondary interpretations of original authors work.

Once you have acquired the literature it needs to be read, but this is not as straightforward as it seems and must be undertaken carefully. There are several 'levels' of reading. The first refers to 'scanning', in which you flip through the paragraphs searching for a structure of headings and subheadings. It also involves reading a few random sentences to get a 'feel' for the grammar and syntax. You may also check the number and frequency of references and obtain a general view of the format quality. The second level refers to reading for meaning and involves studying the content of the paper carefully and making decisions as to what the main arguments are. The main point of the paper needs to be identified and the logic and argumentation needs to be established. The third level of reading refers to reading for sense, which involves taking an overall picture of whether the article makes sense in relation to the analysis of issues, the line of argument, the interpretation of information and the conclusions that are drawn. Finally, the fourth level of reading refers to reading for research. All types of reading are important but it is this last level of reading that requires the greatest skill, and we deal with this next.

Reading for research requires knowledge of the research process and its constituent elements. Furthermore, it is essential that there is an understanding of how these elements interact with, and influence, each other. Therefore, the greater the knowledge of research that you have the more successful you are likely to be in engaging in critical reading for research. The critical reading will involve asking many questions regarding the research process and the structure of the paper that is being read. These questions will include whether the abstract contains all the major elements of the research, whether the introduction does what it is supposed to do and whether the literature is adequate. There will also be questions relating to the aims or hypotheses and whether they were constructed appropriately, and questions as to the appropriateness of the method chosen and its construction. Finally, there will be questions on the presentation of results, the balance of the discussion and the logic of the recommendations and conclusions.

Management of the literature

The management of the literature is a practical issue, but one that carries with it certain elements of professionalism. Let us deal with the practical elements first. We have emphasized the growing amount of literature throughout this section and once one has gone to the trouble of acquiring it, particularly if a cost has been incurred, it needs to be stored and used appropriately. This refers to the practical management of the literature. The articles should be stored in a filing system and you may choose one that suits you best. However, we outline one such system here as a suggestion. On each page, in the top right hand corner, print the first author's name, and *et al.* if necessary, and the year of publication. They can then be stored alphabetically, in a series of subfiles according to the topic areas. The details of each paper should be written on an index card, and this should include the authors' names, date of publication, title of paper, journal, volume number, issue number and page numbers. If this is written as it would be in the reference list, then this makes mistakes less likely. The index cards are also useful for writing important notes on the back of each reference, which can refer to the important points of the paper. Finally, rather than index cards software packages can be used instead. One of these is called *Reference Manager*, which holds a huge number of references in as many subfiles as needed. It can also construct reference lists according to the specific requirements of particular journals.

The final point concerning the management of the literature relates to the question of professionalism. In science, nursing or otherwise, it is important to build personal libraries in order to develop a long-term professional career. As you complete a particular project, whether for a course of study or as a matter of interest, you ought to consider constructing a paper for publication, and therefore the filed papers will be needed in the future. As we begin to publish in specific areas we begin to establish an area of 'expertise' and the files are invaluable for constant referencing. Younger students will recognize you as a valuable source and request copies of specific papers. Papers should also be re-read from time to time: just as in watching a film for a second time we may notice something that we previously missed, so it is with re-reading a book or a paper. In short, part of professionalism involves becoming a recognized source of information on a particular topic and keeping abreast of the ever-expanding knowledge in this area.

Further reading

Hart, C. (1998) *Doing a Literature Review: Releasing the Social Science Research Imagination*. London: Sage.

Hart, C. (2001) *Doing a Literature Search: A Comprehensive Guide for the Social Sciences*. London: Sage.

Whitehead, E. and Mason, T. (2003) *Study Skills for Nurses*. London: Sage.

9.9 Formulating aims, objectives, research questions and hypotheses

In the physical sciences it is often the case in research that we are testing the statistical strength of the causal relationship between two or more variables. In these cases it is clear that a hypothesis must be specific to these anticipated events (if X occurs then the result will be Y). However, in other sciences, including the social sciences, other approaches to setting out the parameters of anticipated events are applied, with some being 'loose' and others more 'tight'. For example, in action research an identified problem, and a consideration that some form of intervention might improve it, is a sufficient starting point (McNiff 1992). In psychological research a structured approach to setting out a research question is considered a basic prerequisite to conducting the research (Russel and Roberts 2001). We in no way wish to be prescriptive and argue for one approach over another, as we would accept most parameters to defining the anticipated events, depending on the type of research being conducted, the context in which it is set, the research design and the preferred outcome. However, in this section we outline the four most commonly employed terms to denote the intention of the research. They are often used interchangeably and in everyday parlance this is not problematic. However, in the sciences they frequently cause students a great deal of confusion, and these are the aims, objectives, research questions and hypotheses. Before we do this, however, we need to deal with where they come from, or at least where they ought to.

Gaps in the literature

It cannot be stressed enough that it is command of the literature that is central to identifying gaps in the knowledge. This command means a breadth and depth of reading in your topic area, and involves reading and re-reading on all 'levels', as mentioned above (9:8). When reading, notes should be taken and questions asked at each stage, such as 'What do the authors mean by that; is that a logical assumption; are there any other explanations for that?' It is advisable to write a short report about the paper, identifying its main points, strengths and weaknesses, and any recommendations regarding future research or limitations of the study. By building up your knowledge of the literature in this way you will be in a position to draw an overall map of the subject area showing, chronologically, the development of ideas in this area. Through this the gaps in knowledge should emerge, and these should be the key areas for further research. While replication has its place in the process of verification it is more usual for one research project to 'grow' out of the work of previous research, which then, in turn, stimulates other research and thus contributes to developing knowledge. It is important that in the formulation of aims, objectives, research questions or hypotheses it is clearly demonstrated that they emerge from the literature. This will add strength to the proposed work, will be logical and in itself ought to show a worthwhile proposed project. We accept that there is a debate within the sociological method of research known as grounded theory (Glaser and Strauss 1967) that suggests that an in-depth literature review of the specific topic area being studied may produce a bias. However, Glaser (1992) argued that the literature review in this methodological approach should be undertaken 'around' the topic rather than focusing on it specifically.

Aims and objectives

Aims and objectives are often used interchangeably in everyday usage, and they are often used interchangeably in scientific circles as well. This is because they are seen as much broader and 'looser' terms than either research questions or hypotheses. Aims have several layers of meaning but it should be noted that they share an overall definitional semantic, and that is they are concerned with an intention to achieve a general end product. The principle involved here pivots on the generalization, which is non-specific and non-precise, and it is an intention, or an attempt to do something. Etymologically, the word aim is related to esteem, which is concerned with value and desire. Therefore, this relationship suggests an overall higher order worth that one wishes to achieve. Thus, aim involves an endeavour that incorporates an estimate as to whether the end product is achievable and what the costs of that achievement might entail. In the word aim we have a value for the end product and also a value for the process of endeavouring to achieve that end product.

We can now interpret the word aim in three ways, First, it is an overall goal, or goal state, towards which a series of events, or behaviours, are orientated. These events, or behaviours, must be purposive and planned, as random, reflexive, involuntary actions would not embody the notion of aim. Second, we can interpret aim as an internal mentalistic idea that represents a symbolic thought, or image, of an end product of directed behaviour. In this sense it is internal to the organism but has links to the external environment via behaviour. Third, aim can refer to the end product in the outside world, which has a relationship to the internal psychic state, which is satisfied when the end product is achieved. Thus, in setting out aims in scientific terms we need to state the general end product of what we wish to achieve, through an intention to do so, which implies that it is valuable, worthwhile and desirable.

Objectives, on the other hand, can be interpreted as more specific strategies, or exercises, within the overall aspiration to achieve the end product. They carry a purpose, which is targeted at a destination and can be viewed as part of the plan or policy to fulfil the achievement. They may be more particular and provide more detail than aims, and may deal with special points, specifications and circumstances by which the aim will be achieved.

Research questions

Sim and Wright (2000) argue that there are three basic types of research questions: (a) exploratory; (b) descriptive; and (c) explanatory. Explanatory questions concern the hypothesis and are dealt with below, and here we focus on the former two. Exploratory research questions are by their nature broad and refer to areas of study that are poorly understood, with relatively little known about that area. Exploratory research questions usually have one or more purposes.

- to explore what may be happening;
- to search for new insights;
- to pose questions;
- to assess phenomena in a different light (Robson 1993).

Box 9.3 Examples of aims, objectives, research questions and hypotheses

- The aim of this research is to investigate the relationship between diet, high cholesterol levels, exercise and heart disease.
- One objective is to establish if increased exercise reduces cholesterol levels.
- A research question is 'do subjects change their diet when diagnosed with heart disease?'
- A hypothesis is that the rate of heart disease will decrease at a greater rate in subjects who have received a health education programme than in subjects who have not received the health education programme. The null hypothesis is that there will be no significant change in the heart disease rate.

Descriptive research questions are concerned with providing insights about particular phenomena under investigation within an established research framework of both method and knowledge. It is usual that previous research has been undertaken and a certain level of theory development achieved, if only through established literature. However, it may be that a fuller descriptive account of certain phenomena within the theoretical framework needs to be established and descriptive research questions are appropriate for this. While research designs within the exploratory phase are usually qualitative, they may well be both qualitative and quantitative in descriptive research questions. This means that the instruments used for data collection are usually more clearly specified.

According to Sim and Wright (2000), within the context of empirical research, a research question should fulfil six basic criteria. First, the research questions should be feasible, in two respects: (a) it should be feasible at a conceptual-empirical level, which means that the concepts and propositions stated in the question should be amenable to testing; and (b) it should be feasible to test it in the real world, given the constraints of resources, time and so on. Second, the research question under study should be interesting. It is difficult to maintain enthusiasm and creativity when the question is uninspiring. Third, the criterion of originality should be clearly identified. This links into identifying gaps in the literature as outlined above in this section. It may be that a previously examined topic is studied via a new method or in a different context, or that the time factor has altered the dynamism. It is necessary to show not that a topic has not been covered, but that the research question shows some element of originality. The fourth criterion is relevance. This will be dependent upon whether the research is applied or basic. In basic research the question may be relevant to furthering our understanding or enlarging our knowledge of theoretical processes. In applied research the questions are more specifically targeted, address specific issues and provide solutions to particular problems. The fifth criterion refers to the theoretical basis of the research question. All research questions should be formulated within a theoretical framework, which refers to the ideas and concepts outlined above (9:5). Even though exploratory research questions may be formulated in sketchy areas they none the less need some element of theory. Finally, research questions need ethical legitimacy in three areas: (a) they should not need designs that threaten the rights or welfare of the subjects/participants; (b) they should not be formulated if the pursuance of the research will be used to the detriment of certain individuals, especially if there is no corresponding benefit to others; and (c) they should not be formulated on the basis of political correctness or merely because they are glamorous.

Hypotheses

Hypotheses are tentative conjectures that are expressed in the form of a causal relation between independent and dependent variables, which can be evaluated following empirical testing. When constructing a hypothesis there is no guarantee that it will be verified: if it is it may be incorporated into the accepted scientific body of knowledge, if it is not then it is rejected and another hypothesis is put forward (Nachmias and Nachmias 1981). Hypotheses may originate from theoretical speculation, directly from observation or intuition from internal thought or from a combination of all these approaches. The important point to note is that the origin of the hypothesis is of little significance and much more important is the method of the testing. Nachmias and Nachmias (1981) have argued that hypotheses share four common features. They are: (a) clear; (b) value-free; (c) specific; and (d) amenable to empirical testing with available research methods.

Hypotheses must be very clearly stated. Many students make hypotheses unclear by not defining the conceptual and operational definitions, as discussed earlier. For accurate empirical testing of a hypothesis all the variables in the hypothesis must be operationally defined. Expert help and the scientific literature are invaluable when constructing hypotheses and defining variables. In social science definitions abound regarding a single concept, as we have seen throughout this book, and reviewing the definitions of the variables that you have chosen will be time well spent. The second common feature is that hypotheses must be value-free. In the physical sciences this may be more easily attainable, as the researcher's own values, biases and subjective preferences can be more easily separated from the operations of, say, molecules. Although it is accepted that some unprofessional scientists may well have attempted to influence certain results. However, notwithstanding this, in the social sciences much of the research is a social activity, and as such, influences and biases may readily appear. Rather than denying them, or pretending that they do not exist, it is better to make them explicit and to be aware of their possible influences.

Hypotheses must be specific. This refers to the necessity to explicate the anticipated relations between the variables in relation to direction, which may be positive or negative, and the conditions under which this is maintained. To state that there is a relationship between X and Y does not give us the required level of specificity, as it can be a positive or negative relationship, or it may change over time, space and the unit of analysis. The fourth common feature is that hypotheses must be testable with available methods. Although interesting hypotheses can be created without testable methods they are doomed to languish in the realms of belief, faith or theory. We may hypothesize that there is a God but without a means of testing this it remains in the domain of a religious belief. What is the scientific point of hypothesizing that the planet Pluto is further away from the Sun than the Earth is without a means of measuring this? Therefore, hypotheses in science are closely related to the methods of testing them and these methods often involve new ways of observation, data collection, data analysis and generalization (Nachmias and Nachmias 1981).

Finally, we will briefly mention several types of hypotheses that are often mentioned in scientific circles. The first is the alternative hypothesis, which is a testable statement proposing the anticipated outcome of the study. It may be based on observations, other studies or previous research. The second is the experimental hypothesis, which states that there will be a difference in a measurable outcome between two conditions that are controlled or observed. The third refers to hypotheses in correlations, which propose that there will be a link between two variables. This requires a clear operational definition of the hypothesis, stating how the outcome can be measured. Fourth is the null hypothesis, in which the alternative hypothesis is contradicted. The findings are then referred to as due to chance and statements such as 'no change', 'no difference', 'no effect' or 'no association' are used. The fifth is a non-directive hypothesis, which is concerned about the prediction of the direction of an effect. These hypotheses usually claim that there will be a difference between conditions in an experiment but the direction, positive or negative, cannot be predicted. They are often referred to as two-tailed. Finally, there are directional, or one-tailed, hypotheses, which predict an outcome in one specified direction: positive or negative, higher or lower, better or worse and so on (Russel and Roberts 2001).

Further reading

Russel, J. and Roberts, C. (2001) *Angles on Psychological Research*. Cheltenham: Nelson Thornes Ltd.

Walliman, N. (2000) *Your Research Project: A Step-by-step Guide for the First-time Researcher*. London: Sage.

9.10 Method

It should be clear by now that the scientific process is logically constructed in a sequential manner with one aspect related to the next. In Part Two of this chapter we have seen that the starting point is to read the literature, and from the literature emerge gaps in the knowledge base. From the gaps we formulate aims, objectives, research questions or hypotheses to be tested. Now comes the crucial decision, which involves designing a method to satisfy the requirements of the aims, objectives, research questions or hypotheses, whether exploratory, descriptive or explanatory. The important point to be emphasized is that the method should be able to produce the correct level of measurability or testability. This leads us into the importance of defining the terms method, design and methodology, which often confuse students. Method refers to the specific technique that is to be used in the execution of a research study. For example, it defines the way in which a sample is chosen, the employment, or construction, of a particular data collection instrument, the way in which the data will be analysed and so on. Design refers to the overall plan or framework of a research study and the logical relationship between each stage. It is the structure into which specific methods are located. One scientific approach may apply a number of different designs depending on the type of research being undertaken. Methodology involves the study of the general principles of investigation and is concerned with epistemological, theoretical and philosophical assumptions that underpin it. It is concerned with whether one design or method is appropriate and whether other designs and methods are not.

Quantitative versus qualitative methods

There are few debates in science that have waged as furiously, for so long and with such little resolution as the entrenched argument about which perspective holds the greatest scientific credibility: quantitative or qualitative research. The pivotal issue lurks in the word *credibility*, and this has a long tradition. The terms science and scientific are historically located in the Renaissance period, with the study of the physical and material worlds from Copernicus (1473–1543) onwards. The study of the laws of physics dominated and became supreme with the establishment of irrefutable universal laws. As the study of the human body developed through medicine and later psychology these disciplines tended to adopt the established credible science of the physical world as their template for understanding the body and mind (9:1). On the other hand, the developing discipline of sociology, despite the early attempts to locate it within the traditional notion of science through the work of Auguste Comte (1798–1857), began to develop 'scientific' principles of their own to explain human nature and social relations (Chapter 2). Interestingly, but not surprisingly, this debate raged throughout this period in philosophy too (Chapter 6).

Ian Dey (1993: 3) gives an excellent introduction to the quantitative and qualitative debate and claims that 'it is easy to exaggerate the differences between qualitative and quantitative analysis, and indeed to counter-pose one against the other'. This has grown commonplace, even among eminent scientists and scientific circles. However, despite these polarized positions there is a recognition that a partnership between the sciences would be more fruitful, and collaboration rather than competition would produce better results. This has been reflected in the increased use of statistics by social scientists and the increased appreciation that statistics require inferences and interpretations. Dey (1993) sums this up simply, by suggesting that quantitative data deal with numbers and qualitative data deal with meanings. Indeed they do, but there is a growing overlap between the two perspectives. Rather than dealing with the divisive elements of this polarized debate we briefly outline the approaches that each perspective takes in dealing with the world and where the approaches overlap in scientific terms.

The first area concerns designs. All sciences design the research method to answer the questions that are posed, and these fall broadly into three basic types: (a) experiments; (b) pre-experiments; and (c) quasi-experiments. The classical experimental design consists of two groups of comparable subjects, which are termed an *experimental group* and a *control group*. Both groups are equivalent as far as is possible (matched), except that the experimental group is exposed to the independent variable while the control group is not. To test the effect of the independent variable both groups are pre-tested, the experimental group is exposed to the independent variable and both groups are post-tested. Scores are then analysed. Pre-experimental designs are weaker, in that the sources of internal and external validity are not controlled for. They tend to fall into three types: (a) the one-shot case study, which involves an observation of a single group, event or situation at one point in time, and inferences drawn from it; (b) the pre-test post-test design, which compares a variable with itself, and two measures of the same variable, one before the event and one after it; and (c) the post-test comparison group design, which relies on post-test measures only but employs a comparison group. Both natural and social scientists employ these types of design, depending upon what is being studied.

However, even a cursory glance at a list of research methods from the qualitative and quantitative perspectives reveals that differences occur, not necessarily in relation to the overall design but in the specifics of the methods of data collection, the types of data to be collected and the ways in which the data are analysed. This brings us to the next quantitative or qualitative hurdle to overcome, and that is the population to be studied.

Population sampling

We saw above in 9:6 that in the physical sciences the emphasis is upon testability and generalizability in the search for universal laws. However, in the social sciences, particularly when undertaking qualitative methods, such concepts as representativeness and generalizability imply a single reality that is independent of the context in which action takes place. When studying human actions many of the qualitative approaches take the view that multiple realities exist, and are reliant on circumstances and contexts (Crabtree and Miller 1992). In biomedical science the concern may well focus on the issue of generalizability in relation to, say, the majority of people with a life-threatening condition responding positively to a particular drug. However, social scientists studying cultural responses to a life-threatening condition are less likely to focus on generalizability and more likely to be concerned with cultural diversity of responses. Rather than embroiling ourselves with which emphasis is more important, we just outline the sampling issues in both quantitative and qualitative perspectives.

In an ideal world sampling would not occur and we would involve everyone in all types of research. However, in the real world this is not practical, so we rely on taking a sample of the total population. In quantitative approaches the emphasis is on the mathematical probability that the sample chosen will represent the total or target population. The *target population* is the total collection of cases that the researcher is interested in and is the group to which the generalization will be made. For example, in a general election the target population is the total number of people over 18 years of age who are eligible to vote. The true election would be 100 per cent turn out. However, when researchers are attempting to gauge which way an election is likely to go they must sample. This brings us to the *accessible population*, which refers to the proportion of the target population that the researcher is able to access for a specific research study. This is often termed the *sampling frame*. In our election study, the sampling frame would be those subjects that the researcher was able to gain access to. The *sample* is the actual selection of the accessible population in a particular study and individual cases are termed *sampling units*. There is usually a difference between the *intended sample* and the *achieved sample*, through refusal, drop-out or incomplete follow-up. Thus, the concern in quantitative research is whether the achieved sample actually represents the target population. In an attempt to achieve this they adopt a number of sampling strategies.

The first is simple random sampling, in which 'units are sampled in such a way that each unit has a known, equal and non-zero chance of being selected' (Sim and Wright 2000: 113). Each selection must be independent, with one unit unable to influence the selection of another. Methods to undertake this include drawing numbered balls out of a box, using tables of random numbers and using computer algorithms to select random numbers. The second is systematic sampling with random start, and involves randomly selecting the first unit and then choosing every *n*th number after that. The selection frame must be exhaustive and can be divided according to the sampling number required. The third is cluster sampling. This is useful when the sampling frame cannot be identified or when the sample units are scattered across a wide geographical area. It involves sampling successively smaller units. The fourth is stratified random sampling, which involves dividing the population into homogeneous subsets and then randomly sampling from these strata. The fifth is quota sampling, which is a non-probability sampling strategy but attempts to attain statistical representativeness. Sampling is undertaken in terms of the units fulfilling specific quotas.

Qualitative, or theoretical, sampling also aims to achieve some degree of representativeness but is less concerned with numbers. Two basic approaches are adopted. The first is called *judgemental sampling*, which refers to the researcher making an informed judgement as to those units that will be relevant to satisfying the aims of the study. This tends to rely on the subject (units) having an extensive knowledge in the specific area under study. The second is *convenience sampling*, which simply relies on the availability of the sampling units. This method is used predominantly when there are constraints of time and resources.

Data collection

In designing a research method it is necessary to choose an approach that answers the questions that are posed. For example, if the question relates to why people predominantly choose the colour red for their car, it is pointless merely to count the number of red cars as opposed to other colours, as this will not answer the question 'why?' Similarly, if we wished to ascertain which colour of car is the most common we would not answer this question by asking people why they have chosen a particular colour. In short, the former question may be better studied qualitatively, while the latter lends itself to a quantitative approach. There is considerable overlap between these approaches and it should be pointed out that both quantitative and qualitative analysts may use methods of data collection from both perspectives. The more important point to focus on, and we make no apology for reiterating it, is that the method should answer the question.

Quantitative approaches involve making scores on one, or more, of four levels of measurement. These are: (a) nominal level, which is the weakest level and simply involves classifying objects or observations into categories; (b) ordinal level, which involves a simple relation between properties, e.g. higher, greater, more difficult, better; (c) interval level, which involves knowing the exact difference between each of these observations, with the distance between them remaining constant, i.e. known scales of, say, distance; and (d) ratio level, which involves known natural zero points, e.g. of weight, time, length or area. These measurements are usually undertaken by a number of methods, including index construction, whereby two or more items yield a composite measure, referred to as an index. For example, the crime rate may be obtained by measuring a selection of offences. Scaling methods may be used in which statements within a question are determined by judges. Examples of this are the Thurstone scales, Likert scales and Guttman scaling. Questionnaires may also be used, which consist of a series of items presented in a written format in a fixed order. For example, tick boxes and yes–no questions are often used. Finally, structured interviews may be employed, which are, in short, face-to-face questionnaires in which the interviewer asks the questions and makes the appropriate recording on the structured interview sheet.

Moving towards outlining more qualitative methods of data collection we would like to reiterate that quantitative analysts may also incorporate some of these methods. The first is the semi-structured interview, which is based on a series of open-ended questions that the subject can answer in their own words. Unstructured interviews may be used where the material is highly sensitive and it requires subtle methods of exploration. Both approaches allow the researcher to probe interesting areas of the discourse. The second is the focus group, which involves a number of people being interviewed at the same time and allows the exploration of subject areas. The group is usually selected on the basis of their 'expertise' in a particular area. Third, the Delphi method may be employed, which is a 'systematic collection and aggregation of informed judgements from a group of experts on specific questions or issues' (Reid 1993: 131). It has a series of stages, with the results of each stage informing the next. Fourth are structured observations, which may be undertaken at a set time within a set situational framework. The observations are clearly defined beforehand and undertaken in a systematic way. Fifth, data may be extracted from records or documents, which may be from extant material such as case notes or from 'live' information obtained by asking subjects to keep a diary. Finally, participant observation may be used, whereby the investigator becomes a member of the group being studied.

Data management and storage

Data management and storage are practical issues and are mainly concerned with protecting the data from contamination and protecting the subjects, or participants, from identification. As mentioned above, quantitative data will usually be in the form of sheets of paper as indexes, questionnaires, scales and so on, and these are known as raw data. Each subject sheet (index, questionnaire etc.) should be given a unique code for the researcher's identification purposes only. No other identification of the subject should be made on the instrument (sheet) and the researcher should ensure that if it is necessary to keep a personal identification of the subject then this is kept under password on computer or kept within a locked cupboard/safe (accessible only to the researcher) within a locked room. Similarly, qualitative data are often in the form of transcripts, audio-tape recordings, field notes, diaries and documents, and these should be treated in the same manner. Once the raw data have been put on the relevant computer database, or analysed by 'hand', the raw data should be destroyed and the tapes erased. It is worth pointing out here that it is a good idea for anonymized raw data to be checked by a supervisor or advisor before destruction.

Managing and storing quantitative data usually involves putting the raw data on to a computer database, usually directly into a statistical program or into a spreadsheet that can be imported into a statistical program later. Modern methods of collecting quantitative data include formatting the instruments so that the answer sheet (tick boxes, scales etc.) can be automatically scanned into the database rather than having to be typed in. However, most small-scale research projects do not have these resources. In any event, the raw data have to be put into the database and once the database has been set up this is usually a reasonably straightforward, if laborious, procedure. Qualitative data are often more varied but with the increasing importance of information technology there are now numerous qualitative research software packages that are employed in storing and analysing the data. Taped recordings will need to be transcribed, either for analysis by 'hand' or for inputting into a qualitative database for computer analysis. Transcription is usually worked out at approximately six to eight hours of transcription per one hour of interview, so clearly it can be time consuming and expensive. There are software programs to store visual data such as photographs and film, and others to record huge amounts of discourse from interviews. There are also programs available whereby one can speak directly into the computer and it will input the words spoken, as printed text. All data stored on computer should be kept under password and must be in compliance with the Data Protection Act. Finally, remember to keep back-up copies of all databases and to make sure that they are stored securely as above. The watchwords are confidentiality, anonymity, data protection, passwords, locked storage and back-up files.

Further reading

Abbott, P. and Sapsford, R. (1998) *Research Methods for Nurses and the Caring Professions*. Buckingham: Open University Press.

Sim, J. and Wright, C. (2000) *Research in Health Care: Concepts, Designs and Methods*. Cheltenham: Stanley Thornes (Publishers) Ltd.

9.11 Analysis

Although we have located this section on analysis in its traditional position – that is, following logically on from data collection and management – it should be emphasized that in the real world of research it should be one of the first considerations, and a major one. At the outset of designing a research study it should be decided how the data are to be analysed and whether they will be quantitative or qualitative, and if undertaken correctly it should indicate the design of data collection, the population, how the data will be managed and so on. It is not acceptable to turn up at a statistician's door, or grounded theorist's floor, with reams of raw data and ask 'How can I analyse this?' Knowledge of the analysis should come well before any data are collected. The term analysis has many connotations, but for our purposes there are two to mention. The first refers to the division, breaking up or deconstruction of a physical or abstract whole into its constituent parts. For example, we may take a piece of rock and analyse it for its constituent chemicals, or the psychology of aggression and examine what factors may contribute towards it. Thus, we analyse from the whole to the parts. The second concerns the reverse analysis; that is, examining individual constituent parts and seeing how they fit together to form a coherent whole. For example, we may analyse the orbits of the individual planets and then fit them together into a theory of gravitation, or we may analyse certain human actions and incorporate them into a theory of, say, courtship. In any event, what are important are the relations between the parts and the whole, and the whole and the parts. The kinds of constituents may be viewed as qualitative, while the amount of each constituent part may be viewed as quantitative. In both, it is a question of interpreting what the relations *mean* to us.

Quantitative analysis

Quantitative analysis incorporates statistics and a statistic refers to a datum that is capable of exact numerical representation. Statistics are concerned with the systematic collection of numerical data and its interpretation. The mathematically, or arithmetically, minded appreciate both the use and limitations of the employment of statistics and we hardly need reminding of the Disraeli quote: 'there are lies, damn lies and statistics'. The reason for this disingenuous view of statistics is that given a little 'creative thinking' we can manipulate the use of statistics to reinforce what we wish to reinforce. Thus, statistics are, and in fact need to be, subjected to interpretation by the researcher and others. Most nurses try to avoid the use of statistics and make the, incorrect, assumption that qualitative analyses are simpler – they rarely are. The avoidance of statistics is usually dependent upon the level of sophistication and complexity of formulae. However, with the use of computers today, it is not necessary to understand the arithmetic that comprises the statistical tests, but it is important to know which one is most appropriate and under which conditions. We will now briefly outline a few of the major statistical approaches and the principles under which they are applied.

Correlations

It is often a quest of research to study the strength of association between two variables, e.g. smoking and lung cancer. To do this the data must be collected on at least the ordinal level of measurement (9:10) and the scores must be recorded on both variables for all cases in the sample. In correlation studies it might be of interest to know if the values on one variable move from low to high with a corresponding move in the same direction on the other variable. For example, higher rates of smoking might correlate with higher rates of lung cancer, and this would be considered a positive correlation. However, if higher rates of smoking corresponded to lower levels of lung cancer then this would be considered a negative correlation. No discernible pattern would be considered as no correlation. The strength of the correlation is known as the coefficient and is represented by a positive or negative sign. Figure 9.2 shows the correlation coefficient scale.

Descriptive statistics

There are two main elements to descriptive statistics: (a) measures of average (central tendency); and (b) measures of dispersion (spread). In analysing measures of average we can use the mode, the median and the mean. The mode refers to the score or value that is represented the most times; if the same score is represented twice it is known as bimodal, and if it is represented three times then it is known as trimodal. The median refers to the middle-most score. This is calculated by rank ordering the scores from the smallest to the largest and then eliminating one score from each end until

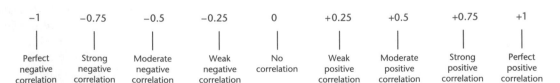

Figure 9.2   The correlation coefficient scale

you are left with one score. If two are left then they are added together and divided by two. The mean, usually called 'the average', is correctly known as the arithmetic mean. This is calculated by adding up all the scores and dividing by the total number of scores.

Measures of dispersion provide us with an index of how spread the data are in relation to the measure of central tendency, and there are four main measures that are used. The *variation ratio*, which is used in conjunction with the mode, can be used with nominal data as well as with continuous data. It is used to calculate the percentage of scores that are not the mode. The *range* is used in conjunction with the median and can be used with any continuous data. The *interquartile range* is also used in conjunction with the median and is a more sensitive measure of dispersion, as it is not affected by extreme scores (outliers). It is the range of the middle 50 per cent of the scores. The *standard deviation* is used in conjunction with the mean, and is the most stringent measure of dispersion. It measures the spread of data around the mean point.

Plotting

Plotting data is a useful way of graphically representing your findings and this is usually undertaken in four ways. The *bar chart* is used for nominal data or plotting average scores for categories. The *x-axis* (horizontal axis) is used for the categories of data and the *y-axis* (vertical axis) is used for the frequency of the occurrences or the average value that is represented. *Histograms* are usually used when the data plotted on the *x*-axis are continuous. *Scattergrams* are used for plotting correlations and the *x*-axis represents one of the numerical measures and the *y*-axis the other. *Frequency polygons*, or line graphs, are used when two sets of data can be directly compared. The *x*-axis should have the scores that have been attained on the task and the *y*-axis should have the frequency of occurrence of the scores.

Non-parametric inferential statistics

These statistical tests are mainly used where the data are nominal or ordinal and they do not make assumptions about the data. They are useful for examining differences, associations and correlations, and allow us to draw certain conclusions from the data being tested. These tests take a step further from descriptive statistics by testing the extent to which two sets of data are distinctly different. They allow the researcher to draw a conclusion as to whether the independent variable is having a true effect on the dependent variable, and following testing there is an accepted hypothesis and a rejected hypothesis. Some non-parametric statistical tests can be seen in Box 9.1.

Parametric inferential statistics

These tests differ from non-parametric tests in a number of ways. First, there is an assumption that the data are normally distributed for the population that is used in the research study. Second, the data are either interval or ratio levels of measurement. Third, the data for both levels of the independent variable have equal variance, or both measured variables have equal variance. Some parametric tests can be seen in Box 9.1, but the three most commonly used ones are the independent *t*-test, the related *t*-test and Pearson's product moment correlation coefficient.

Analysis of variance (ANOVA)

Analysis of variance is a technique in which the total variation associated with recorded scores of an outcome variable is partitioned into distinct components. The analysis tests the significance of each of these components on the total variation. Analysis of variance is used to analyse data from explanatory studies that have several variables under investigation. There are a number of different types of analysis of variance depending on the type of data and experimental design. These include one-way analysis of variance (unrelated), one-way analysis of variance (related), two-way analysis of variance (unrelated), two-way analysis of variance (related) and extensions of analysis of variance.

Qualitative analysis

There are almost as many qualitative analytical approaches as there are researchers undertaking them. However, according to Crabtree and Miller (1992: 17) all these approaches derive from four basic analytic patterns, which fall along a continuum: at one extreme are analytic techniques that are more objective (separate the researcher from the object of research), scientific (valid, reliable, reproducible, accurate and systematic), general (law-like regularities), technical (procedural, mechanical) and standardized (measurable, verifiable). Analytical techniques that share these features are known as quasi-statistical. At the other extreme of the continuum are those subjective qualitative analytic techniques that are considered subjective (emanate from the researcher), intuitive (experience, experimental insight), particular (personal, specific to the context, dependent on the situation), existential (relating to everyday experience), interpretive (related to meaning) and generative (relating to generating theory). These analytical techniques are known as *immersion* or *crystallization* approaches, which represent them on the extreme poles of the continuum. Towards the middle of the continuum are those qualitative analytic techniques that are most commonly used, i.e. editing (more subjective, cut-and-paste type) and template (less subjective, codebook analysis). Although there are differences in analytical approaches to all these techniques, there are a number of general requirements that tend to be needed.

Coding

Coding begins by undertaking a process of reading and re-reading the data many times over. As we mentioned above, re-reading a transcript is likely to reveal something that was missed on the previous reading, so ploughing through the data continuously is likely to provide a rich source of interpretation. As you read, codes and analytic comments can be inserted in the text on the computer. The code may be placed at the beginning of each paragraph and can be distinguished from other strings of words by the use of specific symbols. For example, the code for a particular interlocutor discussing a specific theme could be '@ nurse 136, @ university, @ outpatient, @ conflict'. This gives the researcher a code which can be cross-referenced with other codes as the analysis develops. Analytical interpretations can be entered in the text using '≪ ≫' as brackets and the analyst can insert these as they are reading and re-reading the transcripts/texts. As the analysis develops, and it must be understood here that this is an intensive and time-consuming process, the documents being worked upon should be a complex web of codes and analytical comments. The next stage is category building.

Category building

Category building seems at one level to be a relatively simple matter, and indeed it is if it merely means putting things into piles. However, in qualitative analysis of data we need to be clear as to why a particular comment is placed into a particular category, which means establishing the relations between the comments in the various categories. For example, if we were categorizing shoes, we might put them into piles (subcategories) of colours, or male, female, neutral, or according to type (flat shoes, high-heel shoes, boots, sandals and so on). This would mean that each shoe, in each pile, shares some relation or characteristic that qualifies it to be placed in that pile. With shoes this may be simple, but with qualitative data it raises more difficult issues. First, how do we define an observation of, say, a written comment. Second, how can one observation of a comment be judged to be similar to, related to, another. Clearly, this takes us into the realms of linguistics, semantics, hermeneutics and contexts. Dey (1993: 95) suggested that 'creating categories is both a conceptual and empirical challenge; categories must be "grounded" conceptually and empirically. That means they must relate to an appropriate analytic context, and be rooted in relevant empirical material.' How this is achieved is difficult to explain in so short a space but the starting point is that categories should not be imposed on the data. The categories should emerge from the data and this means reading and re-reading the material.

Splitting and splicing

It is highly likely that the original categorization will need refining, especially if large amounts of data are involved. Therefore, we now need to re-visit each category and re-read the material within it. By doing so we may reveal subcategories within the overall category. This is the process of splitting, and rather than producing more and more categories we can assign codes to the subcategories and maintain them in the overall category formation. Having said that, it may be justified to create another overall category if sufficient evidence is available. Splicing categories means joining categories by inter-weaving the different strands in the analysis. Whereas splitting categories is concerned with greater resolution and detail, splicing provides greater inte-gration and scope. Thus, through splitting and splicing we are refining our thematic analysis until we are satisfied that it is comprehensive and stable.

Linking

Linking data is concerned with how different parts of the data interact or 'hang together'. In qualitative analysis a distinction is drawn between substantive and formal relations. Formal relations are concerned with how things relate to each other in terms of similarity and difference, or not as the case may be. Substantive relations are concerned with how things interact and they may or may not be similar or different. Linking establishes a pathway through these substantive relations.

Triangulation

We finish this section with the issue of triangulation. Triangulation is a term that is used to denote the use of multiple methods of research in an attempt to increase the validity of findings (S. Bradley 1995). It is a term that is 'borrowed' from navigation, whereby one establishes a fixed point by taking bearings from three, or more, compass readings, and establishing where we are by the intersection of these direction lines. In research it involves using different methods to study a particular issue. Crabtree and Miller (1992: 87) argue that 'triangulation refers to both the use of multiple data sources, for example multiple informants, and of multiple methods, such as participant observation and informant interviewing, as well as the use of various records'. This, of course, focuses on data sources, but Crabtree and Miller (1992) also suggest that we can go beyond this to include a triangulation of theoretical perspectives. This includes using methods from both quantitative and qualitative approaches (Denzin 1989). This will involve a process of checking the researcher's interpretation, at each stage of the enquiry, in relation to each specific data source. An example may suffice. Let us say that we wish to study the increase in violence in an accident and emergency (A&E) department and decide to focus on measuring the waiting times before being seen by a doctor. The statistics may show a correlation between the increased waiting times and an increase in violence. However, this may not be the total picture, so we might undertake semi-structured interviews with those who become violent in A&E, and discover that they believe it is not the waiting time that causes the violence but the attitudes of the A&E staff and the way that they are treated while waiting to be seen by a doctor.

This may raise our suspicions and we then use focus groups with the A&E staff, only to discover that they believe that it is the lack of resources, the increased use of alcohol and illicit drugs by those attending A&E and a lack of respect for professionals that reflects the wider societal breakdown of values that is causing an increase in violence. Thus, using different methods, and data sources, we produce a triangulation of results that helps to increase the validity of findings.

Further reading

Crabtree, B. F. and Miller, W. L. (1992) *Doing Qualitative Research*. London: Sage.
Russel, J. and Roberts, C. (2001) *Angles on Psychological Research*. Cheltenham: Nelson Thornes.

9.12 Findings

After all the hard work of designing a study, collecting the data and analysing them, we are now in a position to present our findings. It may seem strange that after all this hard work this is the shortest process to be dealt with! This is because in standard research papers this section is usually one of the shortest, and this is so because we have tended to condense large amounts of information down into a few numbers or illustrations. At least this is the case with quantitative results. The largest section of quantitative data papers follows the results section, and this is the discussion (interpretation) of the results. However, in the presentation of qualitative result, these two sections are often fused.

Presentation of quantitative findings

In these types of research reports the quantitative results are presented in a straightforward, logical and systematic fashion without embellishment, explanation or interpretation. Many students find this section of a research paper the most boring, as findings are presented in a 'cold' and objective manner (the discussion section usually hots things up). What makes them appear 'boring', especially to the untrained eye, is that following their reduction to a series of numbers or graphs, they need explanation to bring them to life. However, let us briefly deal with the basics of quantitative presentation of results. The first point is to keep the commentary short and relevant, and not to drift off into trying to explain them. Second, graphs, charts, illustrations etc. should be kept to a minimum and only those that are meaningful, or at least will be in the discussion section, should be used. In the presentation of statistical results there are a few symbols and numbers that are usually employed, which relate to specific tests. As our example, we use the chi-square test, which is represented by the symbol χ^2. Other tests will use different symbols. The result of a chi-square test is reported as, for example,

$\chi^2 = 3.12$, d.f. $= 2$, $p < 0.05$. We can see that this result falls into three parts. The first is the result of the chi square test $\chi^2 = 3.12$, which is calculated from the data. The second is the symbol d.f. $= 2$, which refers to the degrees of freedom. You do not need to know too much about this at this stage, as statistical tests take it into account. However, the degrees of freedom are the number of subjects minus one $(N - 1)$ or the number of conditions minus one $(C - 1)$. The third symbol, $p < 0.05$, refers to the probability that the findings are not due to chance, and this final figure is arrived at by looking up in a set of tables the previous two figures, i.e. the χ^2 and the d.f., which will then indicate the probability. Computerized statistical packages will do this for you. One other issue to be mentioned is the level of significance, which refers to the extent to which you are prepared to accept that the results occurred by chance (0.05 or 5 per cent).

Presentation of qualitative findings

The presentation of qualitative findings differs considerably, as would be expected, owing to the wide range of data, data collection methods and types of analysis that can be undertaken. There are many terms used to replace the traditional heading of 'results or findings', and these include 'presentation of data', 'producing an account', 'thematic analysis', 'exploration of the data' and so on. However, all approaches share a common feature, and that is they must find a way of summarizing large amounts of data into coherent and concise themes. These themes may be a result of following a series of research stages, or approaches, or they may have emanated from one single study. In any event they should be made explicit, with any linkages established and their relevance to each other stated. As we note above, qualitative results are usually incorporated into the discussion as an interpretation, and this is dealt with in the next section.

Further reading

Campbell, M. J. and Machin, D. (1993) *Medical Statistics: A Commonsense Approach*, 2nd edn. Chichester: John Wiley & Sons.
Dey, I. (1993) *Qualitative Data Analysis: A User-friendly Guide for Social Scientists*. London: Routledge.

9.13 Discussion

Interestingly, the discussion section of a paper is usually the largest part. The question is why? Why is it that a scientific research paper that is structured to be objective and grounded in empirical evidence, through reviewing the literature, formulating hypotheses, designing a method, collecting and analysing data, producing results and establishing facts, then allows a general discussion and subjective interpretation of what has been found? Of course, some would leap to the defence here and claim that the discussion and interpretation of results is part of the scientific process and should be undertaken objectively. This is true. However, without getting embroiled in the philosophical complexities of objectivity versus subjectivity, we can say that it is this area of discussion and interpretation of findings that brings science closer to the experience of being human, and is specifically concerned with what the findings mean to us. If research into the higher mathematics of orbit produced the results that the probability that the orbit of asteroid x would intersect with the orbit of the Earth at the same time and in the same place within less than ten years was $p < 0.0001$, then this would certainly be an interesting finding. However, what does it mean to us as human beings? Thus, the discussion section is both objective and subjective, and should be approached with a view to exposing both elements of the research.

Context of other research

In terms of quantitative research it is customary to discuss the findings of your study in relation to the findings of other research in this field. This is where the earlier literature review comes into its own. If you have done a thorough review of the literature, formulated the index cards and taken brief notes of their main findings, then it is now a relatively easy task to undertake a balanced discussion of the research. It is necessary to break up the discussion into a number of main points that may relate to your own findings. For example, you may write something like the following: 'In this current research we found that the rates of aggression and violence in the A&E were on the increase (p < 0.001) and the reasons given for this were increased waiting times (72 per cent), increased drug and alcohol intake (42 per cent) and lack of resources (22 per cent). This was supported by Green (1990), who reported 68, 38 and 23 per cent respectively. However, it was not supported by Brown's (1994) study, in which she reported bad attitudes of staff in A&E as being accountable for the highest reported cause of increased violence and aggression (76 per cent). It should be noted, however, that the main difference between the studies was that both our current research and that of Green (1990) was conducted in an inner city area, whereas Brown's (1994) study was conducted in a rural setting.' And so on (references are fictitious). Although this is only a short example it gives a flavour of how the balance of studies should emerge. The balance is in relation to the research studies and your own, and the interpretation is your explanation as to why they may or may not support your findings.

In terms of the qualitative research discussion section, as we note above (9:12), the presentation of the data, the analysis and the discussion may well be meshed together to give an indication of how we act, react and interact in the real world. The major problem with qualitative research is the vast amount of data that is usually produced and the need to reduce it to the thematic categories mentioned above (9:12). The presentation of qualitative data may follow the categories that have been identified, and usually employs an example of a question that has been posed, an example of the subject's response and then an interpretation. The interpretation should involve both a grounded explanation (what it may mean in real life) and a theoretical explanation (what it may mean in theory building). Both qualitative and quantitative discussions, or presentations, should address the aims, objectives, research questions or hypotheses that were set for the study, and you should identify whether you met their requirements or not. If not, then you need to explain why. Make sure that the discussion or presentation is very closely related to your analysis and the results that you have produced. There is nothing worse than the production of significant results from a profound analysis, followed by a totally unrelated and rambling discussion or interpretation.

Other discussion elements

The discussion may include other elements, and the ones that we focus on here are: (a) future directions; (b) limitations and modifications; and (c) conclusions and recommendations.

Future directions

Part of the discussion may also include a review of the possible future directions of research in this field, which emerge as a result of your studies. It is important that you do not be too grandiose in this, but ensure that whatever direction you point to is at least a small step further that is both worthwhile and achievable. By identifying future directions you are highlighting the gaps in the current knowledge base, and this is important for two reasons. First, it focuses on the areas that should be studied in order to contribute to the developing theory in this field, and this informs the progression of the human condition, however small. Second, it offers a sensible and logical approach for others to follow, as well as yourself, in order to engage in the next wave of research.

Limitations and modifications

You might wish to incorporate this section within the discussion as a short piece or you might prefer to make this a separate section following on from the discussion. In any event it shows an element of scientific maturity to outline the limitations to your study. All research studies are limited to one degree or another, so do not think that you are courting unjustified criticism by highlighting the limitations. In fact, on the contrary, it is more likely to deflect criticism if you have engaged in self-critique, as an individual author or as a research team. It is highly likely, having gone through the entire research project, that you will be very clear as to the limitations; however, if not then think through the research design and ask yourself a number of questions. For example, was the design appropriate to meet the aims, objectives etc.? Was the sample sufficient? Were any biases introduced? Were the data collected, managed and analysed appropriately? And so on. You can then finish off this section with a series of modifications to improve the next research study. For example, you may identify a limitation to your study as too small a sample, and the modification should be that this should be increased in future studies. This shows that you are able to identify the limitations, learn from your mistakes and correct them for future research.

Conclusions and recommendations

Again, these can be included at the end of your discussion section but equally can be a separate section following on from the limitations. It is important that the conclusions and recommendations come out of your research. If they do not then leave them to someone else to produce. The conclusions should briefly summarize what you have done in your study and you should not add more information at this stage. A brief summary is the best means of covering the central issues of your study. This will make for easy reading and it also leaves the reader with the main points in mind. The recommendations should be clearly stated and reasonable. That is, they should be achievable within a reasonable time-frame and given reasonable resources. A few sensible recommendations are better than an extensive list designed to change the world.

Further reading

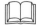

Redman, P. (2001) *Good Essay Writing: A Social Sciences Guide*. London: Sage.

9.14 Writing proposals

On many nursing courses it is a requirement to construct a research proposal. On undergraduate courses this may involve writing a proposal as a form of assignment, which is then presented for marking, but on some postgraduate nursing courses it is a requirement to write a research proposal, seek ethical approval, conduct the research and write up a thesis. The reasons for this focus on nurses undertaking research relates to the move towards evidence-based practice and the need to ensure that nursing care is based on rational scientific approaches rather than personal beliefs or preferences. This is also coupled to the rationalization of the NHS, which recognizes the limited resources and the need to ensure that all health care is delivered effectively and with minimum wastage. It can also be argued that it forms part of the nursing quest towards professionalism and an attempt to keep abreast of our colleagues in the other professions allied to medicine. Constructing proposals is necessary, not only for carrying out research itself, but also for presenting projects or policies to management groups or for attempting to obtain research grants from external bodies. Whatever the reason for constructing a proposal, it should be emphasized that it is often a more time consuming exercise than it would at first appear to be.

Structure and content of a research proposal

Proposals vary considerably in their structure. There is such a wide variety of sources that proposals are submitted to that it is difficult to identify the numerous structures that may be necessary, as each source may have different requirements. Therefore, in this section we have focused on a general structure that tends to be required for submitting *research* proposals, and the student may select their own particular format for their own requirements. In working up a proposal, of any kind, it is worthwhile spending time to ensure that it is as perfect as possible, for two main reasons. First, when writing a proposal you are writing the entire project 'in your head', whether this is a proposal for research or a proposal for a book. Second, it is usually the case that what you write in a proposal can be used in writing up your project after completion. So, the words that you use in a proposal are never 'wasted'. We reiterate that not all proposals require every section that we are about to outline, and many may require extra sections.

Title

The title should make sense and not merely be constructed to attract attention. It should relate to the content of the work and the reader should be able to have a good idea as to what the body of the work is concerned with. In many cases you may be asked for a short title and a long title, so give this some thought and be prepared.

Abstract

This should be succinct, usually between 200 and 300 words, and should be structured carefully. It should be structured according to the project and should flow from one section to the next, as in the project itself. For example, if it is a research proposal then it should cover the structure of the research. Abstracts should summarize the work but should also be comprehensive enough for readers to be clear on the overall project.

Introduction

The introduction should be 'funnel-shaped'. That is, it should start out very broad and finish with a very narrow focus. For example, if a project was being undertaken on violence in the A&E department then the introduction could begin with some general statements about aggression and mankind, moving on to violence in society, followed by contemporary health care settings and the increase in aggression, and closing with violence in the A&E. The introduction should be broad, and it should identify any problems that the project is concerned with.

Background

The background section is usually employed when the context in which the project is being undertaken is unusual or is likely to be unknown for the majority of readers. Specialist areas may need a background section to set the project in context. For example, if research was being undertaken on the health needs of travelling communities it might be beneficial to use a background section to identify the differences between these communities and the health needs of static communities. The reader should have a clearer idea of the need for this particular project after reading the background section.

Literature review

This is one of the most important sections of any project and it cannot be stressed enough that the literature review should be comprehensive. Even if the literature review section is going to be short, the actual review of it should be covered extensively. Seminal works and major publications should be incorporated, as well as related material from a wide variety of sources. The literature review should be logically structured, with a series of subheadings that break up the work into clear, concise and manageable sections. It should also be up to date, with coverage of the very latest material. If recent work has been left out then this will reflect very badly on the overall project. The literature should be managed carefully, with a balanced approach, which is critical without being prejudiced. The literature review should also be used to identify a theoretical or conceptual framework in which you can locate your own project. The literature review should identify any gaps in the knowledge base, which will then logically suggest the need for your own project.

Aims, objectives, research questions and hypotheses

These should emanate from the literature. If the literature review has been undertaken correctly, then the aims etc. should come clearly out of the gaps that have been identified. They should be clearly stated, in as simple terms as possible and with only one relationship established in each hypothesis. They should also be realistic. It is better to have simple aims that can be achieved rather than grand ones that are more likely to fail.

Method

The method section should be appropriate to meet the requirements of the aims etc. It is always helpful if the method itself is explicitly stated; for example, 'an experimental method will be used', or 'for the purposes of this study a grounded theory approach will be adopted'. The method section should incorporate a discussion of the strengths and weaknesses of other methods and the reasons why they have been dismissed in favour of the chosen method. If this is undertaken correctly then this will 'fit' into the aims etc. The method section should be subdivided into a number of subsections. First, the population should be clearly stated. This should include who the subjects will be, how many it is intended to sample, where they are located and how they will be reached. It should also include an explanation as to how the sample has been established and how you have arrived at the numbers stated. You may also establish the inclusion and exclusion criteria, and the details of any matching that is to be undertaken. You may also comment on the issue of the generalizability of your sample to the overall population.

The second subsection of the method section is data collection, and this should include an explanation of the type of data that are to be collected. If they are numbers relating to attitudes on a measurement scale, or audio-taped discourse concerning the policy on asylum seekers, then state this clearly. Simple clear statements are far more beneficial than esoteric and abstruse commentary. The third subsection is the data management component, and this should be explained in terms of what data are being managed, where they will be stored, when they will be transferred on to the computer and the raw data destroyed and how they will be safeguarded. The fourth subsection is data analysis. This should be explained carefully and should fit clearly into the type of data that are collected. Explain clearly how the analysis will achieve the requirements of the aims etc., and what the anticipated outcomes might be. The analysis subsection is an opportunity to show the depth of knowledge that you have, or should have, regarding the research method, and if this subsection is weak then it will suggest an overall weakness to the project.

The final subsection involves ethical issues. Although you may deal with this as a separate section it can be incorporated as a subsection of the method section if preferred. In any event it should mention the various ethics committee approvals that are required, such as local research ethics committee (LREC), multi-site research ethics committee (MREC) and internal committees. Anonymity, and how this will be maintained, should be clearly explicated. The voluntary status of the subjects should be mentioned and the question of informed consent dealt with. The Data Protection Act should be mentioned and how the data are to be secured should be identified.

Results

The results should be clearly stated in a straightforward manner without embellishment. They should link into the data analysis and should be appropriate to the aims etc. The results section is often a bland report in an objective fashion, without explanation or other commentary.

Discussion

In assignments, theses and publications there should be a discussion section. However, if a proposal is being constructed then it is unlikely to have such a section. The discussion should be balanced and deal with both your own results and those of the literature. The discussion should also deal systematically with the aims, objectives etc., and should state whether they have been achieved or not, as the case may be. The discussion is the section of the paper in which you are allowed some degree of subjective interpretation.

Resources required

This section should cover the financial aspects of the proposal and include all materials that will be used. Depending on the requirements of the grant source this section may be very detailed. It should include stationery, office equipment, computer hardware and software, travelling and subsistence, and the employment of any research assistants, secretarial support or other payments. If the project is located in a university there is likely to be university overheads (usually 40 per cent).

Research management

This involves establishing research supervision at the appropriate level and in specialist areas. All research, and other projects, should have supervisors and advisors to ensure a close scrutiny of quality. A research or project steering group should be identified, who are recognized experts in their own field. This group may only meet on two or three occasions, usually at the outset of the project, at an interim level during the project and again at the end. A research working group should also be established, usually two or three people closely involved in the project who will meet on a regular basis and have a hands-on approach. It will involve the lead project manager, any assistants and close workers on the project.

Time-frame

The proposal should have a project time-frame in which the milestones of the project are set out and given a date by which they should be achieved. This should be realistic and include time for holidays, writing up reports and some leeway for emergencies. Be careful with the time-frame, as you are likely to be judged against it.

Conclusions and recommendations

These should be logically drawn from the study and should be realistic and achievable. In a proposed project this section may be entitled 'anticipated outcomes', in which you may outline what benefits there are likely to be from undertaking your project.

References

These should be set out accurately and completely and they are often checked, so be careful with this section. Sloppy referencing usually means a sloppy project.

Appendices

This section should include any material that you have mentioned in the proposal and that is important enough to contribute to the reader's understanding. It may include any measuring instruments that are used or outcomes that have been identified.

We conclude this section with a reiteration of an emphasis, and that is to take time with any proposal to ensure that it is a quality piece of work. This will enhance your chances that your proposal will be accepted.

Further reading

Girden, E. R. (2001) *Evaluating Research Articles from Start to Finish*, 2nd edn. London: Sage.
Rudestan, K. E. and Newton, R. R. (2000) *Surviving Your Dissertation*. London: Sage.

9.15 Conclusions

Nursing has undergone a significant shift in response to the changing societal expectations of health care delivery. Traditionally seen as a practical endeavour alone, nursing is now deeply concerned with establishing its practices in relation to a sound theoretical body of knowledge. The need to produce evidence-based practices has never been so urgent, and nursing courses are now concerned with the processes and content that underpin this knowledge. Limited resources and the increased use of courts following mistakes in health care delivery have provided another impetus for nurses to be accountable for their care. The days of nursing practices, which particular influential nurses might have engaged in, based on personal preferences and myth are now gone. It is important in the development of the nursing profession that contemporary students of this profession are not only aware of the role of science but also skilled in its application. In this chapter on thinking science we have unravelled some of the major issues that contribute to engaging in scientific enquiry. The major thrust of the chapter is concerned with a mental shift in nurses, which moves them from a simple 'hands-on' view of nursing to one that focuses on a scientific approach to nursing care.

10

Thinking writing

10.1 Introduction

Following closely on from the previous chapter on thinking science, we are now concerned with thinking writing. The commonly heard phrase among nursing students – 'I don't want to write, I just want to nurse' – is now, in contemporary health care delivery, yet another anachronism. Again, this is due to a number of factors, including the bureaucratization of the NHS, the professionalization of nursing and the increase in litigation. The writing or, more accurately, recording, of nursing actions is of central importance and it should not be underestimated. Writing is a communication system by which we can transfer our ideas from within us to others in the external world, and through this we can engage in debate and contribute to the development of both theory and practice. Although there are such people as gifted writers, we argue that for the majority of us it is a skill that needs to be developed. It can be seen in a similar vein to driving a car, in which there are a set of skills that need to be practised and then brought together in one overall activity, and a set of rules of the road that need to be learnt and followed. Nurses are asked to write on a daily basis, particularly in relation to outlining what nursing care has been delivered, and this recording is vitally important. However, nurses increasingly need the skills of writing in order to construct assignments, projects, proposals, dissertations and publications of one description or another. Furthermore, nurses are often requested to sit on various committees and are likely to be involved in the construction of official reports. They are also frequently asked to be involved in writing policies and procedures and will need a high level of writing ability to do this. Finally, it should be remembered that many of the documents that nurses write, including dissertations and theses at masters level and above, are public documents. This means that they are accessible by members of the public, usually through university libraries, and should be of a good quality to prevent a diminution of the professional status of nursing.

PART ONE: THEORY

10.2 Referencing

We have seen throughout this book that nursing is moving ever more towards evidence-based practices by underpinning its approach with scientific enquiry, and a major part of this process involves the accurate use of referencing. Referencing is now such a vital aspect of nursing, in both theoretical and practical terms, that its importance cannot be stressed enough. When called upon to outline a nursing care plan, it is no longer acceptable to conjure up an approach that appears merely 'like a good idea at the time'. Now, the patients, the public, the profession and the courts of law require nursing care to be based on evidence, and this evidence must be clearly referenced. Referencing involves identifying the source of the evidence, which must be done extremely accurately, precisely and according to a stringent set of rules.

Timing and types of references

In short, there are three rules regarding when a reference source is needed, and the first is when other people's words have been used. There is nothing wrong with using other people's words, but if you do so, then you need to give credit for them and let the reader know by whom, when and where they were stated. The second rule refers to the production of specific evidence in the form of statements that are often made. For example, we may often hear someone make a comment such as '90 per cent of people say that . . .' or 'most of the people believe . . .', without explaining where the evidence for those comments originates. In the cut and thrust of debate this may be tolerated, but in the written word it is not acceptable without the reference source. The third rule, and closely related to the second, is the use of grand statements. We are all fond of using a grand statement to stress a point but this will need a reference source if it is going to be convincing. For example, a grand statement such as 'nursing is the Cinderella service of health care' would need a reference source, of which there are many.

A glance at a number of journals in the library will very quickly reveal a wide range of referencing styles, and each publishing house has a preferred format. However, we can identify three broad types within which these minor variations are placed. The first is the *legal system*, commonly used in legal circles and in official reports. This system involves the use of footnotes at the bottom of each page on which the reference is used. Explanatory notes are also employed in this manner. The advantages of this method include that the reference is supplied on the page on which it is used, but the main disadvantage is that if used extensively it can break up the flow of reading. The second is the *Vancouver system* of referencing, in which small numbers are used in the text to indicate a reference and these are then placed numerically in the reference list at the back of the paper or book. This system of referencing is more popular in the US literature. The third referencing style is the *Harvard system*, which is more widely used by UK publishing houses and involves putting the names of the authors and the year of publication in the text and listing them alphabetically in the reference list at the back of the paper. As this system is the most commonly used approach in the UK, we focus on it in a little more detail in the next subsection.

The Harvard referencing system

In the Harvard referencing system there are two main elements: (a) using references in the text; and (b) compiling the reference list at the end of the paper, chapter or book. Using references in the text involves two further aspects: first, the use of *primary sources*, which refers to using the original author's work; second, the use of *secondary sources*, which involves using another author's interpretation of an original author's work. It is usually better to deal with primary sources whenever possible. Using primary reference sources in the text involves the following rules. (Please note the references used in this section are fictitious.)

- Actual quotes with author name not used in the sentence require the following: 'quoted text' (Smith 1995: 136). Note the page number quoted (i.e. 136). If two authors had written the quote then the reference would be (Smith and Brown 1995: 136). If three or more authors were involved then it would read (Smith *et al.* 1995: 136).

- Actual quotes with the author's name used in the sentence would require the following: Smith (1995: 136) stated that 'quoted text'. Or, with two authors: Smith and Brown (1995: 136) stated that 'quoted text', and so on. Note that the authors' names are part of the sentence and it would not be grammatically correct without them. Also note that the brackets are used for the date and page numbers only.

- General statements about authors' work but not actual quoted words would require the following (for example): Nursing is now seen as a Cinderella service (Smith 1995). For multiple authors you would have (Smith and Brown 1995) and so on. If more than one reference source was being used in support of this general statement then this might be: Nursing is now seen as a Cinderella service (Smith 1995; Green and Turner 1998; Miller *et al.* 2000). Note that the sources are separated by semi-colons and that they are ordered chronologically.

For secondary sources the rules overlap with those for primary sources, with one explicit difference: citing a reference that is mentioned in another source. In this situation you have read the book that is citing another author's work but you have not actually read that source. This is referenced as Smith (1995, cited in Brown and Green 2000). In this situation you have read Brown and Green's work and cited Smith.

When compiling the reference list, accuracy and precision are the watchwords. They may need to be checked or used by others so they must be able to be tracked down. There are three main reference sources that are used and these are outlined below. However, the reader should be aware that all sources can be referenced and there are set ways in which they should be recorded.

- Complete book. Smith, J. and Jones, M. (2000) *Study Skills*. London: Grimley Publications. Note the authors, date of publication, title with emphasis, place of publication, publisher.
- Chapter in a book. Smith, J. (2000) Diabetic nursing, in C. Brown and J. Williams (eds) *Holistic Nursing*. London: Grimley Publications. Note the author of the chapter, date of publication, title of the chapter, editors, title of the book with emphasis, place of publication and publisher.
- Journal article. Green, A. (2000) What it means to be a nurse in the new millennium, *Journal of Nursing Approaches*, 10(1): 42–54. Note the author, date, title of the paper, journal, volume number, issue number in brackets, page numbers.

Other referencing sources

Any source can be referenced, with the main point being that it should be accurate and the reader should be able to acquire it if needed. Unpublished material can be referenced as long as the author, the title of the work, whose property it is and where it can be accessed are known. Newspaper articles require the name of the newspaper, the year, the title of the article, the author if available, the day and month and the page numbers if possible. Government reports require the Government Office, year, title of the report, command numbers, place of publication and publisher. Videos require title, year, producer, director, length of video, where it is located and its form (e.g. videocassette). The Internet requires the title, the year, names and addresses, the Internet address and when it was accessed.

Further reading

Whitehead, E. and Mason, T. (2003) *Study Skills for Nurses*. London: Sage.

10.3 Construction

Whatever is being written, whether large-scale projects such as a book or small-scale exercises such as writing a letter, it should be thought through first and planned in depth. When you plan out the project it is being constructed within your own mind and if the structure is well designed it is then merely a question of 'filling it in'. However, this emphasizes the importance of planning it thoroughly and meticulously. In building a framework for a project it is a relatively simple matter to adjust the structural elements until one is satisfied with it. However, it should be noted that this is best undertaken *before* we start writing rather than during it. The skeleton of the project will strongly influence how it will look on completion, so time taken at the beginning is valuable time well spent.

The structure of a project is vitally important for a number of reasons. First, a structure will provide a logical progress through a project, which will indicate a beginning, a middle and an end. Second, it will break up large amounts of text into manageable proportions, which will assist readers in taking in the information. Third, a structure will categorize 'types' of text into appropriate sections, which deal with material in distinct ways. For example, the text of the introduction is very different from the text of the results (9:12). Fourth, a structure will provide an interconnectedness of ideas from one element to the next. Fifth, it will allow both the reader and, especially, the author to 'see' the overall argument that is being produced, and the author can write the content in manageable and achievable sections. Finally, a structure will allow the author to plan how many words each section should, and will, have. This is vital when writing for publications that give quite a prescriptive number of words.

Let us now look at constructing a project in a little more detail. The construction of a project, assuming that you have read all the material that you need to, and that you are ready to begin, or at least to think about beginning, to write. The structure of a project should be consistently applied throughout the entire work and the reader should be able to identify where one section, or subsection, fits in the overall project. There is no agreed set structure, but one that is commonly, and effectively, employed utilizes capitals, lower case, bold, underline, italic and indent in a specific format, which provides a clear framework of headings, subheadings and sub-subheadings. An example of this can be seen in Box 10.1.

As we have seen above (9:14), the structure of a research paper is pretty well standard, with an introduction, literature review, aims, method, results, discussion and conclusions. However, other types of papers, reports and projects need to be given a structure of one description or another. In planning out a structure begin with a basic framework of, for example, (a) introduction, (b) background, (c) literature review, (d) main body, (e) proposed plan of work, (f) resources required, (g) anticipated outcomes, (h) conclusions. Remember that these can be changed as you develop your project. Now, within each section identify a number of bullet points that

---

Box 10.1   Example of a structure of a project

TITLE (upper case and bold)
   Introduction (lower case and bold)
   Background (lower case and bold)
   Literature Review (lower case and bold)
      Experimental Studies (lower case and underline)
         Studies with random control (lower case and italicize)
         Studies without randomization (lower case and italicize)
      Quasi-Experimental Studies (lower case and underline)
         Rural populations (lower case and italicize)
         Urban populations (lower case and italicize)
      Anecdotal Evidence (lower case and underline)
         Professionals (lower case and italicize)
         Patients (lower case and italicize)
   Aims and Objectives (lower case and bold)
   Method (lower case and bold)
      Population (lower case and underline)
      Data Collection (lower case and underline)
      Data Management (lower case and underline)
   Resources Required (lower case and bold)
   Ethical Implications (lower case and bold)
   Anticipated Outcomes (lower case and bold)
      Short term (lower case and underline)
      Medium term (lower case and underline)
      Long term (lower case and underline)
   Research Management (lower case and bold)
   Time-frame (lower case and bold)
   References (lower case and bold)

---

may divide up each subsection into a number of paragraphs. Each section can be allotted a number of words.

Further reading

Fairbairn, G. J. and Winch, C. (1996) *Reading, Writing and Reasoning: A Guide for Students*. Buckingham: Open University Press.

10.4 Grammar, syntax and punctuation

Many nurses have a fear of writing and have a crisis of confidence when they need to construct an essay, assignment or project for presentation for others to read. The basis of this trepidation is usually that their grammar, syntax, punctuation and spelling is considered to be weak and they feel somewhat ashamed of their written work. Largely this is unfounded, and it is more usual that it is a question of being a little 'rusty' or lacking in confidence. With modern day information technology and word processing packages, mistakes can be very quickly rectified and there is ample opportunity to practise with writing skills. Writing *is* a skill that can be learnt, practised and reworked until the finished product is satisfactorily completed. In this short section we will not deliver a lesson in English language, but suggest ways in which you can *think* about improving your written word.

Working the words

The basic assumption that we make is that readers of this text are likely to have a sufficient level of education to enable them to write a project, even if English is not the first language in which they have been educated. Therefore, if you have planned out your project, as indicated in the previous sections of this chapter, and have read the required literature, then writing is your next concern. The first thing to overcome is the fear of the blank page, so write, scribble or doodle on the page if this is a problem, to eliminate the starkness of the white sheet of paper. Remember that only you will see the first draft of your work. Therefore, do not worry about grammar or spelling at this early stage of writing. When constructing the paragraph remember that it should have one main point only and whether this is stressed in the first sentence or the middle sentence of the paragraph is a personal choice. The other sentences of the paragraph should support this one main point. Paragraphs should be approximately 200–300 words in length.

Rather than explaining the constituent parts of a sentence, such as a verb, a noun, an adjective, we feel that it would serve better to ask the reader to write a series of sentences to construct a paragraph. It is the reading of the writing that will now prompt you to 'tidy up' the grammar, punctuation and spelling. We consider words, sentences, paragraphs and projects to be like pieces of clay in an overall work of sculpture. This means that we can shape, reshape and mould each part until we are happy with the overall work. Common problems with sentence construction usually relate to the fact that the sentences do not link into each other. One sentence should relate to the next one within an overall paragraph, which reinforces one main point. The single most important point that we wish to stress in relation to improving your writing is to read and re-read your work over and over again in order to see if it can be enhanced in any way. Try out different words by using a thesaurus and manipulate the sentences until you are satisfied with them. Once you have completed your project it is important that you undertake recension; that is, revisit the manuscript for further checking and editing, yet again. It is this process of constantly re-reading one's own work, which we feel nurses are generally poor at, that will improve it considerably. Nurses seem to have, in our experience, a reluctance about re-reading and checking their own work, which is evidenced by spelling mistakes and obvious grammatical errors. No matter how good, or poor, a writer one is, re-reading the work will highlight the common errors and improve the overall quality.

Further reading

Redman, P. (2001) *Good Essay Writing: A Social Sciences Guide*. London: Sage.

10.5 Academic style

When writing assignments, projects, proposals and so on, it is customary to write in a particular style, and this style has distinct elements to it that differentiate it from other modes of writing. We will all be familiar with the writing style of a novel, a letter or a poem, and each will be different from the others. This is also the case with an academic piece of writing, and like the others it has a set of rules that distinguish it from other modes of constructing a written piece of work. The academic style can be summed up as an attempt to bring an objective overview to the topic that is being written about, and is focused on qualification, argumentation and a balanced point of view.

Balance and synthesis

The rules associated with writing in an academic style include a number of simple but important points. The first is concerned with avoiding the use of the personal pronoun 'I'. Although there is a debate regarding this, particularly in sociological circles, in which some argue that it adds an important subjective element based on personal expertise, it remains a taboo in most academic writing. Therefore, avoid using terms such as 'I believe that . . .', 'I think that . . .', 'I said that . . .'. The alternatives to this include 'This author believes that . . .', 'In this writer's opinion . . .'. However, some caution should be noted with this usage, as it can become rather clumsy, and it should be avoided altogether wherever possible.

The second rule concerns the balance and synthesis of argumentation. When constructing an academic piece of work it is important that you do not merely provide evidence in support of your own views, ideas or research findings. Alternative views must be put forward and any other interpretations that may be drawn should be highlighted. Do not think that you are drawing negative attention away from your point of view towards evidence that does not support your ideas, as, on the contrary, you will be showing that you have thought through the alternatives thoroughly. It will strengthen your own point of view if you can show that you have balanced all the arguments and drawn your conclusion from a thorough analysis and synthesis of all the related work. The argument is produced out of the balance of the literature, and will emerge logically if the literature is weighed effectively.

The third rule for the academic style concerns peer review. As we outlined in the previous section (10:4), nurses are, generally, poor at recension of their own texts and they are equally poor at having their work peer reviewed. Once you have produced your manuscript and you have read and re-read it for checking and a final editing, it is important that an appropriate colleague reviews it for you. However, ensure that you do not fall foul of university or college rules regarding the production of your own work for assignments. Notwithstanding this, if you are producing other work that is not part of a course then a peer review is of vital importance. Ensure that the reviewer is of sufficient academic standing to be able to critique your work appropriately, and be prepared to take their comments in good grace. This process will improve the quality of your work.

Further reading

Blaxter, L., Hughes, C. and Tight, M. (1998) *The Academic Career Handbook.* Buckingham: Open University Press.
Redman, P. (2001) *Good Essay Writing: A Social Sciences Guide.* London: Sage.

10.6 Permissions and ethics

Yet another corollary of the massive growth in the literature on health care is the need to reference other people's work, and this needs to be done with great caution (10:2). The use of other authors' work allows you to provide evidence for your own statements, but there are a set of rules that must be complied with. Copyright laws are complicated and serious, so treat others' work with the respect that it deserves. Referencing was covered in section 10:2 and here we briefly reiterate the basics of using others' written prose and expand on using other types of work.

Referencing words

If using the verbatim written words of another's work then you must make sure that you provide the author's name, date of publication and the accurate source of where it has been published. It is customary to use up to approximately 400 words of prose without having to ask permission to use them. However, you must provide a correct reference for the quote. If using longer quotes then you must ask permission to use them from the publisher and in some cases the actual authors themselves. The publisher will usually send you a form on request and you will need to indicate the exact words that you wish to reproduce. It can take several months, so request this early. In some cases publishers may make a charge to grant permission and it can be expensive. To avoid making too many requests to reproduce others' work many authors employ the use of paraphrasing, which involves using your own words to interpret what another author has stated. This free expression of another person's statement needs to do justice to the main essence of what they have said and should maintain the sense of their rendition.

Referencing other types of work

If you are using tables, graphs, illustrations, pictures and so on that other authors have constructed, and you are using them exactly as they have used them, then it is highly likely that you will need to seek their permission as above. Once permission has been granted you will need to acknowledge this with such words as 'reproduced by kind permission of . . .' and also provide the full reference. If you alter it in any way then you will need to provide the full reference and let the reader know that you have changed it in some way with the statement 'adapted from . . .'. If you are in any doubt then it is better to request permission. Finally, we need to point out that although it is a legal matter relating to the laws of copyright, it is also an ethical issue, as the work belongs to someone else. Most authors like to be referenced and in our experience most permissions to reproduce others' work are granted.

Further reading

Baxter, R. (1995) *Studying Successfully*. Richmond: Aldbrough St John Publications.

PART TWO: APPLICATION TO PRACTICE

10.7 Information technology

Like it or loathe it, information technology (IT) is here, and here to stay. IT governs almost every aspect of our lives and health care is no exception. Computers are used as much in GP surgeries as they are in hospital settings, and nurses are called upon to use them in every area of nursing. For many, IT causes fear, alarm and avoidance, while others appear to enjoy every new development. The single most important point that we can make is that avoiding the basics of IT will very quickly lead to another form of illiteracy. Therefore, we emphasize that it is vital that you identify your strengths and weaknesses in relation to IT and address any limitations that you see.

Language

One of the first things that is noted when dealing with IT is the language that is used relating to the component parts, and as with all foreign languages it is a little worrying when we do not understand what is being said to us. Do not be put off by the IT jargon and try to learn what the terms actually mean. There are numerous user-friendly guides to various aspects of IT.

Uses of information technology

As we note above, IT is used widely in health care settings and we outline several uses here. First, there are computer-assisted learning (CAL) programs that will teach students about various aspects of health. The number of these programs is growing daily and nursing students will be expected to work through health-related courses on the computer. Second, the Internet is being increasingly used as a learning tool, and there is a considerable amount of information available on health-related matters. Third, there are communication uses of IT, with shift rotas, diaries and electronic mail used to relay information about staffing issues. Fourth, IT is used for recording information about patient care and can be used for planning what will be done as much as recording what has already happened. Fifth, IT now assists us with analytical packages, both statistical and qualitative, for research purposes. Finally, there are numerous word-processing packages that students are expected to use to write essays, assignments, dissertations and so on. Thus, we can see that the use of IT is varied and most universities, colleges and hospital trusts will have facilities for staff and students to learn the various packages that are available. The most important point to reiterate is that avoiding the issue will not assist you in any way and will only compound the problem. Therefore, addressing any weaknesses in relation to the use of IT is central to developing one's career.

Further reading

Thede, L. Q. (1999) *Computers in Nursing: Bridges to the Future.* Philadelphia: Lippincott.

Barbercheck, M., Cookmeyer, D. and Wayne, M. (2001) *Women, Science and Technology: A Reader in Feminist Science Studies.* London: Routledge.

10.8 Outlines

As we point out above (10:3), constructing projects, of any description, is a vital component of professional development. At the outset of your career it may seem somewhat outlandish to suggest that you may be involved in writing policies for a professional organization or writing a report that will be presented in court. However, many nurses go on to be involved with these tasks and are becoming increasingly involved in many other areas in which the skills of writing are important. It may be that you will need to write a project for a management group, for a research grant or for an educational body, and most certainly you will be called upon to write an essay, dissertation or assignment on the courses that you attend. In producing an outline of any project it is important to plan the structure and to ensure that all the main points are covered (10:3).

Frameworks

Whatever the project it should be stressed that the important issue is to be very clear as to what the requirements are in relation to the body to which the project is being submitted. For example, if you are writing an essay for a particular course then make sure that you know what the course requirements are in relation to the submission of essays. If they call for 3000 words then you are normally allowed plus or minus 10 per cent. Therefore, your essay needs to be in the range of 2700–3300. This will then need to be structured accordingly. While a PhD thesis in the social sciences will need to be around 80,000 words, a proposal to a management body may be fewer than 1000. Management proposals are often structured with the use of numbered headings, such as 1: Introduction, 2: Background and so on. Managers are extremely busy and have much reading to do, and therefore prefer short, sharp and concise proposals of two or three pages only, with supportive material as appendices.

It is important, in any project, to be very clear and concise, and to 'grab' the reader's attention by highlighting the salient points. A 'snappy' proposal is usually more successful than one that is detailed to the point of pedantry. It is the important points that need to be stressed and not the detail – unless the detail is what is required. A well known saying in student life is 'find out what they want and give it to them'.

Further reading

Crème, P. and Lea, M. R. (1997) *Writing at University: A Guide for Students.* Buckingham: Open University Press.

10.9 Presentation skills

It should be clear by now that nurses are often called upon to construct projects pertaining to their professional practice in many areas of health care delivery. These may be delivered at, for example, management groups, conferences or educational settings, and the presentation of these projects is a fundamentally important one. Good ideas and good projects may not be accepted if they are poorly presented, and knowing how to present a project may be the difference between success or failure. If you have constructed a project, or contributed towards its production in some way, then it is a part of you, and it will reflect on you, both as a person and as a professional. Therefore, time spent on ensuring that your project is as perfect as it can be is time well spent. Remember that a project with a poor structure, lots of spelling mistakes and bad grammar will reflect you in a bad light, just as a well structured project with close attention to detail and lots of recension will reflect you in a good light.

Presenting written projects

Take time to check a written project and allow yourself at least three readings for checking purposes. Make sure that there is a consistency of structure throughout the project and that it has a logical series of headings and sub-headings. It is usually the little inconsistencies that highlight the lack of careful checking. For example, left margins may alter on different pages or indented quotes may differ from one to the next. References are a main source of inconsistency and these should be checked rigorously for consistency of approach. Every comma, full stop, colon etc. should be carefully scrutinized. As we mentioned above (9:14, 10:2), the spelling should be checked and this should be done by reading it yourself, and not relying solely on the computer spell-checker. This is because the computer will not realize that the word 'form' is a misspelling of 'from'. Similarly, the computer grammar-check should not be solely relied on and in no way replaces the careful reading of each sentence to ensure that it is as correctly structured as it can be. One final point to note in the presentation of written projects is not to go 'over the top' with symbols, illustrations or fonts. That is, do not make your project look infantile with outlandish colouring, large font sizes and a single heading on a single page. These attempts to 'pad out' the project and impress the reader simply do not work and, in fact, detract significantly from your project.

Personal presentations

Again, nurses are often called upon to make a personal presentation of their projects by making a short speech in support of it, and while there are certainly gifted orators who ooze confidence, for most of us it is a question of ensuring that a few basic rules are followed and doing our best. Confidence is usually acquired by the experience of public speaking, so the more you do it, the more confidence you will develop. It is preferred if you do not read from a script but *ad lib* from prompts, such as bullet points on an overhead projector or *Powerpoint* (computer presentation software). Speak slowly and clearly, and remember that it is better to say too little than too much. Look around the room and not just at one person, and it is better to stand up while speaking rather than to speak sitting down. The skills of personal presentations are many and it is not expected that all nurses will have all these skills. However, it is becoming increasingly necessary to acquire the basics, and a good way of achieving this is to recognize someone whom you consider to be a good presenter and to emulate their skills.

Further reading

Bolton, G. (2000) *Reflective Practice Writing and Professional Development*. London: Sage.

Tomey, A. M. (2000) *Guide to Nursing Management and Leadership*, 6th edn. St Louis: Mosby.

10.10 Library use

Libraries are central sources of information for most people in health care settings and this is true for clinicians wishing to keep abreast of developments, academics undertaking research, educationalists wishing to teach others or managers interested in effective service delivery. As we have noted above (1:2, 9:8, 10:1), with the expanding growth in the amount of literature that is available to us we can become swamped with the sheer volume of literature. Fortunately, there are now computerized systems that manage much of this material, including both electronic books and journals and the referencing systems of the library itself. Libraries have become daunting places, particularly the larger libraries of universities and colleges, and as the IT has grown so have the systems that store and control this information.

Overcoming fear of libraries

Overcoming the fear of libraries must be undertaken as soon as the problem is identified and should not be avoided until time is running out. Most libraries will run regular introductory courses or are happy to show the interested person the basics of getting started. It is important to know such things as opening times and courses that are available within the library. Acquire a library card as soon as possible and make sure that you understand how many books can be taken out at any one time and for how long. You will also need to know the fining system, as fines can be quite expensive. Ensure that you know how to order and reserve books and how to order journal articles. Computers govern much of the library work so make sure that you know what is available and how you can access it. You will probably be given a computer password, which must be safeguarded. Photocopying is likely to be necessary at some stage; therefore, understand the system, the cost and the rules associated with copyright laws. Spend time in the library and know where your most often needed book sections and journals are kept, and visit them regularly to cover new material.

If there is a fear of the library, or at least a sense of being daunted by the amount of information that is available, it is important that this tension is overcome early and made to work for you rather than against you. It is sometimes useful to approach large libraries initially with a specific focus and to be selective as to the systems that you wish to use. Allocate a certain amount of time to visit the library and stick to it, and if you have developed a good filing and indexing system (9:8) then you will feel more in control of the information that is being gathered. Working through the tracking systems of the library will give you confidence, so start modestly with the books and journals that are available on the shelves before moving on to computer databases such as *Medline* and *CINAHL* (9:8). For many people, libraries are a joy to visit, and even 'home' to some, so if you have any element of fear regarding it then visit it often and it will quickly become familiar to you.

Further reading

Whitehead, E. and Mason, T. (2003) *Study Skills for Nurses*. London: Sage.

10.11 Preparing to write

With all that has been said regarding the need to construct written projects and the amount of information that usually needs to be tracked down, acquired and read, plus the need to ensure that the writing that is presented is of a good quality, it may seem surprising that the actual moment of putting the first few words on paper is often the most difficult. Let us assume that you have spent considerable time preparing yourself by synthesizing all the relevant material, that you have planned out the project with a logical structure and appropriate loading of words and that you are now ready to begin writing. It may even be that a deadline is looming and that time is beginning to run out. The question now is: what problems contribute towards a person not writing?

Avoidance strategies

Avoidance strategies are wide and varied, with many being uniquely specific to each individual and related to their own personality and context. However, there are a few common avoidance strategies that most of us share, and we outline a small number to emphasize the point. Most of us have been in the situation in which we are ready to begin penning some words only to find that when we sit down at the desk, or we are about to sit down, we find that we have said something to ourselves like 'I will just tidy the drawer and then I will start' or 'I will just sharpen all the pencils and then begin', and we will engage in almost any mundane task rather than start to write. These are avoidance strategies and they can be numerous, such as 'It's coming up to Christmas, I will start in the New Year', 'I will start on Monday after the weekend', 'I will start when the kids have gone back to school'. They may include starting 'after mowing the lawn, doing the shopping, feeding the dog'. The point is that they *are* avoidance strategies and you need to be able to identify what yours are, as it is in the identification process that the solution to them lies. If you are about to sit down and write and find you are saying to yourself 'I will just . . . and then I will begin' and you realize that this is an avoidance strategy, then you can turn this around to make it a reward for yourself. You can do this by saying to yourself that 'No, this is an avoidance strategy and I will write one sentence/paragraph/page, and then I will – sharpen the pencils, tidy the drawer, do the shopping etc.' The identification of an avoidance strategy should make you feel guilty and then you can turn it around into a reward.

When sitting down to begin writing many people are fearful of the blank page. That is, they feel that they just cannot get started and find the starkness of the clean white page somewhat off-putting (10:4). As we note above, to overcome this we suggest that you draw something on the page, doodle on it or scribble some nonsense words down. In fact write anything on it that will break the purity of the blank page. Remember that only you will see the first draft of what you produce; therefore, you can always erase it, add to it or subtract from it as you proceed to edit it. Your editing and the peer review process will improve the quality further. Finally, we emphasize that you need to reward yourself for writing and give yourself a daily and weekly target (remember days off), and when you have written the required number of words per day and week, then give yourself a treat for doing so. Thus, writing will not be punishing, but rewarding.

Further reading

Crème, P. and Lea, M. R. (1997) *Writing at University: A Guide for Students*. Buckingham: Open University Press.

10.12 Conclusions

In this chapter on thinking writing we have stressed the theoretical aspects of writing or, more accurately, the mental procedures that contribute to the writing process. This is not to say that there are not practical aspects to writing, as of course there are. However, the practical skills can be acquired in many forums and, although in this book we have attempted to balance theory and practice, we have been more concerned about the theory of practice rather than the practical skills themselves. Thus, for us, the theory of writing is concerned with how we think about approaching the practice of writing, with its fears and confidences and problems and solutions. Modern day nurses are being called upon to construct projects in many and varied areas of health care practice, and this is likely to continue. Therefore, the importance of identifying if we have skills deficits in this area cannot be stressed enough. Of course, addressing these deficits is central to our personal development, as well as contributing to the advancement of the nursing profession itself.

11

Conclusions and recommendations

11.1 Introduction

In writing this book we aimed to offer the student material that they could draw upon to give a structure to their thoughts on various aspects of nursing. The student should now be able to analyse nursing practices from differing perspectives and with a wide range of analytical tools. This should bring a focus to their thoughts and enable them to *think nursing*; that is, not to think *about* someone who is nursing but to think as a nurse from a nurse's perspective. This involves being able to draw upon all the perspectives in the book and bring them to bear on nursing practice.

We began the main chapters of this book with sociology in Chapter 2. The rationale for this was that, in our opinion, nursing is predominantly a social action and it is difficult to separate out the practice of nursing from the human interaction of helping someone in need. The main perspectives in sociology were set out to reveal how they are employed to understand the social world, and this was then applied to certain elements of nursing practice. Chapter 3 dealt with human psychology and its relationship to nursing. The study of psychology has long played a part in nursing studies, as it has an extended tradition in terms of mind–body dualism, and as the body (or mind) becomes ill or disordered it can have an impact on the mind (or body). Few nurses have not had to deal with a person's psychological state, in relation to emotions and feelings, when they have become ill, diseased or injured, and are in pain.

Anthropology was the focus of Chapter 4, as nursing may be viewed as a cultural group with its own set of rules and regulations, and sanctions and punishments should they be broken. Nursing is also embellished with rites and rituals, both in terms of practice and in the emblems of uniform. Anthropological perspectives were employed to illuminate some of these nursing traditions. Chapter 5 dealt with public health, which has a long-standing tradition in the history of health care and remains a central concern today. Disease and ill-health in the population are closely related to social issues of poverty, poor housing, unemployment and so on, and can have a huge draw on health care resources. Public health is a major concern for all of us, as contagious diseases can ravage whole populations if not checked.

Philosophical perspectives are not usually a mainstay of nurse education, yet they are closely related to medical ethics and moral conduct. Therefore, Chapter 6 outlined the main philosophical perspectives as related to the practice of nursing, and it became clear that they were highly relevant in many areas of patient care. Chapter 7 focused on economics and its relationship to health. Increasingly health care workers are being called upon to influence how the service is delivered, and they need to understand at least the basics of economic theory. A realization that health resources are a finite entity means that their deployment and management need to be both effective and efficient.

While some believe that health care should be separated from politics, others believe that health care *is* politics, and Chapter 8 focused on these issues. The main political positions and structures were highlighted in relation to health care services in contemporary society. Part Two of the chapter dealt with how politics impinge on health care practice both positively and negatively. Nurses often find the notion of science and scientific principles either irrelevant or difficult to understand. However, in modern day health care services, where the focus is upon evidence-based practice, science is now central to nursing practice. In Chapter 9 we outlined the main scientific principles that nurses tend to have the most difficulty with and showed how they link into the notion of providing evidence for nursing care. Finally, Chapter 10 outlined the main areas for constructing a written report, whether in terms of a research report, an essay or an assignment. Nurses are becoming increasingly called upon to construct written reports and these need to be of a significantly high quality to ensure a high standard of professionalism. It is an area that often causes those unused to writing some degree of trepidation.

While we were writing this book a number of recommendations emerged, for us, in relation to *thinking nursing*. These are: first, the development of reflective practice should be encouraged; second, creative thinking should be focused upon in relation to putting ideas about practice into action; third, the importance of drawing on various scientific, and even artistic, perspectives should be stressed; fourth, the march of science should be embraced; and, fifth, the process of thinking, alongside the natural tendency of nurses to want to practise, should be a central component of our personal and professional development.

Further reading

Abbott, P. and Sapsford, R. (1997) *Research into Practice: A Reader for Nurses and the Caring Professions*. Buckingham: Open University Press.

11.2 Reflective practice

Reflective practice is closely associated with thinking, and its influence in nursing has grown significantly since such scandals as the case of Beverly Allitt, the nurse who killed a number of young children while they were in hospital, the Bristol heart surgery disgrace and the Alder Hey Hospital organ retention policy. In the ensuing inquiries it was felt that staff, both medical and nursing, ought to have raised questions relating to 'suspicions' regarding certain practices. Reflection calls on nurses, as well as others, to consider aspects of their own practice, as well as that of others who are involved in delivering patient care. Reflection is based on the ability of the human mind to 'bend back' on itself and to think about thinking (2:6). It is not a cursory thought about something that has happened but a conscious process, employed in a systematic way, which can be done in isolation but is often undertaken with others. The majority of nurses who are asked to engage in reflective practice are also encouraged to have a reflective mentor who they can meet in order to explore the major issues that emerge from the reflection.

In reflective practice a nurse is asked to think of a recent situation or event that has occurred, which has caused them some concern or worry. This may be a minor occurrence, such as a difficult encounter with a colleague, who perhaps was impolite, or it may be a major event such as the death of a patient, which may be causing an element of grief. The important point is that the situation should be causing, at least, some measure of tension. From this position the thinking is focused on both the internal feelings that are generated by the nurse regarding the event and the external factors involved in the event itself. The relationship between the internal and external factors should be explored and analysed in relation to how both internal and external factors make you 'feel'. This should then reveal what the real issues are that make you sense an element of discomfiture about the situation that is being reflected upon. The next stage is to explore what alternative actions could be implemented to ensure that the situation does not occur again or it does not have the same outcome. In short, it focuses on how practice can be changed.

Reflective practice is a skill that has a number of subskills to it, and these can be learnt and brought together as an overall process to help to identify what practices may need changing. Thus, reflective practice is not only an important aspect in developing oneself but also important in developing our profession. Of course, the fact that it is focused on situations or events that cause some degree of tension means that it is highly likely to be uncomfortable for some nurses to undertake. This is so particularly when our own role in the situation is being examined, and also when we are planning to change some aspect of our behaviour. However, emphasizing the point that reflective practice is being undertaken on an aspect of nursing/medical practice that may be contributing to bad patient care should give us the impetus to overcome our discomfiture. Furthermore, the more that we undertake reflective practice the more secure we will become with doing it. It is now a part of our professional practice and we must adopt a professionally mature stance towards this. Through *thinking* we are helping to eradicate poor quality services and contributing towards improved patient care.

Further reading

Taylor, B. (2000) *Reflective Practice: A Guide for Nurses and Midwives*. Buckingham: Open University Press.

11.3 Ideas in action

Most people can come up with a good idea, although we often hear people say the opposite. A common phrase that we hear from students is that they cannot think of an idea for research, for a project, or for a paper, and that they have nothing to say on a particular topic or issue. However, if nothing else, this book has shown that there is a wealth of perspectives that can be employed to view a nursing action or enlighten a nursing situation. The conditions for thinking can be created in a number of different ways, and the first, and most enjoyable, is probably the one that involves relaxation. There are few of us who have not enjoyed the company of others who are involved in similar work as ourselves, over a cup of tea, a meal or even a glass of wine. In these situations, when discussing work related matters, light-hearted discussion can take the mind into all manner of new directions. Some of these may be ridiculous, but some may have a spark of potential. These should not be dismissed, but should be noted and recalled for later scrutiny in the cold light of day. This book was conceived in the waiting lounge of an airport during a three-hour flight delay, although its birth took almost three years. There are many more formal ways of creating ideas, through brainstorming, listening to others, having meetings and even paying attention to the moans and groans of both yourself and others. Again, there are few of us who have not got a complaint or point of view concerning a particular issue, development or proposed change in nursing, and underlying this will be an idea. This idea should be scrutinized objectively as well as subjectively to reveal its possible development for some form of action. This action phase is a more difficult step to take.

The second aspect of ideas in action concerns the action itself; that is, putting the ideas into action. While we may state that most people can come up with an idea, we cannot make the claim that most people put that idea into action. In fact, the opposite appears to be the case: most people who do have an idea do not go on to do something about it. There may be many reasons for this, ranging from apathy and lack of confidence in oneself to obstruction and lack of motivation in others. However, overcoming these hurdles is important if the ideas are to come to fruition. The strategies for doing this include: first, think the idea through carefully and identify its strengths and weaknesses; second, establish who will gain and who will lose, as this is important when sabotage appears as a problem; third, plan out what you intend to do and try to establish who or what the hurdles are, and how you will overcome them; fourth, as you proceed to act on your idea and you are meeting problems, then plan strategies to overcome, circumnavigate or circumscribe them. Whatever the reason why the idea is not developing into action, the single most important thing to do is to *identify* what that reason is.

The third, and final, component of ideas in action involves completion. If most people can have an idea, but few of those put the idea into action, then even fewer of these see the project through to completion. The main reasons for this are similar to those in the action phase above, and require a similar approach to overcome them. The central message is to think about ways of pursuing the action and aim to have identifiable and achievable targets.

Further reading

Komaromy, C. (2001) *Dilemmas in UK Health Care*. Buckingham: Open University Press.

11.4 Perspective thinking

We have emphasized throughout this book the importance of drawing on various perspectives in thinking about nursing, and thinking needs knowledge and training if it is to be undertaken effectively. Employing perspective thinking involves having a wide and varied amount of knowledge concerning many areas of life from which you can draw in analysing a particular situation. Narrow mindedness, bigotry and prejudice are the worst enemies of perspective thinking, but unfortunately are also the most commonly met. The need to broaden thinking horizons, especially one's own, is easily stated, but the practice is more difficult, and although this book is an attempt to help, it is one small step in what can be understood as a greater quest. In terms of nursing, there has been a long-standing effort to establish a specific body of knowledge that is unique to nursing, particularly in the post-Second World War era. The proliferation of nursing models throughout the 1960s and 1970s is testimony to this. However, a unique body of nursing knowledge remains elusive, and it is now questionable whether it actually exists. It is more likely that nursing will continue to be based on the numerous disciplines that it has always been based on, such as anatomy and physiology, and, in our view, the perspectives outlined in this book. As nursing develops it will draw on numerous disciplines and professional bodies of knowledge, and through this growth it will extend in complexity. Nurses will expand their repertoire of thinking skills to bring ever more highly tuned analytical skills to bear on the intricate area between nursing practice and patient care.

Although we have made a strong case for employing the perspectives in this book, we cannot suggest that they are the only ones. In fact, on the contrary, there are many more areas of human life that can contribute to an understanding of nursing. Seen in its widest sense, nursing can be understood as a relationship between human tragedy and human helping. Tragedy, since Aristotelian times, has been seen as part of the human condition, as a natural contrast to the joy of life. Misfortune, as illness, disease and injury, is a tragic human state in relation to health and happiness. Human history is also replete with the kindness of giving through helping those in need. Any tragedy – for example, an earthquake – always involves those helping to search for survivors, as it is an inherent human trait to assist. We also accept, of course, that it is also a human trait to hurt others, but this adds to the complexity of the human condition. We emphasize that there are many other areas of life that are helpful for understanding nursing and these perspectives may also include art, poetry, literature and drama, as these often reflect the contrast between tragedy and joy. Examples of human suffering and human helping are often the central theme of these perspectives and may be useful in bringing a different view to nursing. It is a question of widening your knowledge base and broadening your thinking perspective in relation to nursing practice and patients' needs.

Further reading

Scambler, G. (2001) *Health and Social Change: A Critical Theory*. Buckingham: Open University Press.

11.5 Future expansion

We have seen that health care is not a static concept but an ever-changing developmental, and dynamic, state of affairs that responds to both factors internal to itself and external factors from society. While we can look back into the past to examine such things as the history of medicine and nursing, and we can also identify the state of health care delivery that is occurring today, it is, of course, more difficult to look into the future and attempt to 'see' how it might be configured at some time hence. However, what we can do is to take some historical and contemporary indicators and identify how they offer 'signposts' to the future. The first 'signpost' that we would point out is the medicalization of life. Alongside the march of science is the march of medicine. More and more aspects of human life are coming under the focus of the medical 'gaze'. From the beginnings of life through *in vitro* fertilization to the frontiers of death through life-support technology, and from the way that we breathe, talk, eat, sit, sleep and so on to the way that we think, feel, are happy, are sad, treat ourselves, treat others and so on, we are scrutinized by medical means. We only need to recall the relatively recent human genome project to appreciate the ever-expanding 'gaze', and where medicine goes, nursing tends to eventually follow.

The second signpost is the expansion of information technology (IT). Although there has been a significant surge in IT over the past few decades, which is unlikely to be sustained at this pace indefinitely, we can anticipate that there will be a slower but consistent growth in IT in the future. This will most certainly have an impact on many areas of health care delivery but we restrict ourselves to mentioning two: communication and surveillance. The first major impact in health care will continue to be related to how information on health care matters will be stored, managed and employed. This will range from the growing literature surrounding the many professional disciplines to information on patient care. Growing concerns abound in relation to how much information is stored on computers about all of us, and not just patients, and who has access to that information and for what purposes. None the less, this expansion looks set to continue. The second major impact that IT has on health care relates to the increase in surveillance. By surveillance we refer to how technology has assisted medicine (as well as other disciplines) in mapping and investigating the human body. From the development of the early speculums and probes, which penetrated only a few inches inside the human body, to the fibre-optics that now slide into previously unseen areas of living tissue, technology reveals the most sacred parts of the body. Even the last bastion, the brain, is succumbing to the advancement of technology through the various scanning techniques that have been, and will continue to be, developed.

The third 'signpost' to be mentioned concerns three elements: first, the challenge of new diseases that affect us; second, the re-emergence of old diseases; and, third, the numerous diseases that continue to ravage many communities because of ignorance, poverty or politics. We saw with HIV that this new disease brought with it stigma and prejudice alongside the suffering that accompanies the condition. An old disease, tuberculosis, is on the increase in the UK, and this has brought with it an examination of the living conditions in which this disease thrives and a questioning as to why these conditions should prevail in a supposedly modern world. There are many conditions, particularly in Third World countries, that could be eradicated given the appropriate resources, but factors such as the lack of investment in research by corporations, who do not encourage it for various reasons, war, politics and poverty prevent this. As we note above, what the future holds is difficult to 'see' but clearly a starting point must be a good deal of *thinking* about the problems of our world and their possible solutions.

Further reading

Gerrish, K., Husband, C. and Mackenzie, J. (1996) *Nursing for a Multi-Ethnic Society*. Buckingham: Open University Press.

11.6 Consequences of 'Thinking'

Clearly this book has been concerned with *thinking*, but we hope that we have balanced this by pointing out the importance of practice. Practice is, of course, central to the process of nursing, as without practice patients would not receive the care that they ought to. Practice is, therefore, vital in the delivery of a quality health care product. However, what we have argued is that practice without thinking will lead to a dire situation in which few, if any, of those involved in the clinical team, including the patient, will benefit. Therefore, the importance of thinking is stressed in relation to nursing practice, rather than as an activity that stands alone. Having said that, we point out that it is unlikely that nursing practice will develop if thinking does not accompany it. Rather than focusing on the negative aspects of not undertaking a thinking strategy, we conclude this book on a more positive note by briefly pointing out the positive consequences of *thinking nursing*.

The first consequence of thinking refers to the improvement in practice. Examining practice through thinking will reveal many issues and raise many questions, and through the analysis of these with the appropriate methods, and the identification of strategies for creating change, practice ought to improve. Thinking about nursing in a critical way is often difficult, but if undertaken rigorously it will highlight our own role and function within the process of care delivery. The second consequence of thinking involves the impact on the individual who is undertaking it. In terms of your own mental capacity, and creative ability, thinking analytically enhances academic skills, opens minds and reveals many insights that otherwise would remain hidden. It helps to create an ability to balance arguments and offer alternative interpretations where others may remain bigoted and narrow minded. The third consequence is the balance that thinking brings to both personal and professional development. The ability to think will create the pioneering spirit and put individuals at the forefront of nursing practice, and put the nursing profession alongside the other professions in the delivery of health care. All these other professions are involved in critical analysis of their practices, as well as having robust research programmes. Nursing must also proceed along these lines. The fourth, and final, consequence of thinking involves the notion that thinking begets thinking. Once the process of analysis of practice is under way, through a systematic approach, and insights have been made, there is an almost unstoppable progression of scrutiny. If the profession of nursing prioritizes patient care above all else then this can only be supported and enhanced through the process of *thinking nursing*.

Glossary of terms

Action research: social science research in which the role of the researcher is involved and interventionist. The research is joined with action to plan, implement and monitor change as an ongoing process.

Aetiology: the science relating to the cause of disease.

Alienation: the estrangement of individuals from their self-fulfilment through the necessity of having to work.

Anomie: a social condition in which there is a breakdown of the values and norms that govern social interaction and leads to conflict.

Apocryphal: of doubtful authenticity.

Ascites: free fluid in the peritoneal cavity causing the abdomen to become distended.

Asthma: paroxysmal dyspnoea characterized by wheezing and difficulty in exhaling.

Axiomatic: generally held proposition without absolute proof; self-evident.

Base: the economic base of society consisting of the relations between people and the means of production.

Bourgeoisie: in capitalist societies this term denotes the property owners who control the means of production.

Capitalism: an economic arrangement in which capital accumulates in the hands of private businesses based on wage labour by a working force.

Chronologically: arrangement of events according to dates or times of occurrence.

Circadian rhythms: one of the body's natural clocks that has a cycle of about 24 hours.

Class consciousness: a term to denote an individual's sense of his or her belonging to a particular social group.

Conflict: in sociological terms societies develop through transformations made out of conflicts.

Conscience collective: an external normative prescription or social fact that compels individuals to act in certain ways. Rather than seeing the typical conscience as internal to the individual, Durkheim believed that the conscience collective lay in the social.

Consequentialism: the assessment of the rightness of an action based on the value of the outcomes (consequences).

Culpable: blameworthy.

Defence mechanisms: involuntary or unconscious mental processes that protect the person against painful psychological effects.

Deontology: an ethical theory that takes duty as the basis of morality.

Depersonalization: a non-specific state in which the person feels that he or she has lost his or her personal identity, and feels strange and unreal.

Dialectical materialism: dialectics is concerned with developments that emerge out of conflicts and in this sense is linked to the driving force of materials.

Disseminated strongyloidiasis: infection with a genus of the nematode worm.

Electra complex: a Freudian psychological conflict occurring in the phallic stage in which the daughter desires the father and resents the mother.

Engram: a hypothesized biochemical change occurring in the brain as a result of external stimuli. It is purported to be the manifestation of memory.

Ensoulment: in religious beliefs when the soul is infused into the body.

Epistemic: a term relating to a body of knowledge acquired through scientific principles.

Epistemology: the study of the theory of knowledge.

Etymology: the study of the derivation and meaning of words.

Exchange value: consists of the quantity of another commodity against which it can be exchanged in conditions of equilibrium.

Existentialism: a twentieth-century philosophical perspective that stresses subjectivity, free will and individuality. The emphasis is upon personal decisions rather than social pressures.

Exogamous: marrying outside of the tribe.

Gestalt: a German term that has no direct English translation. However, the term is used to refer to unified wholes, total structures, holistic versions etc. that are greater than the sum of the individual parts, and that cannot be revealed by simply analysing those parts.

Hedonists: persons who believe that happiness is the sole and proper aim of human action.

Hermeneutic: this refers to the theory and method of interpreting human action, whether through observation of behaviour or through text, music, folklore etc.

Homophobic: negative attitudes towards homosexuals or homosexuality.

Iatrogenesis: additional problems or complications brought about through the application of medicine.

Identification: a mental process whereby an individual unconsciously behaves or imagines themselves behaving as if they were the person with whom they have an emotional tie.

Idiographic: relating to the concrete, individual or unique. Opposite of nomothetic.

Latent function: in functionalism it refers to the unrecognized and unintended consequences of social interaction.

Manifest function: in functionalism it refers to the recognized and intended consequences of social interaction.

Maxim: a generally held truth or proposition derived from science or experience; a rule of conduct.

Metaphysics: this has meant many things to many people from the early Greeks onwards. In short, it can be understood as an attempt to characterize reality, or pure existence, as a whole entity rather than as a conglomerate of subdivided parts.

Moiety: one of two parts or divisions of something.

Monistic: the philosophical theory that argues that there is only one true substance.

Moral principle: behaviours judged with respect to rightness and wrongness.

Multiple sclerosis: a disease of the nervous system that, although slow in onset, ultimately renders the person paralysed and suffering from tremors.

Normative: the establishment of a standard by the prescription of rules.

Nomothetic: relating to the abstract, universal or general. Opposite of idiographic.

Nosology: a branch of medicine that is concerned with the systematic description and classification of diseases and disorders.

Oedipus complex: a Freudian psychological conflict occurring in the phallic stage in which the son desires the mother and feels a sense of rivalry and threat from the father.

Oligarchy: a small group of people in control of a country or state.

Oligopoly: a market structure in which there are only a few firms, which are able to erect barriers against the entry of new firms in competition.

Palliative: an agent that relieves but does not cure a condition.

Paris Club: a group composed of world government officials and World Bank members set up to assess the need for debt relief in developing countries. They work closely with the IMF.

Passive consumption: an indoctrination into the uncritical acceptance of a social order through discipline, rules and regulation.

Patrilineal: of kinship descent through the male line.

Pleasure principle: an early and primitive id function that seeks to satisfy any need, directly or by fantasy.

Pluralism: this refers to the view that the world is actually constructed of many entities that are unique to themselves.

Prima facie: at first sight.

Proletariat: the working classes.

Rationality: a belief that knowledge can be gained by reason alone.

Reality principle: the recognition of the real environment by the child and the limitations imposed on their desires.

Recension: this refers to the re-reading of text to correct it. It is a term that is derived from the times when parchments were written by hand and needed constant revision.

Reification: the process of treating abstract concepts as if they were 'real' entities.

Secular: earthly, of the world, rather than divine or heavenly.

Sentience: the capacity to receive stimuli; the primitive limit of consciousness.

Shamanism: a religious belief in many aboriginal tribes of Asia and North American Indians. The central figure is the shaman, who is the medicine man, sorcerer and seer, and is believed to be able to make contact with the spirit world.

Shop steward: a person elected in a factory to represent the workers in negotiations with management.

Superstructure: social levels of society founded on the economic base, including law, family, church and ideologies.

Surplus value: the value that remains when the basic subsistence of the workers has been subtracted from the value that they have produced.

Teleology: the study of final causes, or the means, design or purpose of achieving a final state.

Totem: a totem refers to a plant, animal or object that is the accepted symbolic representation of a particular group, clan or tribe. Totems usually have a historic relationship that deals with the association between man and nature.

Use value: the direct value applied to a commodity in terms of its use.

Utility: in economics this refers to the amount of satisfaction that we get out of a product.

Verstehen: the German word for understanding. In sociology it has become the procedure by which researchers access the meanings of those who are being studied. Hence, it is often translated as empirical understanding.

Volition: exercise of the will.

References

Abdussalam, M. and Kaferstein, F. (1996) Food beliefs and taboos, *World Health*, 2: 10–12.

Abercrombie, N., Hill, S. and Turner, B. S. (1980) *The Dominant Ideology Thesis*. London: Allen & Unwin.

Acheson, D. (1998) *Independent Inquiry into Inequalities in Health Report*. London: Stationery Office.

Adair, J., Deuschle, K. and McDermott, W. (1957) Patterns of health and disease among the Navahos, *Annals of the American Academy of Political Social Science*, 311: 86.

Adams, J. F. (2001) Highlights from the hill: needlestick prevention and reduction in medical errors, *ORL Head and Neck Nursing*, 19(1): 20–1.

Adorno, T. W., Frenkel-Brunswick, E., Levinson, J. D. and Sanford, R. N. (1950) *The Authoritarian Personality*. New York: Harper and Row.

Ainsworth, M., Blehar, M., Waters, E. and Wall, S. (1978) *Patterns of Attachment: A Psychological Study of the Strange Situation*. Hillsdale, NJ: Erlbaum.

Ajzen, I. and Fishbein, M. (1977) Attitude–behaviour relations: a theoretical analysis and review of empirical research, *Psychological Bulletin*, 84: 888–918.

Akinleye, J. O. (1991) The impact of hierarchy on communication and decision-making among administrators, physicians, and nurses: a survey of two hospitals, Unpublished PhD, Howard University.

Alexander, J. C. (1985) *Neofunctionalism*. London: Sage.

Allsop, J. (1995) *Health Policy and the NHS towards 2000*, 2nd edn. London: Longman.

Alspach, G. (1998) Patient advocacy: have we ascended to new heights or fallen to new depths?, *Critical Care Nursing*, 18(4): 17–19.

Altman, I. (1975) *The Environment and Social Behaviour*. San Francisco: Brooks Cole.

Andersen, Y. (1994) European nurses take lead in quality assurance, *International Nursing Review*, 4(1): 13–16.

Anderson, P. (1976) *Considerations on Western Marxism*. London: New Left Books.

Anonymous (1988) Euthanasia: what you think, *Nursing Times*, 84(33): 38–9.

Anonymous (1997) News in mental health nursing: myths abound concerning depression in the elderly, *Journal of Psychosocial Nursing and Mental Health Service*, 35(6): 6–7.

Anonymous (1999a) Caveat in obtaining consent to organ donations, *Regan Report on Nursing Law*, 39(12): 2.

Anonymous (1999b) Care of patients and subterfuge, in equal parts, *Lancet*, 354(9192): 1743.

Anonymous (1999c) Maternal death and the medical model, *Practising Midwife*, 2(2): 4–5.

Arblaster, G., Brooks, D., Hudson, R. and Petty, M. (1990) Terminally ill patients' expectations of nurses, *Australian Journal of Advanced Nursing*, 7(3): 34–43.

Archer, J. (1999) *The Nature of Grief: The Evolution and Psychology of Reactions to Loss*. London: Routledge.

Ardagh, M. (1999) Resurrecting autonomy during resuscitation: the concept of professional substituted judgement, *Journal of Medical Ethics*, 25(5): 375–8.

Armstrong, F. (2001) Defending wages and conditions, *Queensland Nurse*, 20(4): 4–7.

Aron, R. (1977) *The Opium of the Intellectuals*. Westport, CT: Greenwood Press.

Asbridge, J. (2002) A new organisation with a new purpose, *Nursing and Midwifery Council News*, Spring: 3.

Asch, S. E. (1952) *Social Psychology*. Englewood Cliffs, NJ: Prentice Hall.

Ashton, J. (ed.) (1992) *Healthy Cities*. Milton Keynes: Open University Press.

Ashton, J. and Seymour, H. (1988) *The New Public Health*. Milton Keynes: Open University Press.

Atkinson, R. C. and Shiffrin, R. M. (1968) Human memory: a proposed system and its control processes, in K. W. Spence and J. T. Spence (eds) *The Psychology of Learning and Motivation, Volume 2*. London: Academic Press.

Atkinson, R. C. and Shiffrin, R. M. (1971) The control of short-term memory, *Scientific American*, 224: 82–90.

Azar, B. (2000) What's in a face?, *Monitor on Psychology*, 31(1): 44–5.

Baber, Z. (2001) Colonizing nature: scientific knowledge, colonial power and the incorporation of India into the modern world-system, *British Journal of Sociology*, 52(1): 37–58.

Baggott, R. (2000) *Public Health: Policy and Politics*. London: Macmillan.

Bailey, C. (1995) Nursing as therapy in the management of breathlessness in lung cancer, *European Journal of Cancer Care*, 4(4): 184–90.

Baillie, L. (1993) A review of pain assessment tools, *Nursing Standard*, 7(23): 25–9.

Baines, B. K. and Norlander, L. (2000) The relationship of pain and suffering in a hospice population, *American Journal of Hospice and Palliative Care*, 17(5): 319–26.

Bandura, A. (1982) The psychology of chance encounters and life paths, *American Psychologist*, 37: 747–55.

Bannock, G., Baxter, R. E. and Davis, E. (1987) *Dictionary of Economics*. London: Penguin.

Banton, M. (1988) *Racial Consciousness*. London: Longman.

Banton, M. (1994) *Discrimination*. Buckingham: Open University Press.

Banyard, P. and Hayes, N. (1994) *Psychology: Theory and Application*. London: Chapman and Hall.

Baron, R. A. and Byrne, D. (2000) *Social Psychology*, 9th edn. Boston: Allyn and Bacon.

Basu, J. (2001) Access to primary care: the role of race and income, *Journal of Health and Social Policy*, 13(4): 57–73.

Bateson, G. and Mead, M. (1942) *Balinese Character: A Photographic Analysis*. New York: New York Academy of Sciences.

Bauer, P. T. (1971) *Dissent on Development*. London: Weidenfeld and Nicolson.

Bauman, S. L. (1997) Contrasting two approaches in a community-based nursing practice with older adults: the medical model and Parse's nursing theory, *Nursing Science Quarterly*, 10(3): 124–30.

Baumrind, D. (1973) The development of instrumental competence through social-ization, in A. D. Pick (ed.) *Minnesota Symposia on Child Development, Volume 7*. Minneapolis: University of Minneapolis Press.

Beaglehole, R. and Bonita, R. (1997) *Public Health at the Crossroads: Achievements and Prospects*. Cambridge: Cambridge University Press.

Beardshaw, J., Brewster, D., Cormack, P. and Ross, A. (1998) *Economics: A Student's Guide*, 4th edn. Harlow: Pearson Education.

Bee, H. (2000) *The Developing Child*, 9th edn. Boston: Allyn and Bacon.

Bell, D. and Kristol, I. (1981) *The Crisis in Economic Theory*. New York: Basic Books.

Berkeley, G. (1948) *The Works of George Berkeley*. Edinburgh: Thomas Nelson.

Bernstein, B. (1975) *Class, Codes and Control*. London: Routledge and Kegan Paul.

Berridge, V. (1999) *Health and Society in Britain since 1939*. Cambridge: Cambridge University Press.

Bertero, C. M. (1998) Transition to becoming a leukaemia patient: or putting up barriers which increase patient isolation, *European Journal of Cancer Care*, 7(1): 40–6.

Bevan, A. (1961) *In Place of Fear*. London: MacGibbon and Kee.

Beveridge, W. H. (1931) *Unemployment*. London: Longman.

Beveridge, W. H. (1942) *Social Insurance and Allied Services (The Beveridge Report)*, Cmnd 6404. London: HMSO.

Beveridge, W. H. (1943) *The Pillars of Society*. New York: Macmillan.

Beveridge, W. H. (1944) *Full Employment in a Free Society*. London: Allen & Unwin.

Beveridge, W. H. (1945) *Why I Am a Liberal*. London: Jenkins.

Beynon, C. and Laschinger, H. K. (1993) Theory-based practice: attitudes of nursing managers before and after educational sessions, *Public Health Nursing*, 10(3): 183–8.

Bhagat, K., Mamutse, G. and Jonsson, K. (2000) Investigation of ascites: are we doing enough? *Central African Journal of Medicine*, 46(4): 221–3.

Biley, A. M. (1995) The experience of hospitalisation for physically disabled patients, *British Journal of Therapy and Rehabilitation*, 2(2): 61–4.

Billig, M., Condor, S., Edwards, D., *et al.* (1988) *Ideological Dilemmas: A Social Psychology of Everyday Thinking*. London: Sage.

Black, H. K. (2001) Jake's story: a middle-aged, working-class man's physical and spiritual journey toward death, *Quality Health Research*, 11(3): 293–307.

Blackburn, R. (1993) *The Psychology of Criminal Conduct: Theory, Research and Practice*. New York: John Wiley.

Blakemore, K. (1998) *Social Policy: An Introduction*. Buckingham: Open University Press.

Blane, D. (1989) Preventive medicine and public health: England and Wales 1870–1914, in C. J. Martin and B. V. McQueen (eds) *Readings for a New Public Health*. Edinburgh: Edinburgh University Press.

Blumer, H. (1969) *Symbolic Interactionism: Perspective on Method*. Englewood Cliffs, NJ: Prentice Hall.

Bock, P. K. (1980) *Rethinking Psychological Anthropology: Continuity and Change in the Study of Human Action*. New York: W. H. Freeman and Co.

Bonita, R. and Beaglehole, R. (2000) Reinvigorating public health, *Lancet*, 356(9232): 787–8.

Bottomore, T. and Nisbet, R. (1978) Structuralism, in T. Bottomore and R. Nisbet (eds) *A History of Sociological Analysis*. London: Heinemann.

Bottorf, J. L. (1990) Persistence in breastfeeding: a phenomenological investigation, *Journal of Advanced Nursing*, 15(2): 201–9.

Bourdieu, P. (1986) *Distinction: A Social Critique of Judgements of Taste*. London: Routledge and Kegan Paul.

Bourdieu, P. (1988) *Language and Symbolic Power*. Cambridge: Polity Press.

Bourdieu, P. and Passeron, J.-C. (1977) *Reproduction: In Education, Society and Culture*. London: Sage.

Bowlby, J. (1969) *Attachment and Loss, Volume 1: Attachment*. Harmondsworth: Penguin.

Bowlby, J. (1973) *Attachment and Loss, Volume 2: Separation*. Harmondsworth: Penguin.

Bowlby, J. (1980) *Attachment and Loss, Volume 3: Loss, Sadness and Depression*. London: Hogarth Press.

Bracco, D., Favre, J. B., Bissonnette, B. *et al.* (2001) Human errors in a multidisciplinary intensive care unit: a 1-year prospective study, *Intensive Care Medicine*, 27(1): 137–45.

Bradley, L. A. (1995) Chronic benign pain, in D. Wedding (ed.) *Behaviour and Medicine*, 2nd edn. St Louis, MO: Mosby-Year Book.

Bradley, S. (1995) Methodological triangulation in healthcare research, *Nurse Researcher*, 3(2): 81–9.

Brandt, R. B. (1983) A defence of utilitarianism, *Hastings Center Report,* 13: 40.

Brennan, T. (1988) Controversial discussions and feminist debate, in N. Segal and E. Timms (eds) *The Origins and Evolution of Psychoanalysis*. New Haven, CT: Yale University Press.

British Medical Association (1984) *The Handbook of Medical Ethics*. London: British Medical Association.

British Medical Association (1989) *Hazardous Waste and Human Health*. Oxford: Waste Regulation Authority.

Brosnan, C. A. and Swint, J. M. (2001) Cost analysis: concepts and application, *Public Health Nursing*, 18(1): 13–18.

Brown, B., Nolan, P. and Crawford, P. (2000) Men in nursing: ambivalence in care, gender and masculinity, *International History of Nursing Journal*, 5(3): 4–13.

Brulde, B. (2001) The goals of medicine: towards a unified theory, *Health Care Annals*, 9(1): 15–23.

Bruner, J. S. (1983) *Child's Talk: Learning to Use Language*. Oxford: Oxford University Press.

Brunswick, N., Wardle, J. and Jarvis, M. J. (2001) Public awareness of warning signs for cancer in Britain, *Cancer Causes Control*, 12(1): 33–7.

Buck, D. J., Malik, S., Murphy, N. *et al.* (2001) Ethnic classification in primary dental care and dental health service research: time to pause for thought, *Primary Dental Care*, 8(2): 83–7.

Bull, F. C., Eyler, A. A., King, A. C. and Brownson, R. C. (2001) Stages of readiness to exercise in ethnically diverse women: a US survey, *Medical Science and Sports Exercise*, 33(7): 1147–56.

Burnard, P. (1995) Conference characters, *Nursing Standard,* 10(12): 42–3.

Burton, N. W. and Turrell, G. (2000) Occupation, hours worked, and leisure-time physical activity, *Preventative Medicine*, 31(6): 673–81.

Buxton, V. (1998) Behind the blockade: the Cuban health care system, *Nursing Times*, 94(38): 30–1.

Byrne, D. (1999) *Social Exclusion*. Buckingham: Open University Press.

Callon, M. (1998) *The Laws of the Market*. Oxford: Blackwell.

Campbell, D. T. and Stanley, J. C. (1963) *Experimental and Quasi-experimental Designs for Research*. Chicago: Rand McNally.

Campbell, I. D. and Rader, A. D. (1999) Community-informed consent for HIV testing and a continuum of confidentiality, *Tropical Doctor*, 29(4): 194–5.

Candilis, P. J. and Appelbaum, K. L. (1997) Physician-assisted suicide and the

Supreme Court: the Washington and Vacco verdicts, *Journal of the American Academy of Psychiatry and the Law*, 25(4): 595–606.

Carlson, J. G. and Hatfield, E. (1992) *Psychology of Emotion*. Fort Worth, TX: Harcourt Brace Jovanovich.

Chalmers, A. F. (1999) *What Is This Thing Called Science?* Buckingham: Open University Press.

Chan, C. (2000) A study of health services for the Chinese minority in Manchester, *British Journal of Community Nursing*, 5(3): 140–7.

Chapple, A., Ling, M. and May, C. (1998) General practitioners' perceptions of the illness behaviour and health needs of South Asian women with menorrhagia, *Ethnicity and Health*, 3(1/2): 81–93.

Chase, S. K. (1995) The social context of critical care clinical judgement, *Heart and Lung: Journal of Critical Care*, 24(2): 154–62.

Chisholm, D., Dolhi, C. and Schreiber, J. (2000) Creating occupation-based opportunities in a medical model clinical practice setting, *Occupational Therapy Practice*, 5(1): 1–8.

Chodorow, N. (1978) *The Reproduction of Mothering*. Berkeley: University of California Press.

Chodorow, N. (1988) *Psychoanalytic Theory and Feminism*. Cambridge: Polity Press.

Chomsky, N. (1957) *Syntactic Structures*. The Hague: Mouton.

Chomsky, N. (1965) *Aspects of the Theory of Syntax*. Cambridge, MA: MIT Press.

Chomsky, N. (1968) *Language and Mind*. New York: Harcourt Brace Jovanovich.

Christman, J. (ed.) (1989) *The Inner Citadel: Essays on Individual Autonomy*. Oxford: Oxford University Press.

Clarke, A. (1998) Professional update. 'What happened to your face?' Managing facial disfigurement, *British Journal of Community Nursing*, 3(1): 13–16.

Coburn, D. (1999) Phases of capitalism, welfare states, medical dominance and health care in Ontario, *International Journal of Health Services*, 29(4): 833–51.

Cohen, F. and Lazarus, R. (1979) Coping with the stress of illness, in G. C. Stone, F. Cohen and N. E. Ader (eds) *Health Psychology: A Handbook*. San Francisco: Jossey-Bass.

Cohen, M. R. (2001) Medication errors, *Nursing*, 31(4): 14.

Collins, C. (1996) Medical model vs social model of care, *Canadian Nursing Home*, 7(3): 17–19.

Collins, H. (1992) *The Equal Opportunities Handbook: A Guide to Law and Best Practice in Europe*. Oxford: Blackwell.

Conrad, P. and Schneider, J. (1992) *Deviance and Medicalization: From Badness to Sickness*. Philadelphia: Temple University Press.

Corless, I. B., Nicholas, P. K. and Nokes, K. M. (2001) Clinical scholarship: issues in cross-cultural quality-of-life research, *Journal of Nursing Scholarship*, 33(1): 15–20.

Corner, J. (1997) Beyond survival rates and side effects: cancer nursing as therapy: the Robert Tiffany lecture, *Cancer Nursing*, 20(1): 3–11.

Cortis, J. D. (2000) Caring as experienced by minority ethnic patients, *International Nursing Review*, 47(1): 53–62.

Cowan, M. J., Pike, K. C. and Budzynski, H. K. (2001) Psychosocial nursing therapy following sudden cardiac arrest: impact on two-year survival, *Nursing Research*, 50(2): 68–76.

Crabtree, B. F. and Miller, W. L. (1992) *Doing Qualitative Research*. London: Sage.

Craig, P. M. and Lindsay, G. M. (2000) *Nursing for Public Health*. Edinburgh: Churchill Livingstone.

Crespo, C. J., Smit, E., Andersen, R. E., Carter-Pokras, O. and Ainsworth, B. E. (2000) Race/ethnicity, social class and their relation to physical inactivity during leisure time: results from the Third National Health and Nutrition Examination Survey, 1988–1994, *American Journal of Preventative Medicine*, 18(1): 46–53.

Crist, P. H., Davis, C. G. and Coffin, P. (2000) The effects of employment and mental health status on the balance of work, play/leisure, self-care, and rest, *Occupational Therapy in Mental Health*, 15(1): 27–42.

Crouch, C. (1982) *Trade Unions: The Logic of Collective Action*. Glasgow: Fontana.

Dababneh, A. J., Swanson, N. and Shell, R. L. (2001) Impact of added rest breaks on the productivity and well being of workers, *Ergonomics*, 44(2): 164–74.

Dalton, J. A. (1989) Nurses' perceptions of their pain assessment skills, pain management practices, and attitudes toward pain, *Oncology Nursing Forum*, 16(2): 225–31.

D'Anglure, B. S. (1996) Lévi-Strauss, Claude, in A. Barnard and J. Spencer (eds) *Encyclopedia of Social and Cultural Anthropology*. London: Routledge.

Daniel, W. W. (1991) *Biostatistics: A Foundation for Analysis in the Health Sciences*, 5th edn. New York: John Wiley.

Daponte, B. O. and Garfield, R. (2000) The effect of economic sanctions on the mortality of Iraqi children prior to the 1991 Persian Gulf War, *American Journal of Public Health*, 90(4): 546–52.

Davidhizar, R. E. and Brownson, K. (1999) Literacy, cultural diversity, and client education, *Health Care Manager*, 18(1): 39–47.

Davidson, D. (1984) *Inquiries into Truth and Interpretation*. Oxford: Oxford University Press.

Davies, S. (1996) *Big Brother*. London: Macmillan.

Davis-Floyd, R. E. (1987) The technological model of birth, *Journal of American Folklore*, 100: 479–95.

Day, P. and Klein, R. (1991) Political theory and policy practice: a case of general practice, 1911–1992, Paper presented at the Political Studies Association Conference, Lancaster.

Day, W. (2000) Relaxation: a nursing therapy to help relieve cardiac chest pain, *Australian Journal of Advanced Nursing*, 18(1): 40–4.

de Beauvoir, S. (1949) *The Second Sex*. London: Jonathan Cape.

Denzin, N. K. (1970) *The Research Act*. Chicago: Aldine.

Denzin, N. K. (1989) *Interpretive Interactionism*. Newbury Park, CA: Sage.

Des Jardin, K. E. (2001) Political involvement in nursing: politics, ethics and strategic action, *Association of Operating Room Nursing Journal*, 74(5): 613–15, 617–18, 621–6.

Dey, I. (1993) *Qualitative Data Analysis: A User-friendly Guide for Social Scientists*. London: Routledge.

Dickenson, D. and Johnson, M. (eds) (1993) *Death, Dying and Bereavement*. London: Sage/Open University Press.

Donaldson, R. J. and Donaldson, L. J. (1998) *Essential Public Health Medicine*. Plymouth: Petroc Press.

Donohue, J. (1998) 'Wrongful living': recovery for a physician's infringement on an individual's right to die, *Journal of Contemporary Health Law and Policy*, 14(2): 391–419.

Donovan, T. (2001) The stigma of terminal cancer, in T. Mason, C. Carlisle, C. Watkins and E. Whitehead (eds) *Stigma and Social Exclusion in Healthcare*. London: Routledge.

Dooks, P. (2001) Diffusion of pain management research into nursing practice, *Cancer Nursing*, 24(2): 99–103.

Dougherty, M. C. and Tripp-Reiner, T. (1985) The interface of nursing and anthropology, *Annual Review of Anthropology*, 14: 219–41.

Downe, S. (2000) Something will turn up . . . at a rural maternity station, I met my vocation, *Midwifery Matters*, 87: 4.

Downes, D. and Rock, P. (1989) *Understanding Deviance*, 2nd edn. Oxford: Oxford University Press.

Doyle, Y. (1991) A survey of the cervical screening service in a London district, including reasons for attendance, ethnic responses and views on the quality of the service, *Social Science and Medicine*, 32(8): 953–7.

Drever, J. (1964) *A Dictionary of Psychology*. Harmondsworth: Penguin.

Dube, S. C. (1955) *Indian Village*. London: Routledge and Kegan Paul.

Duck, S. (1988) *Relating to Others*. Milton Keynes: Open University Press.

Dummett, M. (1978) *Truth and Other Enigmas*. London: Duckworth.

Dumpe, M. L., Herman, J. and Young, S. W. (1998) Forecasting the nursing workforce in a dynamic health care market, *Nursing Economics*, 16(4): 170–9.

Duncan, S. M. (1996) Empowerment strategies in nursing education: a foundation for population-focused clinical studies, *Public Health Nursing*, 13(5): 311–17.

Durham, M. (1991) *Sex and Politics*. London: Macmillan.

Durkheim, E. (1893) *The Division of Labour*. Glencoe, IL: Free Press (1960 edn).

Dworkin, G. (1988) *The Theory and Practice of Autonomy*. Cambridge: Cambridge University Press.

Dyck, I. and Jongbloed, L. (2000) Women with multiple sclerosis and employment issues: a focus on social institutional environments, *Canadian Journal of Occupational Therapy*, 67(5): 337–46.

Eagleton, T. (1996) *The Illusions of Postmodernism*. Oxford: Blackwell.

Earman, J. (1986) *A Primer on Determinism*. Dordrecht: Reidal.

Easton, D. (1966) Alternative strategies in theoretical research, in D. Easton (ed.) *Varieties of Political Theory*. Englewood Cliffs, NJ: Prentice Hall.

Ekman, P. (1980) *The Face of Man*. New York: Garland.

Eliason, M. J. and Gerken, K. C. (1999) Attitudes shown by nursing college students, staff, and faculty towards substance abuse, *Journal of Substance Use*, 4(3): 155–63.

Elliott, S. (2001) Woven into the community, *Community Practitioner*, 74(11): 413–14.

Elshtain, J. (1987) *Women and War*. New York: Basic Books.

Epsing-Anderson, S. (1990) *Three Worlds of Welfare Capitalization*. Cambridge: Polity Press.

Erikson, E. (1963) *Childhood and Society*. New York: W. W. Norton.

Esser, J. K. (1998) Alive and well after 25 years: a review of groupthink research, *Organizational Behavior and Human Decision Processes*, 73(2/3): 116–41.

Evans, J. (1995) *Feminist Theory Today: An Introduction to Second-wave Feminism*. London: Sage.

Faries, J. E., Mills, D. S., Goldsmith, K. W., Phillips, K. D. and Orr, J. (1991) Systematic pain records and their impact on pain control: a pilot study, *Cancer Nursing*, 14(6): 306–13.

Farnworth, L. (1998) Doing, being, and boredom, *Journal of Occupational Science*, 5(3): 140–6.

Farrell, G. A. and Gray, C. (1992) *Aggression: A Nurse's Guide to Therapeutic Management*. London: Scutari Press.

Farrell, M. and Corrin, K. (2001) The stigma of congenital abnormalities, in T. Mason, C. Carlisle, C. Watkins and E. Whitehead (eds) *Stigma and Social Exclusion in Healthcare*. London: Routledge.

Ferguson, S. L. (2001) An activist looks at nursing's role in health policy development, *Journal of Obstetric, Gynecologic and Neonatal Nursing*, 30(5): 546–51.

Fernando, S. (1991) *Mental Health, Race and Culture*. London: Billing and Sons.

Festinger, L., Riecken, H. W. and Schachter, S. (1956) *When Prophecy Fails*. Minneapolis: University of Minneapolis Press.

Festinger, L. (1957) *A Theory of Cognitive Dissonance*. Evanston, IL: Row Peterson.

Figert, A. E. (1996) *Women and the Ownership of PMS*. New York: Aldine de Gruyter.

Finer, S. (1952) *The Life and Times of Sir Edwin Chadwick*. London: Macmillan.

Firestone, S. (1970) *The Dialectics of Sex: The Case for Feminist Revolution*. New York: Morrow.

Fisher, B. H. and Strauss, A. L. (1978) Interactionism, in T. Bottomore and R. Nisbet (eds) *A History of Sociological Analysis*. London: Heinemann.

Flatt, S. (1998) By the book . . . dealing with people with different religious beliefs, *Nursing Standard*, 12(46): 18.

Fletcher, J. (1966) *Situation Ethics*. Philadelphia: Westminster Press.

Flew, A. (1979) *A Dictionary of Philosophy*. London: Macmillan.

Foolchand, M. K. (2000) The role of the Department of Health and other key institutions in the promotion of equal opportunities, multi-cultural and anti-racist issues in nurse education, *Nurse Education Today*, 20(6): 443–8.

Foucault, M. (1967) *Madness and Civilization: A History of Insanity in the Age of Reason*. London: Tavistock.

Foucault, M. (1973) *The Birth of the Clinic: An Archaeology of Medical Perception*. London: Tavistock.

Fouere, T., Maire, B., Delpeuch, F. *et al.* (2000) Dietary changes in African urban households in response to currency devaluation: foreseeable risks for health and nutrition, *Public Health Nutrition*, 3(3): 293–301.

Frank, J. D. (1977) Nature and functions of belief systems: humanism and transcendental religion, *American Psychologist*, 32: 555–9.

Frazer, W. M. (1950) *A History Of Public Health: 1834–1939*. London: Bailliere Tindall and Cox.

Freeden, M. (2000) Ideology, in *Routledge Encyclopedia of Philosophy*. London: Routledge.

Freud, S. (1913) *Totem and Taboo*. New York: Norton (1950 edn).

Freud, S. (1920) Beyond the pleasure principle, in J. Strachey (ed.) *The Complete Psychological Works of Sigmund Freud, Volume 18*. London: Hogarth Press.

Fried, C. (1978) *Right and Wrong*. Cambridge, MA: Harvard University Press.

Friedman, M. (1962) *Capitalism and Freedom*. Chicago: Chicago University Press.

Froggatt, K. (1997) Signposts on the journey: the place of ritual in spiritual care, *International Journal of Palliative Nursing*, 3(1): 42–6.

Funnel, R., Oldfield, K., and Speller, V. (1995) *Towards Healthier Alliances*. London: Health Education Authority.

Galambos, C. M. (1998) Preserving end-of-life autonomy: the Patient Self-Determination Act and the Uniform Health Care Decisions Act, *Health and Social Work*, 23(4): 275–81.

Galbraith, J. K. (1963) *American Capitalism*. London: Penguin.

Galbraith, J. K. (1970) *The Affluent Society*, 2nd edn. London: Penguin.

Gallison, M. (1992) Confronting the medical model: a hermeneutic view of the quest for health care by gay men with HIV and AIDS. Unpublished PhD, University of Washington.

Ganguly-Scrase, R. (2000) Globalisation and its discontents: an Indian response, *Journal of Occupational Science (Australia)*, 7(3): 138–47.

Gardner, H. (1985) *Frames of Mind: The Theory of Multiple Intelligences*. London: Paladin.

Garfinkel, H. (1986) *Ethnomethodological Studies of Work*. London: Routledge and Kegan Paul.

Gaskins, S. T. (1994) G.I. nurses at war: gender and professionalization in the Army Nurse Corp during World War II, Unpublished PhD, University of California, Riverside.

Gauker, C. (1990) How to learn language like a chimpanzee, *Philosophical Psychology*, 3: 31–53.

Gelbart, M. (1999) A fetching little lilac number, *Nursing Times*, 95(15): 26–7.

Gendron, C. (1999) Transcending death: the search for eternity, *Canadian Nurse*, 95(8): 38–40.

General Medical Council (1985) *Professional Conduct and Discipline: Fitness to Practice*. London: General Medical Council.

George, V. and Wilding, P. (1985) *Ideology and Social Welfare*. London: Routledge and Kegan Paul.

Ger, L., Ho, S. and Wang, J. (2000) Physicians' knowledge and attitudes toward the use of analgesics for cancer pain management: a survey of two medical centers in Taiwan, *Journal of Pain and Symptom Management*, 20(5): 335–44.

Ghusn, H. F., Teasdale, T. A. and Skelly, J. R. (1998) Limiting treatment in nursing homes: differences in knowledge and attitudes of nursing homes, *Annals of Long Term Care*, 6(1): 16–23.

Gibbons, E. and Garfield, R. (1999) The impact of economic sanctions on health and human rights in Haiti, 1991–1994, *American Journal of Public Health*, 89(10): 1499–504.

Giddens, A. (1973) *The Class Structure of the Advanced Societies*. London: Hutchinson.

Giddens, A. (1989a) *Sociology*. Cambridge: Polity Press.

Giddens, A. (1989b) *Consequences of Modernity*. Cambridge: Cambridge University Press.

Giddens, A. (1999) *Runaway World: How Globalisation Is Reshaping Our Lives*. London: Profile Books.

Gillon, R. (1986) *Philosophical Medical Ethics*. Chichester: John Wiley & Sons.

Glaser, B. G. (1992) *Emergence versus Forcing: Basics of Grounded Theory Analysis*. Mill Valley, CA: Sociology Press.

Glaser, B. G. and Strauss, A. (1967) *The Discovery of Grounded Theory*. Chicago: Aldine.

Glass, C. (1995) Addressing psychosexual dysfunction in neurological rehabilitation settings, *Journal of Mental Health*, 4(3): 251–60.

Glover, J. (1988) *Causing Death and Saving Lives*. London: Penguin.

Goetsch, V. L. and Fuller, M. G. (1995) Stress and stress management, in D. Wedding (ed.) *Behavior and Medicine*, 2nd edn. St Louis, MO: Mosby-Year Book.

Goffman, E. (1959) *The Presentation of Self in Everyday Life*. London: Longman.

Goffman, E. (1961) *Asylums*. Harmondsworth: Penguin Books.

Goffman, E. (1964) *Stigma: Notes on the Management of Spoiled Identity*. Englewood Cliffs, NJ: Prentice Hall.

Goffman, E. (1990) *Stigma: Notes on the Management of Spoiled Identity*. London: Penguin.

Goldberg, R. T. (1987) The right to die: the case for and against voluntary passive euthanasia, *Disability, Handicap and Society*, 2(1): 21–39.

Gomm, R. and Davies, C. (2000) *Using Evidence in Health and Social Care*. London: Sage.

Gorer, G. and Rickman, J. (1949) *The People of Great Russia: A Psychological Study*. London: Cressett.

Gramsci, A. (1971) *Selections from the Prison Notebooks*. London: New Left Books.

Graves, R. (1986) *New Larousse Encyclopedia of Mythology*. London: Guild Publishing.

Gray, A. J. (2001) Attitudes of the public to mental health: a church congregation, *Mental Health, Religion and Culture*, 4(1): 71–9.

Greer, G. (1970) *The Female Eunuch*. London: Verso.

Gregory, R. L. (1983) Visual illusions, in J. Miller (ed.) *States of Mind*. London: BBC Productions.

Griffiths, A. and Wall, S. (1999) *Applied Economics: An Introductory Course*, 8th edn. Harlow: Pearson Education.

Griffiths, P. (1999) Physician-assisted suicide and voluntary euthanasia: is it time the UK law caught up? *Nursing Ethics*, 6(2): 107–17.

Griffiths, R. (1983) *NHS Management Enquiry*. London: DHSS.

Gross, R. (2001) *Psychology: The Science of Mind and Behaviour*, 4th edn. London: Hodder and Stoughton.

Guildford, J. P. (1967) *The Nature of Human Intelligence*. New York: McGraw-Hill.

Gutman, S. A. (1999a) The transition through adult rites of passage after traumatic brain injury: preliminary assessment of an occupational therapy intervention, *Occupational Therapy International*, 6(2): 143–58.

Gutman, S. A. (1999b) Alleviating gender role strain in adult men with traumatic brain injury: an evaluation of a set of guidelines for occupational therapy, *American Journal of Occupational Therapy*, 53(1): 101–10.

Hagland, M. (1996) Power to the patient, *Hospitals and Health Networks*, 70(20): 24–6.

Hall, E. T. (1963) A system for the notation of proxemic behaviour, *American Anthropologist*, 65: 1003–26.

Hall, S. and Gieben, B. (1992) *Formations of Modernity*. Cambridge: Polity Press.

Hall, S. and Olahfimihan, D. (1999) Killing them softly: the plight of sick children in sanctions-hit Iraq, *Nursing Times*, 95(34): 18.

Hallenbeck, J. L. (2000) Terminal sedation: ethical implications in different situations, *Journal of Palliative Medicine*, 3(3): 313–20.

Hall-Long, B. (2001) Running for elective office: one nurse's adventure in campaigning, *Policy, Politics and Nursing Practice*, 2 (2): 149–56.

Halsey, A. H. (1993) *British Social Trends since 1900*. London: Macmillan.

Ham, C. and Hill, M. (1984) *The Policy Process in the Modern Capitalist State*. Brighton: Harvester.

Hancock, T. (1999) Future directions in population health, *Canadian Journal of Public Health*, 90(suppl. 1): S68–70.

Handysides, S. (1993) Taking babies' temperatures: science versus social taboos in battle over Baby Check, *British Medical Journal*, 307(6905): 673–5.

Harlow, H. F. (1949) Formation of learning sets, *Psychological Review*, 11: 456–65.

Harnack, L. J., Rydell, S. A. and Stang, J. (2001) Prevalence of use of herbal products by adults in the Minneapolis/St Paul, Minn, metropolitan area, *Mayo Clinical Proceedings*, 76(7): 688–94.

Harris, M. I. (2001) Racial and ethnic differences in health care access and health outcomes for adults with type 2 diabetes, *Diabetes Care*, 24(3): 454–9.

Harris, M. R., Graves, J. R., Solbrig, H. R., Elkin, P. L. and Chute, C. G. (2000) Embedded structures and representations of nursing knowledge, *Journal of the American Medical Information Association*, 7(6): 539–49.

Hartman, R. L. (1992) Value hierarchies and influence structures of practicing professional nurses, Unpublished PhD, Columbia University Teachers College.

Harvey, D. (1990) *The Condition of Postmodernity*. Oxford: Blackwell.

Harvey, J. (1988) *Modern Economics*, 5th edn. London: Macmillan.

Hasseler, M. (2001) Effects of health political measures on health and well-being of women postpartum and their newborns, *Pflege*, 14(2): 6–7.

Hawkins, L. H. and Armstrong-Esther, C. A. (1978) Circadian rhythms and night shift working in nurses, *Nursing Times*, 4 May: 49–52.

Hayek, F. A. (1949) *Individualism and Economic Order*. London: Routledge and Kegan Paul.

Hayek, F. A. (1960) *The Constitution of Liberty*. London: Routledge and Kegan Paul.

Hayek, F. A. (1967) *Studies in Philosophy, Politics and Economics*. London: Routledge and Kegan Paul.

Hebb, D. O. (1949) *The Organization of Behaviour*. New York: Wiley.

Held, D., McGrew, A., Goldblatt, D. and Perraton, J. (1999) *Global Transformations: Politics, Economics and Culture*. Cambridge: Polity Press.

Hellings, P. and Howe, C. (2000) Assessment of breastfeeding knowledge of nurse practitioners and nurse-midwives, *Journal of Midwifery and Women's Health*, 45(3): 197–201, 264–70.

Helman, C. G. (2000) *Culture, Health and Illness*. Oxford: Butterworth-Heinemann.

Henderson, L. J. (1935) Physician and patient as a social system, *New England Journal of Medicine*, 212: 819–23.

Hennessy, D. (1997) The shape of things to come, *Nursing Times*, 93(27): 36–8.

Her Majesty's Stationery Office (1983) *The Independent Inquiry into Inequalities in Health Report*. London: HMSO.

Her Majesty's Stationery Office (1998) *Our Healthier Nation*. London: HMSO.

Hewison, A. (1999) Tales of the expected: nursing myths, *Nursing Times*, 95(1): 32–3.

Hibbert, C. (1987) *The English: A Social History*. Bury St Edmonds: Book Club Associates.

Higgs, Z. R., Bayne, T. and Murphy, D. (2001) Health care access: a consumer perspective, *Public Health Nursing*, 18(1): 3–12.

Hirst, P. Q. and Thompson, G. (1996) *Globalization in Question: The International Economy and the Possibilities of Governance*. Cambridge: Polity Press.

Ho, Y. P., To, K. K., Au-Yeung, S. C. *et al.* (2001) Potential new antitumor agents from an innovative combination of demthylcantharidin, a modified traditional Chinese medicine, with a platinum moiety, *Journal of Medical Chemistry*, 44(13): 2065–8.

Hodges, J. L. and Lehmann, E. L. (1964) *Basic Concepts of Probability and Statistics*. San Francisco: Holden-Day.

Hogg, C. (1999) *Patients, Power et Politics: From Patients to Citizens*. London: Sage.

Holden, P. and Littlewood, J. (1991) *Anthropology and Nursing*. London: Routledge.

Holland, W. and Stewart, S. (1990) *Screening in Health Care: Benefit or Bane?* London: NPHT.

Holmes, H. B. (1992) A call to heal medicine, in H. B. Holmes and L. M. Purdy (eds) *Feminist Perspectives in Medical Ethics*. Bloomington: Indiana University Press.

Honigsbaum, F. (1992) *Who Shall Live and Who Shall Die?* London: King's Fund College.

Horn, J. L. and Cattell, R. B. (1967) Age differences in fluid and crystallised intelligence, *Acta Psychologica*, 26: 107–29.

Hughes, R. and McGuire, G. (2001) Delayed diagnosis of disseminated strongyloidiasis, *Intensive Care Medicine*, 27(1): 310–12.

Hugman, R. (1999) Ageing, occupation and social engagement: towards a lively later life, *Journal of Occupational Science*, 6(2): 61–7.

Hunt, G. (1994) *Ethical Issues in Nursing*. London: Routledge.

Hutton, W. (1995) *The State We're In*. London: Vintage.

Iddi, A. (1999) Mind the gap: how what we do differs from what we say, in F. Porter, I. Smyth and C. Sweetman (eds) *Gender Works*. Oxford: Oxfam.

Illich, I. (1973) *Deschooling Society*. Harmondsworth: Penguin.

Illich, I. (1990) *Limits to Medicine. Medical Nemesis: The Exploration of Health*. London: Marion Boyars.

Ingelfinger, F. (1980) Arrogance, *New England Journal of Medicine*, 303: 1507–11.

Ison, S. (2000) *Economics*. Harlow: Pearson Education.

Izard, C. E. (1994) Basic emotions, relations among emotions, and emotion-cognition relations, *Psychological Bulletin*, 115: 561–5.

Jackson, C. (1991) Female circumcision: should angels fear to tread? *Health Visitor*, 64(8): 252–3.

Jambunathen, J. and Bellaire, K. (1996) Evaluating staff of crisis prevention/intervention techniques: a pilot study, *Issues in Mental Health Nursing*, 17(6): 541–58.

Janis, I. L. (1982) *Groupthink*, 2nd edn. Boston: Houghton Mifflin.

Jones, E. E., Farina, A., Hastorf, A. H. *et al.* (1984) *Social Stigma: The Psychology of Marked Relationships*. New York: Free Press.

Jones, B. (1987) *Political Issues in Britain Today*. Manchester: Manchester University Press.

Jonsson, H. and Andersson, L. (1999) Attitudes to work and retirement: generalization or diversity? *Scandinavian Journal of Occupational Therapy*, 6(1): 29–35.

Joshi, B. S. and Kaul, P. N. (2001) Alternative medicine: herbal drugs and their critical appraisal. Part 1, *Progressive Drug Research*, 56: 1–76.

Kagan, C., Evans, J. and Kay, B. (1986) *A Manual of Interpersonal Skills for Nurses: An Experimental Approach*. London: Harper and Row.

Kane, R. (1996) *The Significance of Free Will*. New York: Oxford University Press.

Kant, I. (1785) *The Moral Law: Groundwork of the Metaphysic of Morals*. London: Routledge (1948 edn).

Karch, A. M. and Karch, F. E. (2001) Practice errors: 'clean' vs 'sterile', *American Journal of Nursing*, 101(4): 25.

Keddy, B., Gregor, F., Foster, S. and Denney, D. (1999) Theorizing about nurses' work lives: the personal and professional aftermath of living with healthcare reform, *Nursing Inquiry*, 6 (1): 58–64.

Kee, C. C., Minick, P. and Connor, A. (1999) Nursing student and faculty attitudes toward people who are homeless, *American Journal of Health Behavior*, 23(1): 3–12.

Kendall, S. (ed.) (1998) *Health and Empowerment Research and Practice*. London: Arnold.

Kent, B. (1996) *Virtues of the Will: The Transformation of Ethics in the Late Thirteenth Century*. Washington, DC: Catholic University of America Press.

Kerckhoff, A. C. (1974) The social context of interpersonal attraction, in T. L. Huston (ed.) *Foundations of Interpersonal Attraction*. New York: Academic Press.

Kerckhoff, A. C. and Davis, K. E. (1962) Value consensus and need complementarity in mate selection, *American Sociological Review*, 27: 295–303.

Keynes, J. M. (1936) *The General Theory of Employment, Interest and Money*. London: Macmillan.

Kim, H. S. (1998) Structuring the nursing knowledge system: a typology of four domains, *Scholarly Inquiry for Nursing Practice*, 12(4): 367–88.

Kim, S., Moon, S. and Popkin, B. M. (2000) The nutrition transition in South Korea, *American Journal of Clinical Nutrition*, 71(1): 44–53.

King, M., Speck, P. and Thomas, A. (1994) Spiritual and religious beliefs in acute illness: is this a feasible area of study, *Social Science and Medicine*, 38(4): 631–6.

Kissane, D. W., Street, A. and Nitschke, P. (1998) Seven deaths in Darwin: case studies under the Rights of the Terminally Ill Act, Northern Territory, Australia, *Lancet*, 352(9134): 1097–102.

Klein, M. (1990) *Determinism, Blameworthiness and Deprivation*. Oxford: Oxford University Press.

Kletz, T. A. (1980) Benefits and risks: their assessment in relation to human need, *Endeavour*, 4: 46–51.

Koehler, S., Ramadan, R. and Salter, M. (1999) Do not resuscitate (DNR), *Journal of the Oklahoma State Medical Association*, 92(7): 316–19.

Koestler, A. (1970) *The Act of Creation*. London: Pan Books.

Krause, E. A. (1977) *Power and Illness: The Political Sociology of Health and Medical Care*. New York: Elsevier.

Krieger, N. (2000) Refiguring 'race': epidemiology, racialized/biology, and biological expressions of race relations, *International Journal of Health Services Planning, Administration and Evaluation*, 30(1): 211–16.

Kubler-Ross, E. (1970) *On Death and Dying*. London: Tavistock Publications.

Kuhn, T. S. (1970) *The Structure of Scientific Revolutions*, 2nd edn. Chicago: University of Chicago Press.

Kuiper, R. (2000) A new direction for cognitive development in nursing to prepare the practitioners of the future, *Nursing Leadership Forum*, 4(4): 116–24.

Lacan, J. (1977) *Ecrits*. London: Tavistock.

Lange, F. A. (1967) *History of Materialism*. New York: Basic Books.

Lash, S. and Urry, J. (1987) *The End of Organized Capitalism*. Cambridge: Polity Press.

Last, J. M. (1995) *A Dictionary of Epidemiology*, 3rd edn. Oxford: Oxford University Press.

Laswell, H. D. (1948) The structures and function of communication in society, in L. Bryson (ed.) *Communication of Ideas*. New York: Harper.

LeDoux, J. E. (1997) Emotion, memory, and the brain, *Scientific American Mysteries of the Mind Special Issue*, 7(1): 68–75.

Lemert, E. (1972) *Human Deviance: Social Problems and Social Control*. Englewood Cliffs, NJ: Prentice Hall.

Lenin, V. I. (1951) *Imperialism, as the Highest Stage of Capitalism*. Moscow: Progress Publishers.

Lee, D. and Newby, H. (1987) *The Problem of Sociology*. London: Hutchinson.

Lévi-Strauss, C. (1962) *Totemism*. London: Merlin Press.

Lévi-Strauss, C. (1964) *Introduction to a Science of Mythology*. London: Cape.

Lévi-Strauss, C. (1966) *The Savage Mind*. New York: Viking Press.

Levy, M. J. (1952) *The Structure of Society*. Princeton, NJ: Princeton University Press.

Lewin, K. (1951) *Field Theory in Social Science*. New York: Harper.

Lewontin, R. (1982) *Human Diversity*. London: W. H. Freeman.

Liaschenko, J. and Fisher, A. (1999) Theorizing the knowledge that nurses use in the conduct of their work, *Scholarly Inquiry for Nursing Practice*, 13(1): 29–41.

Lindstrom, M., Hanson, B. S. and Ostergren, P. O. (2001) Socio-economic differences in leisure-time physical activity: the role of social participation and social capital in shaping health related behaviour, *Social Science and Medicine*, 52(3): 441–51.

Lipsey, R. G. and Harbury, C. (1988) *First Principles of Economics*. London: Weidenfeld and Nicolson.

Littlewood, J. (2000) Anthropology and children's nursing, *Journal of Child Health Care*, 4(4): 154–6.

Lobo, F. (1998) Social transformation and the changing work-leisure relationship in the late 1990s, *Journal of Occupational Science*, 5(3): 147–54.

Lobo, F. (1999) The leisure and work occupations of young people: a review, *Journal of Occupational Science*, 6(1): 27–33.

Lockwood, D. (1956) Some remarks on 'The Social System', *British Journal of Sociology*, 8(2): 218–32.

Locsin, R. C. (2001) The culture corner: nursing practice and the preoccupation with power over death, *Holistic Nursing Practice*, 15(2): 1–3.

Logan, W. P. D. (1950) Mortality in England and Wales from 1848 to 1947, *Population Studies*, 4: 132–78.

Lohr, J. M. and Staats, A. (1973) Attitude conditioning in Sino-Tibetan languages, *Journal of Personality and Social Psychology*, 26: 196–200.

Lorber, J. (1994) *Paradoxes of Gender*. New Haven, CT: Yale University Press.

Lorenz, K. (1966) *On Aggression*. London: Methuen.

Louis, R. (1992) Passive taboos, *Nursing Times*, 88(45): 37–9.

Lovejoy, J. C., Champagne, C. M., Smith, S. R., de Jonge, L. and Xie, H. (2001) Ethnic differences in dietary intakes, physical activity, and energy expenditure in middle-aged, premenopausal women: the Health Traditions Study, *American Journal of Clinical Nutrition*, 74(1): 90–5.

Lowy, E. and Ross, M. W. (1994) 'It'll never happen to me': gay men's beliefs, perceptions and folk constructions of sexual risks of HIV transmission, *AIDS Education and Prevention*, 6(6): 467–82.

Lukacs, G. (1971) *History and Class Consciousness*. London: Merlin Press.

Lyotard, J.-F. (1979) *The Postmodern Condition: A Report on Knowledge*. Manchester: Manchester University Press.

McArdle, E. (2001) Communication impairment and stigma, in T. Mason, C. Carlisle, C. Watkins and E. Whitehead (eds) *Stigma and Social Exclusion in Healthcare*. London: Routledge.

McCann, E. (2000) The expression of sexuality in people with psychosis: breaking the taboos, *Journal of Advanced Nursing*, 32(1): 132–8.

McCarthy, T. R. and Minnis, J. (1994) The health care system in the United States, in U. K. Hoffmeyer and T. R. McCarthy (eds) *Financing Health Care*. Dordrecht: Kluwer.

McCormack, B. (1993) How to promote quality of care and preserve patient autonomy, *British Journal of Nursing*, 2(6): 338–41.

McCourt, F. (1997) *Angela's Ashes: A Memoir of Childhood*. London: Flamingo.

McCrea, F. B. (1983) The politics of menopause: the 'discovery' of a deficiency disease, *Social Problems*, 31(1): 111–22.

McGuire, A. J., Henderson, J. and Mooney, G. (1988) *The Economics of Health Care*. London: Routledge.

McIlroy, J. (1995) *Trade Unions in Britain Today*, 2nd edn. Manchester: Manchester University Press.

McIntosh, I. B., Swanson, V., Power, K. G. and Rae, C. A. L. (1999) General practitioners' and nurses' perceived roles, attitudes and stressors in the management of people with dementia, *Health Bulletin*, 57(1): 35–40.

McKeown, M. and Stowell-Smith, M. (1998) Language, race and forensic psychiatry: some dilemmas for anti-discriminatory practice, in T. Mason and D. Mercer (eds) *Critical Perspectives in Forensic Care*. London: Macmillan.

McNiff, J. (1992) *Creating a Good Social Order through Action Research*. Poole: Hyde Publications.

Madanipour, A., Cars, G. and Allen, J. (eds) (1998) *Social Exclusion in European Cities*. London: Jessica Kingsley.

Maes, S. and van Elderen, T. (1998) Health psychology and stress, in M. W. Eysenck (ed.) *Psychology: An Integrated Approach*. London: Longman.

Mahony, C. (1999) Hemmed in, *Nursing Times*, 95(15): 24–5.

Mahony, C. (2001) Alan's 15-minute spin cycle, *Nursing Times*, 97(22): 13.

Malinowski, B. (1926) *Myths in Primitive Psychology*. London: Kegan Paul, Trench, Tubner.

Mallik, M. (1998) Advocacy in nursing: perceptions and attitudes of the nursing elite in the United Kingdom, *Journal of Advanced Nursing*, 28(5): 1001–11.

Mannheim, K. (1960) *Ideology and Utopia*. London: Routledge and Kegan Paul.

Marsh, I. (1986) *Sociology in Focus: Crime*. London: Longman.

Marsh, I., Keating, M., Eyre, A. *et al.* (1996) *Making Sense of Society: An Introduction to Sociology*. London: Longman.

Martins, E. L., Alves, R. N. and Godoy, S. A. F. (1999) Feelings and reaction of nurses in the face of death, *Revista Brasileira de Enfermagem*, 52(1): 105–17.

Mashazi, M. I. and Roos, S. D. (2000) The utilization of a midwifery obstetrical unit (MOU) in a metropolitan area, *South African Journal of Nursing*, 23(4): 98–106.

Maslow, A. (1968) *Towards a Psychology of Being*, 2nd edn. New York: Van Nostrand Reinhold.

Maslow, A. (1970) *Motivation and Personality*, 2nd edn. New York: Harper & Row.

Mason, J. K. and McCall-Smith, R. A. (1983) *Law and Medical Ethics*. London: Butterworth.

Mason, T. (1993) Seclusion as a cultural practice in a special hospital, *Educational Action Research*, 1(3): 411–23.

Mason, T. and Chandley, M. (1999) *Managing Violence and Aggression: A Manual for Nurses and Health Care Workers*. Edinburgh: Churchill Livingstone.

Mason, T., Carlisle, C., Watkins, C. and Whitehead, E. (2001) *Stigma and Social Exclusion in Healthcare Settings*. London: Routledge.

Mastro, J. V., Burton, A. W., Rosendahl, M. and Sherrill, C. (1996) Attitudes of elite athletes with impairments toward one another: a hierarchy of preference, *Adapted Physical Activity Quarterly*, 13(2): 197–210.

Mauss, M. (1954) *The Gift*. New York: Free Press.

Mazur, L. J., De Ybarrondo, L., Miller, J. and Colasurdo, G. (2001) Use of alternative and complementary therapies for pediatric asthma, *Texas Medicine*, 97(6): 64–8.

Mead, G. H. (1934) *Mind, Self and Society*. Chicago: University of Chicago Press.

Meadows, S. (1993) *The Child as Thinker*. London: Routledge.

Meadows, S. (1995) Cognitive development, in P. E. Bryant and A. M. Colman (eds) *Developmental Psychology*. London: Longman.

Medical Services Review Committee (1962) *A Review of the Medical Services in Great Britain (the Porritt Report)*. London: Social Assay.

Meier, E. (1999) Legislation to address privacy related to medical records, *Oncology Nursing*, 14(5): 7.

Mercer, D. and McKeown, M. (1997) Pornography: some implications for nursing, *Healthcare Analysis*, 5(1): 56–61.

Meyer, J.-R. (1988) The fate of the mentally ill in Germany during the Third Reich, *Psychological Medicine*, 18: 575–81.

Merton, R. K. (1957) *Social Theory and Social Structure*. New York: Free Press.

Michels, R. (1962) *Political Parties: A Sociological Study of the Oligarchical Tendencies of Modern Democracy*. New York: Free Press.

Milgram, S. (1974) *Obedience to Authority*. New York: Harper & Row.

Miller, D. (1999) *Market, State and Community: Theoretical Foundations of Market Socialism*. Oxford: Oxford University Press.

Millett, K. (1970) *Sexual Politics*. London: Virago Press.

Mill, J. S. (1991) *On Liberty, in Collected Works of John Stuart Mill, Volume 18*. London: Routledge.

Millerson, G. L. (1964) *The Qualifying Association*. London: Routledge and Kegan Paul.

Milne, R. (1992) Competitive tendering for support services, in E. Beck, S. Lonsdale, S. Newman and D. Patterson (eds) *In the Best of Health*. London: Chapman & Hall.

Miner, H. (1956) Body ritual among the Nacirema, *American Anthropologist*, 58(3): 503–7.

Moghaddam, F. M., Taylor, D. M. and Wright, S. C. (1993) *Social Psychology in Cross-cultural Perspective*. New York: Freeman & Co.

Mohan, J. and Woods, K. (1985) Restructuring health care: the social geography of public and private health care under the British Conservative government, *International Journal of Health Services*, 15: 197–215.

Money, M. (2000) Shamanism and complementary therapy, *Complementary Therapies in Nursing and Midwifery*, 6(4): 207–12.

Moore, L. E. (1997) False distinctions: the legal and ethical issues surrounding court-ordered caesarean section, *Midwifery Matters*, 75: 19–22.

Moore, W. E. (1979) Functionalism, in T. Bottomore and R. Nisbet (eds) *A History of Sociological Analysis*. London: Heinemann.

Moore, W. W. (1991) Corporate culture: modern day rites and rituals, *Healthcare Trends and Transition*, 2(4): 8–13, 32–3.

Moos, R. and Houts, P. (1968) The assessment of the social atmosphere of psychiatric wards, *Journal of Abnormal Psychology*, 73: 595–604.

Morgan, D. (1991) *Discovering Men*. London: Routledge.

Morris, J. (1974) *Conundrum*. Oxford: Oxford University Press.

Morris, S. (1998) *Health Economics for Nurses: An Introductory Guide*. London: Prentice Hall Europe.

Morrison, E. (1990) The tradition of toughness: a study of nonprofessional nursing care in psychiatric settings, *Image: Journal of Nursing Scholarship*, 22(1): 32–8.

Moscovici, S. (1984) The phenomenon of social representations, in R. M. Farr and S. Moscovici (eds) *Social Representations*. Cambridge: Cambridge University Press.

Moskop, J. C. (1999) Informed consent in the emergency department, *Emergency Medicine Clinics of North America*, 17(2): 327–40.

Mulhall, A. (1996) *Epidemiology of Nursing and Health Care*. London: Macmillan.

Munro, R. (1999) The battle for hearts and minds: is user involvement, reform of community care, or the medical model of mental health the key? *Nursing Times*, 95(12): 16.

Munro, R. (2001) Nurses are caught in the crossfire, *Nursing Times*, 97(22): 14.

Murata, P., Hayakawa, T., Satoh, K. *et al.* (2001) Effects of Dai-kenchu-to, a herbal medicine, on uterine and intestinal motility, *Physiotherapy Research*, 15(4): 302–6.

Murstein, B. I. (1976) The stimulus-value-role theory of marital choice, in H. Grunebaum and J. Christ (eds) *Contemporary Marriage: Structures, Dynamics and Therapy*. Boston: Little & Brown.

Murstein, B. I. (1987) A clarification and extension of the SVR theory of dyadic parting, *Journal of Marriage and the Family*, 49: 929–33.

Myles, M. (1981) *Textbook for Midwives*. London: Macmillan.

Nachmias, C. and Nachmias, D. (1981) *Research Methods in the Social Sciences*. London: Edward Arnold.

Neale, J. M. and Liebert, R. M. (1986) *Science and Behavior: An Introduction to Methods of Research*, 3rd edn. Englewood Cliffs, NJ: Prentice Hall.

Nichols, T. and Beynon, H. (1977) *Living with Capitalism*. London: Routledge & Kegan Paul.

Nicoll, L. H. (2001) *Nurses' Guide to the Internet*. Philadelphia: Lippincott.

Nicolson, J. (1995) Feminism and psychology, in J. A. Smith, R. Harré and L. van Langenhove (eds) *Rethinking Psychology*. London: Sage.

Nightingale, F. ([1860] 1980) *Notes on Nursing: What It Is and What It Is not*. London: Churchill Livingstone.

Novek, J., Bettess, S., Burke, K. and Johnston, P. (2000) Nurses' perceptions of the reliability of an automated medication dispensing system, *Journal of Nursing Care Quality*, 14(2): 1–13.

Nyman, D. J. and Sprung, C. L. (2000) End-of-life decision making in the intensive care unit, *Intensive Care Medicine*, 26(10): 1414–20.

Oakley, A. (1985) *Sex, Gender and Society*. Aldershot: Gower Publishing in association with New Society.

O'Connell, S. (2000) Pain? Don't give it another thought, *The Independent Review*, 16 June: 8.

Oddy, D. J. (1970) Working class diets in the late 19th century, *Britain Economic History Review*, 23: 314–22.

O'Dowd, A. (2000) One-stop shop for sexual health, *Nursing Times*, 96(34): 10–11.

OECD (1992) *The Reform of Health Care: A Corporate Analysis of Seven OECD Countries*. Paris: OECD.

Olson, L. L. (1993) Commentary on assessing organizational culture: a planning strategy, *Nursing Scan in Administration*, 8(4): 10–11.

Orr, J. (1988) The porn brokers, *Nursing Times*, 84(20): 22.

Osman, L. (1998) Health habits and illness behaviour: social factors in patient self-management, *Respiratory Medicine*, 92(2): 150–5.

Owen, D. (1984) Medicine, morality and the market, *Canadian Medical Association Journal*, 130: 1341–5.

Packman, J. and Kirk, S. F. L. (2000) The relationship between nutritional knowledge, attitudes and dietary fat consumption in male students, *Journal of Human Nutrition and Dietetics*, 13(6): 389–95.

Parker, A. and Bhugra, D. (2000) Attitudes of British medical students towards male homosexuality, *Sexual Relationship Therapy*, 15(2): 141–9.

Parsons, T. (1937) *The Structure of Social Action*. New York: McGraw-Hill.

Parsons, T. (1951a) *The Social System*. New York: Free Press.

Parsons, T. (1951b) *Towards a General Theory of Action*. Boston, MA: Harvard University Press.

Parsons, T. (1964) *Social Structure and Personality*. New York: Free Press.

Parsons, T. (1969) *Sociological Theory and Modern Society*. New York: Free Press.

Parsons, T. (1971) *The System of Modern Societies*. Englewood Cliffs, NJ: Prentice Hall.

Parsons, T. and Shils, E. A. (1962) *Toward a General Theory of Action*. New York: Harper & Row.

Pascall, G. (1997) *Social Policy: A New Feminist Analysis*. London: Routledge.

Pavlov, I. P. (1927) *Conditioned Reflexes*. Oxford: Oxford University Press.

Payne, C. (2000) Medical model perspective of psychosocial and behavioural aspects of diabetic foot complications, *Australian Journal of Podiatric Medicine*, 34(2): 55–60.

Payne, D. (2000) Fresh image for new century ... public attitudes to nursing, *Nursing Times*, 96(1): 5.

Peacock, J. L. (1986) *The Anthropological Lens: Harsh Light, Soft Focus*. Cambridge: Cambridge University Press.

Peat, J. (2001) *Health Science Research: A Handbook of Quantitative Methods*. London: Sage.

Petty, R. E. and Cacioppo, J. T. (1981) *Attitudes and Persuasion: Classic and Contemporary Approaches*. Dubuque, IA: Brown.

Piaget, J. (1963) *The Origins of Intelligence in Children*. New York: W. W. Norton.

Piesik, C. (1998) Identifying women victims of domestic violence in the emergency department, *Physician Assistant*, 22(10): 18, 20, 23–4.

Piliavin, J. A., Dovidio, J. F., Gaertner, S. L. and Clark, R. D. (1981) *Emergency Intervention*. New York: Academic Press.

Pink, T. (1996) *The Psychology of Freedom*. Cambridge: Cambridge University Press.

Pomeroy, V. M., Niven, D. S., Barrow, S., Faragher, E. B. and Tallis, R. C. (2001) Unpacking the black box of nursing and therapy practice for post-stroke shoulder pain: a precursor to evaluation, *Clinical Rehabilitation*, 15(1): 67–83.

Popper, K. (1980) *The Logic of Scientific Discovery*. London: Unwin Hyman.

Porritt, J. (1990) *Where on Earth Are We Going?* London: BBC Books.

Porter, F., Smyth, I. and Sweetman, C. (1999) *Gender Works*. Oxford: Oxfam.

Potter, J. (1996) Attitudes, social representations and discursive psychology, in M. Wetherell (ed.) *Identities, Groups and Social Issues*. London: Sage/Open University Press.

Prior, M., Smart, D., Sanson, A. and Oberklaid, F. (2001) Longitudinal predictors of behavioural adjustment in pre-adolescent children, *Australian and New Zealand Journal of Psychiatry*, 35(3): 297–307.

Purdy, L. M. (1992) A call to heal medicine, in H. B. Holmes and L. M. Purdy (eds) *Feminist Perspectives in Medical Ethics*. Bloomington: Indiana University Press.

Quinn, F. M. (1994) The demise of curriculum, in J. Humphreys and F. M. Quinn (eds) *Healthcare Education: The Challenge of the Market*. London: Chapman & Hall.

Rambur, B. and Mooney, M. M. (1998) A point of view: why point-of-care places are not free market places, *Nursing Economics*, 16(3): 122–4.

Ramsay, R. and de Groot, W. (1977) A further look at bereavement. Paper presented at EATI conference, Uppsala. Cited in P. E. Hodgkinson (1980) Treating abnormal grief in the bereaved, *Nursing Times*, 17 January: 126–8.

Rappaport, J. (1984) Studies in empowerment: introduction to the issue, *Prevention in Human Services*, 3: 1–7.

Rathus, S. A. (2002) *Psychology in the New Millennium*, 8th edn. Fort Worth, TX: Harcourt College Publishers.

Reber, A. S. (1985) *The Dictionary of Psychology*. London: Penguin.

Reddy, M. (2000) Economics of ageing in Pacific Islands, *Asia Pacific Disability Rehabilitation Journal*, 11(2): 43–50.

Reed, J. and Watson, D. (1994) The impact of the medical model on nursing practice and assessment, *International Journal of Nursing Studies*, 31(1): 57–66.

Register, N., Eren, M., Lowdermilk, D., Hammond, R. and Tully, M. R. (2000) Knowledge and attitudes of pediatric office nursing staff about breastfeeding, *Journal of Human Lactation*, 16(3): 210–15.

Reid, N. (1993) *Health Care Research by Degrees*. Oxford: Blackwell Scientific.

Reissman, C. K. (1983) Women and medicalization: a new perspective, *Social Policy*, 14(1): 3–18.

Richman, J. (1987) *Medicine and Health*. London: Longman.

Richman, J. (1989) Psychiatric ward cultures revisited: implications for treatment regime, Paper presented to the British Sociological Association Annual Conference.

Rinn, W. E. (1991) Neuropsychology of facial expression, in R. S. Feldman and B. Rine (eds) *Fundamentals of Nonverbal Behaviour*. Cambridge: Cambridge University Press.

Ritzer, G. (1997) *The McDonaldization Thesis: Explorations and Extensions*. London: Sage.

Robb, N. (1997) Death in a Halifax hospital: a murder case highlights a profession's divisions, *Canadian Medical Association Journal*, 157(6): 757–62.

Roberts, K. J. (1999) Patient empowerment in the United States: a critical commentary, *Health Expectations*, 2(2): 82–92.

Roberts, H. (2001) Accra: a way forward for mental health care in Ghana?, *Lancet*, 357(9271): 1859.

Robinson, D. and Reed, V. (1998) *The A–Z of Social Research Jargon*. Aldershot: Ashgate.

Robson, C. (1993) *Real World Research: A Resource for Social Scientists and Practitioner-researchers*. Oxford: Blackwell.

Rogers, R. R. (2000) Identity revisited in the new technological culture, *Medical Law*, 19(3): 381–7.

Rollman, G. B. (1998) Culture and pain, in S. S. Kazarian and D. R. Evans (eds) *Cultural Clinical Psychology: Theory, Research and Practice*. New York: Oxford University Press.

Rose, M. J., Reilly, J. P., Pennie, B. *et al.* (1997) Chronic low back pain rehabilitation programs: a study of the optimum duration of treatment and a comparison of group and individual therapy, *Spine*, 22: 2246–53.

Rosenberg, M. J. and Hovland, C. I. (1960) Cognitive, affective and behavioural components of attitude, in M. J. Rosenberg, C. I. Hovland, W. J. McGuire, R. P. Abelson and J. W. Brehm (eds) *Attitude Organization and Change: An*

Analysis of Consistency among Attitude Components. New Haven, CT: Yale University Press.

Ross, W. D. (1930) *The Right and the Good*. Oxford: Oxford University Press.

Royal College of Midwives (2000) Position paper 23: racism and the maternity services, *Royal College of Midwives Journal*, 3(11): 342–4.

Rubin, Z. (1973) *Liking and Loving*. New York: Holt, Rinehart & Winston.

Runciman, W. G. (1990) How many classes are there in contemporary society?, *Sociology*, 24: 377–96.

Russel, J. and Roberts, C. (2001) *Angles on Psychological Research*. Cheltenham: Nelson Thornes.

Ryan, A. (1970) *The Philosophy of the Social Sciences*. London: Macmillan.

Ryan, W. (1971) *Blaming the Victim*. London: Orbach & Chambers.

Ryan, A. (1973) *The Philosophy of Social Explanation*. Oxford: Oxford University Press.

Sabiston, J. A. and Laschinger, H. K. (1995) Staff nurse work empowerment and perceived autonomy: testing Kanter's theory of structural power in organisations, *Journal of Nursing Administration*, 25(9): 42–50.

Salladay, S. A. (1998) Ethical problems. Mental retardation: questions about consent, *Nursing*, 28(6): 72.

Sapir, E. (1929) The study of linguistics as a science, *Language*, 5: 207–14.

Sarvimaki, A. (1994) Science and tradition in the nursing discipline: a theoretical analysis, *Scandinavian Journal of Caring Sciences*, 8(3): 137–42.

Sawley, L. (2001) Perceptions of racism in the health service, *Nursing Standard*, 15(19): 33–5.

Sayers, J. (1986) *Sexual Contradiction: Psychology, Psychoanalysis and Feminism*. London: Tavistock.

Scambler, A. and Scambler, G. (1993) *Menstrual Disorders*. London: Routledge.

Scambler, G. (ed.) (1997) *Sociology As Applied To Medicine*, 4th edn. London: W. B. Saunders.

Scambler, G. and Higgs, P. (1998) *Modernity, Medicine and Health: Medical Sociology towards 2000*. London: Routledge.

Schachter, S. (1959) *The Psychology of Affiliation: Experimental Studies of the Sources of Gregariousness*. Stanford, CA: Stanford University Press.

Schutz, A. (1970) *On Phenomenology and Social Relations*. Chicago: University of Chicago Press.

Scott, J. (1979) *Corporations, Classes and Capitalism*. London: Hutchinson.

Scruton, R. (1982) *A Dictionary of Political Thought*. London: Macmillan.

Segall, M. H., Dasen, P. R., Berry, J. W. and Poortinga, Y. H. (1990) *Human Behavior in Global Perspective: An Introduction to Cross Cultural Psychology*. New York: Pergamon.

Selye, H. (1956) *The Stress of Life*. New York: McGraw-Hill.

Shaddox, C. C. (1999) The martyrdom and myth of Edith Cavell, *Connecticut Nursing News*, 72(1): 7–9.

Sharpe, S. (1994) *Just Like a Girl*. Harmondsworth: Penguin.

Shaughnessy, P. (2001) Not in my back yard: stigma from a personal perspective, in T. Mason, C. Carlisle, C. Watkins and E. Whitehead (eds) *Stigma and Social Exclusion in Healthcare*. London: Routledge.

Sherwin, S. (1984) A feminist approach to ethics, *Dalhousie Review*, 64(4): 703–13.

Siegler, M. (1982) Confidentiality in medicine: a decrepit concept, *New England Journal of Medicine*, 307: 1518–21.

Sim, J. and Wright, C. (2000) *Research in Health Care: Concepts, Designs and Methods*. Cheltenham: Stanley Thornes (Publishers) Ltd.

Simon, J. (1978) *Basic Research Methods in Social Science*, 2nd edn. New York: Random House.

Simpson, G. and Kenrick, M. (1997) Nurses' attitudes toward computerization in clinical practice in a British general hospital, *Computers in Nursing*, 15(1): 37–42.

Skinner, B. F. (1957) *Verbal Behavior*. New York: Appleton-Century-Crofts.

Skorupski, J. (2000) Morality and ethics, in *The Concise Routledge Encyclopedia of Philosophy*. London: Routledge.

Sloman, J. (2001) *Essentials of Economics*. London: Prentice Hall.

Smale, M. (2001) The stigmatisation of breast-feeding in stigma and social exclusion in healthcare, in T. Mason, C. Carlisle, C. Watkins and E. Whitehead (eds) *Stigma and Social Exclusion*. London: Routledge.

Smart, J. J. and Williams, B. (1973) *Utilitarianism: For and Against*. Cambridge: Cambridge University Press.

Smith, E. M., Brown, H. O., Toman, J. E. P. and Goodman, L. S. (1947) The lack of cerebral effects of D-tubo-curarine, *Anaesthesiology*, 8: 1–14.

Social Exclusion Unit (1999) *Teenage Pregnancy*. London: HMSO.

Solomon, R. (1993) *The Passions: Emotions and the Meaning of Life*. Indianapolis: Hackett.

Solomon, R. and Higgins, K. (1993) *The Age of German Idealism*. London: Routledge.

Somjee, G. (1991) Social change in the nursing profession in India, in P. Holden and J. Littlewood (eds) *Anthropology and Nursing*. London: Routledge.

Sontag, S. (1983) *Illness as Metaphor*. London: Penguin.

Spearman, C. (1927) The doctrine of two factors, in S. Wiseman (ed.) *Intelligence and Ability*. Harmondsworth: Penguin (1967 edn).

Stacy, M. (1988) *The Sociology of Health and Healing*. London: Unwin Hyman.

Stanmer, W. (1975) Reflections on Durkheim and aborigine religion, in W. Pickering (ed.) *Durkheim on Religion*. London: Routledge and Kegan Paul.

Stanton, H. A. and Schwartz, M. S. (1954) *The Mental Hospital: A Study of Institutional Participation in Psychiatric Illness and Treatment*. New York: Basic Books.

Stasser, G. (1999) A primer of social decision scheme theory: model of group influence, competitive model-testing, and prospective modelling, *Organizational Behavior and Human Decision Processes*, 80(1): 3–20.

Statham, J. (1986) *Daughters and Sons: Experiences of Non-sexist Childrearing*. Oxford: Blackwell.

Sternberg, R. J. (1977) *Intelligence, Information Processing and Analogical Reasoning: The Componential Analysis of Human Abilities*. Totowah, NJ: Erlbaum.

Sternberg, R. J. (1985) *Beyond IQ: A Triarchic Theory of Human Intelligence*. Cambridge: Cambridge University Press.

Stockwell, F. (1972) *The Unpopular Patient*. London: Royal College of Nursing.

Strange, M. L. and Ezzell, J. R. (2000) Valuation effects of health cost containment measures, *Journal of Health Care Finance*, 27(1): 54–66.

Strauss, R. (1957) The nature and status of medical sociology, *American Sociological Review*, 22: 200–4.

Strawson, G. (1986) *Freedom and Belief*. Oxford: Clarendon Press.

Stroebe, W. (2000) *Social Psychology and Health*, 2nd edn. Buckingham: Open University Press.

Strydom, M., Greeff, M. and Nel, A. (2000) Guidelines for implementation in the education–learning situation regarding tuberculosis, *South African Journal of Nursing*, 23(4): 82–9.

Sullivan, J. and Rogers, P. (1997) Cognitive behavioural nursing therapy in paranoid psychosis, *Nursing Times*, 93(2): 28–30.

Suominen, T., Muinonen, U., Valimaki, M. *et al.* (2000) HIV and AIDS: knowledge and attitudes of home nursing staff, *Hoitotiede*, 12(4): 184–94.

Sweeney, K. (2001) Introduction, in M. Dixon and K. Sweeney (eds) *A Practical Guide to Primary Care Groups and Trusts*. Oxford: Radcliffe Medical Press.

Swinton, J. (2000) Reclaiming the soul: a spiritual perspective on forensic nursing, in D. Robinson and S. Hood (eds) *Forensic Nursing and Multidisciplinary Care of the Mentally Disordered Offender*. London: Jessica Kingsley.

Tadele, F. (1999) Men in the kitchen, women in the office? Working on gender issues in Ethiopia, in F. Porter, I. Smyth and C. Sweetman (eds) *Gender Works*. Oxford: Oxfam.

Tasiemski, T., Bergstrom, E., Savic, G. and Gardner, B. P. (2000) Sports, recreation and employment following spinal cord injury: a pilot study, *Spinal Cord*, 38(3): 173–84.

Tayler, C. and McLeod, B. (2001) Linking nursing pain assessment, decision-making and documentation, *Canadian Oncology Nursing Journal*, 11(1): 28–32.

Thede, L. Q. (1999) *Computers in Nursing: Bridges to the Future*. Philadelphia: Lippincott.

Thom, A. (1989) Who decides?, *Nursing Times*, 85(2): 35–6.

Thompson, J. (1982) *Sociology*. London: Heinemann.

Thurston, W. E., Burgess, M. M. and Adair, C. E. (1999) Commentary: ethical issues in the use of computerized databases for epidemiological and other health research, *Chronic Diseases of Canada*, 20(3): 127–31.

Thurstone, L. L. (1935) *The Vectors of the Mind*. Chicago: University of Chicago Press.

Tilah, M. (1996) The medical model to the management model: power issues for nursing, *Nursing Praxis in New Zealand*, 11(2): 16–22.

Tinnelly, K., Kristjanson, L. J., McCallion, A. and Cousins, K. (2000) Technology in palliative care: steering a new direction or accidental drift?, *International Journal of Palliative Nursing*, 6(10): 495–500.

Tolman, E. C. (1948) Cognitive maps in rats and man, *Psychological Review*, 55: 189–208.

Tones, K. and Telford, S. (1994) *Health Education: Effectiveness, Efficiency and Equity*. London: Chapman and Hall.

Tong, R. (1993) *Feminine and Feminist Ethics*. Belmont, CA: Wadsworth.

Townsend, P. and Davidson, N. (eds) (1988) *Inequalities in Health: The Black Report*. London: Penguin.

Townsend, P. and Davidson, N. (eds) (1992) *The Black Report*, 2nd edn. London: Penguin.

Tradewell, G. (1996) Rites of passage: adaptation of nursing graduates to a hospital setting, *Journal of Nursing Staff Development*, 12(4): 183–9, 224.

Tran-Duc-Thao, T. (1951) *Phenomenology and Dialectical Materialism*. Paris: Gordon and Breach (1971 edn).

Trevelyan, G. M. (1973) *English Social History: A Survey of Six Centuries*. London: Longman.

Turner, B. S. (1987) *Medical Power and Social Knowledge*. London: Sage.

Turner, B. S. (1990a) *Theories of Modernity and Postmodernity*. London: Sage.

Turner, B. S. (1990b) *Medical Power and Social Knowledge*. London: Sage.

Tylor, E. (1871) *Primitive Culture*. New York: Harper Row (1958 edn).

Underwood, S. M. (2000) Minorities, women, and clinical cancer research: the charge, promise, and challenge, *Annals of Epidemiology*, 10(8, suppl.): 3–12.

United Kingdom Central Council (1999) *The Continuing Professional Development Standard*. London: UKCC.

United Nations Environment Programme (1999) *Global Outlook 2000*. Nairobi: UNEP.

van den Berghe, P. L. (1978) *Race and Racism*. Chichester: Wiley.

van Gennep, A. (1960) *The Rites of Passage*. London: Routledge and Kegan Paul.

Vernon, P. E. (1950) The hierarchy of ability, in S. Wiseman (ed.) *Intelligence and Ability*. Harmondsworth: Penguin.

Vivian, J. and Brown, R. (1995) Prejudice and intergroup conflict, in M. Argyle and A. M. Colman (eds) *Social Psychology*. London: Longman.

Vundule, C., Maforah, F., Jewkes, R. and Jordan, E. (2001) Risk factors for teenage pregnancy among sexually active black adolescents in Cape Town: a case control study, *South African Medical Journal*, 91(1): 73–80.

Vygotsky, L. (1934) *Thought and Language*. Cambridge, MA: MIT Press (1962 edn).

Wadsworth, M. E., Montgomery, S. M. and Bartley, M. J. (1999) The persisting effect of unemployment on health and social well-being in men early in working life, *Social Science and Medicine*, 48(10): 1491–9.

Walker, A. and Walker, C. (eds) (1997) *The Growing Divide: A Social Audit 1979–87*. London: Child Poverty Action Group.

Walker, M. (1989) Moral understanding: alternative 'epistemology' for a feminist ethics, *Hypatia*, 4(2): 15–28.

Wallace, A. F. C. (1966) *Religion: An Anthropological View*. New York: Random House.

Warren, V. L. (1992) Feminist directions in medical ethics, in H. B. Holmes and L. M. Purdy (eds) *Feminist Perspectives in Medical Ethics*. Bloomington: Indiana University Press.

Warshaw, C. (1993) Domestic violence: challenges to medical practice, *Journal of Women's Health*, 2(1): 73–80.

Watson, J. B. (1913) Psychology as the behaviorist views it, *Psychological Review*, 20: 158–77.

Weber, M. (1904) *The Protestant Ethic and the Spirit of Capitalism*. London: Allen and Unwin (1976 edn).

Weber, M. (1922) *The Theory of Social and Economic Organisation*. New York: Free Press (1964 edn).

Weber, M (1968) *Economy and Society*. Berkeley: University of California Press.

Webster, C. (1988) *The Health Services since the War, Volume 1: Problems of Healthcare before 1957*. London: HMSO.

Webster, C. (1998) *The NHS: A Political History*. Oxford: Oxford University Press.

Wecht, C. H. (1998) The right to die and physician-assisted suicide: medical, legal and ethical aspects, *Medicine and Law*, 17(3): 477–91.

Wedgeworth, R. L. (1998) The reification of the 'pathological' gambler: an analysis of gambling treatment and the application of the medical model to problem gambling, *Perspectives in Psychiatric Care*, 34(2): 5–13.

Weedon, C. (1987) *Feminist Practice and Post-structuralist Theory*. Oxford: Blackwell.

Wells, W. (1997) *Review of Cervical Cancer Screening Service and Kent and Canterbury Hospital, NHS Trust*. London: NHSE South Thames.

West, E., Barron, D. N., Dowsett, J. and Newton, J. N. (1999) Hierarchies and cliques in the social networks of health care professionals: implications for the design of dissemination strategies, *Social Science and Medicine*, 48(5): 633–46.

Westphal, M. (1984) *God, Guilt, and Death: An Existential Phenomenology of Religion*. Bloomington: Indiana University Press.

Wheen, F. (2000) *Karl Marx*. London: Fourth Estate.

Whiteford, G. (2000) Occupational deprivation: a global challenge in the new millennium, *British Journal of Occupational Therapy*, 63(5): 200–4.

Whitehead, E. (2001) Teenage pregnancy: on the road to social death, *International Journal of Nursing Studies*, 38: 437–46.

Whitehead, E., Mason, T., Carlisle, C. and Watkins, C. (2001) The changing dynamic of stigma, in T. Mason, C. Carlisle, C. Watkins and E. Whitehead (eds) *Stigma and Social Exclusion in Healthcare*. London: Routledge.

Whitehead, E. and Mason, T. (2003) *Study Skills for Nurses*. London: Sage.

Whiting, J. and Child, I. L. (1953) *Child Training and Personality: A Cross-cultural Study*. New Haven, CT: Yale University Press.

Whorf, B. L. (1956) *Language, Thought and Reality*. Cambridge, MA.: MIT Press.

Wilkinson, I. (2001) Dollar$ & ene: common cent$: one-armed economists and the invisible hand, *Clinical Leadership and Management Review*, 15(4): 261–3.

Will, J., Self, P. and Datan, N. (1976) Maternal behaviour and perceived sex of infant, *American Journal of Orthopsychiatry*, 46(1): 135–9.

Williams, M. (1995) Challenging nursing myths and traditions, *British Journal of Theatre Nursing*, 5(9): 8–11.

Williams, S. S. and Semanchuk, L. T. (2000) Perceptions of safer sex negotiation among HIV– and HIV+ women at heterosexual risk: a focus group analysis, *International Quarterly of Community Health Education*, 19(2): 119–31.

Willis, P. (1977) *Learning to Labour: How Working Class Kids Get Working Class Jobs*. London: Saxon House.

Wilshaw, G. (1997) Integration of therapeutic approaches: a new direction for mental health nurses?, *Journal of Advanced Nursing*, 26(1): 15–19.

Wilson, L. E. (1989) An analysis of selected variables influencing the acceptance of an innovation (autonomous nursing units) by nurses in an acute care, Unpublished PhD, University of Pennsylvania.

Winter, R. (1989) *Learning from Experience*. London: Falmer Press.

Wirsing, R. G. (1981) *Protection of Ethnic Minorities*. London: Pergamon Press.

Wirth, L. (1931) Clinical sociology, *American Journal of Sociology*, 37: 49–66.

Wolfgang, M. E. and Ferracutti, F. (1967) *A Subculture of Violence*. London: Tavistock.

Woller, W., Kruse, J., Schmitz, N. and Richter, B. (1998) Determinants of high risk illness behavior in patients with bronchial asthma, *Psychotherapy, Psychosomatic Medical Psychology*, 48(3/4): 101–7.

Wollstonecraft, M. (1792) *A Vindication of the Rights of Women: With Strictures on Political and Moral Subjects*. Harmondsworth: Penguin (1975 edn).

Wong, F. K. Y., Lee, W. M. and Mok, E. (2001) Educating nurses to care for the dying in Hong Kong: a problem based-learning approach, *Cancer Nursing*, 24(2): 112–21.

Wood, W. (2000) Attitude change: persuasion and social influence, *Annual Review of Psychology*, 51: 539–70.

Woolfenden, S. R., Williams, K. and Peat, J. (2001) Family and parenting interventions in children and adolescents with conduct disorder and delinquency aged 10–17, *Cochrane Database of Systematic Reviews*, 2: CD003015.

World Bank (1993) *Investing in Health*. Geneva: World Bank.

World Health Organization (1959) *Expert Committee on Health Statistics*. Geneva: WHO.

World Health Organization (1977) *Health for All by the Year 2000*. Geneva: WHO.

World Health Organization (1985a) *Targets for Health for All*. European Health for All Series No. 1. Copenhagen: WHO Regional Office for Europe.

World Health Organization (1985b) *Targets for All: Targets in Support of the European Regional Strategy for All*. Copenhagen: WHO.

World Health Organization (1986a) *Ottawa Charter for Health Promotion*. Geneva: WHO.

World Health Organization (1986b) *Healthy Cities Workshop*. Lisbon: WHO.

World Health Organization (1995) *Implementation of the Global Strategy for Health for All by the Year 2000*. Geneva: WHO.

Wright, E. (1984) *Psychoanalytic Criticism: Theory in Practice*. New York: Methuen.

Yafchak, R. (2000) A longitudinal study of economies of scale in the hospital industry, *Journal of Health Care Finance*, 27(1): 67–89.

Young, A. (1990) *Femininity in Dissent*. London: Routledge.

Zammuner, V. L. (1987) Children's sex-role stereotypes: a cross-cultural analysis, in P. Shaver and C. Hendrich (eds) *Sex and Gender*. London: Sage.

Zborowski, M. (1952) Cultural components in response to pain, *Journal of Social Issues*, 8: 16–30.

Zillman, D. (1979) *Hostility and Aggression*. Hillsdale, NJ: Erlbaum.

Zimbardo, P. G. and Leippe, M. (1991) *The Psychology of Attitude Change and Social Influence*. New York: McGraw-Hill.

Index